THE
FOUR
PILLARS OF
HEALING

THE
FOUR
PILLARS OF
HEALING

*How the New Integrated Medicine—the Best
of Conventional and Alternative
Approaches—Can Cure You*

LEO GALLAND, M.D.

Random House • New York

The name of every patient in this book has been changed. Certain identifying characteristics of some patients have been changed as well.

All rights reserved under International and Pan-American Copyright Conventions. Published in the United States by Random House, Inc., New York, and simultaneously in Canada by Random House of Canada Limited, Toronto.

Library of Congress Cataloging-in-Publication Data
Galland, Leo.
The four pillars of healing: how the new integrated medicine—the best of conventional and alternative approaches—can cure you / Leo Galland.
p.   cm.
Includes bibliographical references and index.
ISBN 0-679-44888-8
1. Holistic medicine.   2. Medicine—Philosophy.   I. Title.
R733.G35   1997   610—dc21   96-49729

Random House website address: http://www.randomhouse.com/
Printed in the United States of America on acid-free paper
24689753

First Edition

For Christopher

ACKNOWLEDGMENTS

I wish to thank Harold Evans at Random House for understanding my message of healing and encouraging me to pursue its publication. I am grateful to Betsy Rapoport, whose guidance and brilliant editing helped to shape the structure of this book. Henry Dunow, my agent, provided me with invaluable advice. Peter Riva helped me focus my ideas during preliminary drafts of two chapters. For their enthusiasm and generous help in bringing this work to fruition, I thank Nola Beldegreen, Lisa Gleicher, Connie Brothers, Marcia Kelly, Erika and Hank Holzer, Marlo Thomas, David Fenton, Billy Crook, Stephen Levine, Marty Lee, Steve Barrie, Jeff Bland, Sid Baker, Nancy Epstein, Peter Sturtevant, Jessica Guff, Michele Squitieri, and Annie Berthold-Bond. Thanks also to the energetic people of Random House for their hard work and commitment, especially Carol Schneider, Pamela Cannon, Alexa Cassanos, Kimberly Burns, Clara Sturak, Miranda Brooks, John Rambow, and Dennis Ambrose. I would like to thank the patients who graciously allowed me to share their stories.

My wife, Christina, and my children, Jonathan, Jefferson, Christopher, and Jordan, gave their love and support throughout the long journey that led to the writing of this book. Christina and Jonathan read and reread the manuscript at every stage in its evolution, contributing insight and wisdom.

CONTENTS

IN RESTAURO

With its cold, marble floors, gray walls, and cavernous ceiling, the room reminded me of a ward in the old Bellevue Hospital, where I'd spent my medical internship. The patients here, blighted and broken, lay silently in rows, tended with a reverence I had never seen in any hospital. Most were very old, four hundred to seven hundred years old, medieval altarpieces and Renaissance paintings sent from museums and churches to this hospital for sick works of art, *Laboratori di Restauro,* on the grounds of a fortress near the center of Florence. Botticelli's *Coronation of the Virgin,* ready for discharge after ten years of painstaking restoration, stood leaning against a wall. Forty years it had spent on its back in the damp and musty basement of the Uffizi Gallery, its vibrant colors hidden by a brown scum of dust and mold, smelling like aged cheese and peeling so badly from a prior restoration that the picture would have fallen in flakes had it remained upright. Nearby, a Raphael Madonna awaited her return to the Palazzo Pitti. In a far room stood a ceiling-high crucifix, painted by Giotto in 1296, recently admitted from the Church of Santa Maria Novella. I had looked for it in the church's sacristy the week before and found only its photograph and the familiar sign, IN RESTAURO (In Restoration), which confounds art lovers throughout Italy. Today I was able to climb the scaffolding and inspect

Giotto's masterpiece face to face. To stand in the mysterious place where *restauro* actually happens filled me with such excitement that I found it hard to concentrate on the purpose of my visit.

The enemies of paintings are also the enemies of people: physical injury, bacteria, fungi, and air pollution, which hastens the ravages of time and of light. Successful art restoration requires detailed scientific support, the reason why *Restauro* seems more like a hospital than a studio. Before 1500, most paintings were made with a mixture of egg yolk, vinegar, and plant and mineral pigments applied over several layers of aged gypsum and parchment-glue to pieces of wood stuck together with cheese and limestone. Left undisturbed and protected from light, these are the most permanent paintings that humankind has yet invented. Their colors don't darken with age, as do those of oil paintings, but shine out brightly when the grime of centuries is removed. They were rarely left undisturbed, however. Varnishing, overpainting, cosmetic trimming, and botched restoration have joined forces with microbial parasites to damage them all. Even *Mona Lisa*, an oil painting whose colors have dimmed from their initial liveliness to a murky gloom, had a swatch of her panel sliced off in the seventeenth century to accommodate a new frame, distorting Leonardo's complex perspective.

The technicians of *Restauro* use X ray, ultrasound, and infrared thermography to define the layers of a painting, detect revisions, and discover the artist's original charcoal sketch. Minute fragments of paint and priming are removed for microscopic and chemical analysis and microbial culture. Under high magnification, the color of paint fractures into its component primary pigments. Blue azurite and red cinnabar are revealed from purple, the richness of color directly related to the coarseness of granules in the paint. The chemistry of restoration must distinguish mineral pigments from plant dyes and the curious lake pigments formed from lac, dead insects mummified in the sap of living trees. Chemical assay can reveal the artist's original intent. Blue salts of copper, limestone, and ammonia lose ammonia to turn green with age. Precise analysis suggests the proper treatments. Old varnishes, if their composition is known, can now be safely removed with tailor-made enzymes rather than with corrosive solvents. White lead, darkened by the sulfur in air pollution, can be blanched by hydrogen peroxide, with no harm to other pigments. Mold growth can be removed mechanically; no chemical methods have been found that are both effective and safe.

It was the mold problem that first led me to *Restauro* on a wintry morning in 1990, to consult with the laboratory's microbiologists, Iseta Tosini and Maria Rizzi, who were searching for a safe antifungal. I went there to help them by drawing upon my experience with natural antibiotics. I left enriched by a vision of their work that raised my hopes for my own profession.

Art restoration owes so much to medical technology that restoration directors often compare their work to medical care. *Laboratori di Restauro* is like a multispecialty group practice: each "patient" has a primary physician coordinating a team of specialists in surgery, infectious disease, and environmental health, drawing on the support of radiologists and clinical chemists. In *Restauro*, however, unlike in medicine, the primary physician is always the senior member of the team, because she alone has the training to treat the whole patient. Attention to the patient as a whole is so distinctly missing in contemporary medical care that physicians and patients have much to learn from *Restauro*.

While Florentine restorers rely heavily on scientific techniques to gather information about the state of their patients, they acknowledge science as a servant that helps them uncover the unique attributes of each work as it has changed over time. Their primary guide to its application is an unfaltering awareness of the individuality of each piece. Guido Botticelli, senior restorer of frescoes for *Restauro*, expressed his view succinctly: ". . . every chapel is different, with different problems which require different solutions. Every *fresco* is different, even if they happen to be in the same chapel."[1]

Understanding individuality is a perplexing task for science. Scientists study individual events to discover general principles, which can then be applied to other events. The validity of their conclusions is established by *replicating* their findings under controlled conditions. Medical scientists are, therefore, most comfortable when analyzing the similarities and differences between groups of patients. Artists, on the other hand, use general principles, like the rules of perspective, to create unique works that derive their value from being *irreplicable*. In the art of medicine, every patient is approached as an individual, biologically and psychologically unique. General principles—sometimes validated by the methods of science—are applied to each case, solely for the purpose of better understanding the unique characteristics of each patient. Sadly, in most medical practice today, the bond between art and science has been severed. The art of medicine lies dying of malnutrition, recognized only in the "bedside manner" of a good physician or the dexterity of a skillful surgeon. The science of medicine has lost its human face, deformed by the massive technology it has spawned. I have spent most of my life searching for an antidote, a patient-centered medicine, in which the power of science is harnessed to the plow of art, so that medical care becomes *restauro* for sick people.

When I entered medical school in 1964, I knew the profession was ailing, but I thought its sickness resulted mainly from greed. I believed that doctors moved into narrow specialties and ordered excessive numbers of tests and procedures solely for monetary reasons. It took me years to see that doctors were doing this because they were following a fundamentally flawed blueprint. In this blueprint, sickness is understood as mechanical breakdown and the patient is a broken machine. Each type of breakdown is considered distinct, so distinct that it can be given its own disease-name and its own disease-code and can be fully described and understood as an independent entity, with no relation to the person who is sick or the environment in which the sickness occurs. "What *disease* does this patient have?" is the primary clinical question. Its answer dictates the treatment to be prescribed—treatment for the disease, not the patient.

Like all my contemporaries, I received my clinical training in hospitals, observing patients who were acutely, often critically, ill. We were taught from the catechism of modern biological science, which preaches that the best way to understand anything is to break it down into its component parts and to study each part intensively. The ideology that promotes this approach to solving problems is called *reductionism*. Within its conceptual framework, specialization is a pathway to deeper understanding. The narrower the vision, the deeper it penetrates. The power of the specialist reinforces the grasp of reductionist thinking, because specialists tend to ask only questions that can be answered by the tools they possess.

My patients taught me the limits of medical reductionism. Their problems could never be fully explained by their "diseases." There was always something strange or quirky that separated each person's illness from the textbook case. Sometimes, there was little correlation between the patient's pain or distress and the pathology that could be measured.[2] Often, the response to treatment was unpredictable, each patient behaving like the subject of a unique experiment. The care of patients taught me that disease-entities are merely abstractions, the shadows cast by each individual's struggle to maintain health in a hostile world.[3]

I learned from patients that medicine's greatest challenges are not posed by the questions that most clinical research attempts to answer. They are posed by the frustrations of general physicians who are responsible for the primary care of patients. Researchers and specialists have the luxury of confining their activities to those aspects of patient care that fit into the theory of diseases. They can ignore concerns that lie outside the domain of the specific disease or pass them on to another specialist.

At a time when the best and the brightest of students were in record numbers deserting primary patient care for specialty training, I sought to invigorate primary care by elevating its status within the hierarchy of medical education, and spent several years pursuing this goal within the State University of New York. I finally concluded that a generation would pass before the training of primary physicians was likely to be a central goal of medical education and that engaging in the struggle would teach me a great deal about academic politics but little about the needs of patients.

Two decades ago, I left a full-time academic career to establish a general practice in a small town in Connecticut. As I describe in Chapter Two, there I developed a habit that taught me more about patients than did eight years of schooling and residency training and five years of teaching. I began phoning patients that I hadn't seen for several months to inquire about how they were feeling and what they were doing to take care of themselves. I was constantly impressed by the huge extent of individual differences in response to the same kind of treatment. I also realized that most of the accepted therapies for chronic ailments did little to improve the quality of a patient's life or health.

Frustrated by the obvious limitations of conventional therapeutics, I explored alternative strategies, beginning with the study of nutrition, psychology, and therapeutic exercise. I was amazed to discover that although so much of medical relevance within these disciplines was already known and published, little had been incorporated into the practice of medicine. My effort to integrate these fields into health care led me back into training and research and eventually into a unique specialty that is patient-oriented, not disease-oriented. For the past fourteen years, I have worked intensively with people who pose diagnostic dilemmas or are considered to be treatment failures. Most have seen numerous medical specialists, and many have consulted a variety of alternative health practitioners. In attempting to help these patients, I have moved beyond conventional notions of diagnosis and treatment to explore aspects of the patient's lives that had previously been ignored: dietary, environmental, interpersonal. I have gained new insight into the importance of our "inner environment"—the microbial ecology of the intestinal tract—in supporting or undermining health. I have lectured extensively in order to share what I've learned with other health practitioners and have been repeatedly gratified to hear, from practitioners and patients I had never met, that these teachings had allowed them to substantially improve their health or their ability to help others.

My most startling discovery has been that the concepts of greatest importance for enhancing therapeutic efficacy are not really new. They flourished in different times and in different places, and have been neglected by contemporary medicine because they failed to support the theory of diseases. Current research in basic and applied science revitalizes these concepts and allows their application with greater certainty and competence than ever before. These concepts comprise the foundation of the Hippocratic tradition, which dominated Western medicine until the eighteenth century.

In *The Four Pillars of Healing*, I'll begin by explaining the origins of Western medicine, origins that have much in common with traditional medicine all over the world. In Chapter One, "Eclipse of the Patient," I'll describe the historical reasons for the gradual demise of Hippocratic medicine and the ascendancy of the theory of diseases. In Chapter Two, "Medical Odyssey," I'll recall those pivotal experiences in my own education and training that led me to reject disease theory and apply science to the Hippocratic model. Chapter Three describes the system of *patient-centered diagnosis*, which is at the heart of my work, and explains how I apply it to individual patients. What doctors call a disease is in fact a pattern of symptoms, signs, behaviors, and pathological changes in the tissues of the body that appears coherent to the practi-

tioner. The anatomy of each patient's illness can be accurately described by examining the *triggers, mediators,* and *risk factors* that provoke her disease. Chapter Four, "The Four Pillars of Healing,"
introduces the four components of a therapeutic program that supports
a return to health: the power of relationship, the elements of a healthy
lifestyle, the importance of environmental hygiene, and the complexities of detoxification. I'll explore the science that underlies each of
these pillars in the next four chapters, with specific recommendations
for how you can apply them to safeguard your own health and recover
from illness. Chapter Nine reexamines the nature of infection with a
focus on the so-called emerging diseases that have recently received so
much public attention. The concept of the "war on infection" and the
availability of antibiotics have fostered a critical misconception of our
relationship with microbes. Infectious disease is ecological failure, not
invasion, so I discuss individual strategies for restoring symbiosis. I'll
conclude with a look to the future. As our unbalanced medical care system begins to topple of its own weight, held upright only by bureaucratic restraints and tethers, a great opportunity exists for radical reform.
The science of medicine must be vigorously applied to the Four Pillars
of Healing, so that they also become the pillars of standard clinical
practice.

THE
FOUR
PILLARS OF
HEALING

1

ECLIPSE OF
THE PATIENT

All ancient systems of healing, however much they differ among themselves, share with one another a common skein that divides them from modern clinical medicine. They all approach sickness as a problem of balance and relationship, the result of disharmony between the sick person and his environment rather than the product of specific diseases. To the traditional healer, disease itself has no reality independent of the person who is sick and the web of relationships of which he is part. By understanding how this universal wisdom was displaced from the conceptual basis of modern Western medicine, we can learn how to restore it.

DISEASE AS DISHARMONY

For tribal cultures as varied in time and place as biblical Canaan, the Australian bush, Africa's Serengeti Plain, and the Navajo reservations of Arizona, the critical relationships that underlie sickness are ethical, moral, or spiritual. Sickness results from transgression, the entire tribe or family is involved in healing, and retribution or atonement is the ultimate medicine. The healer's main goal is to reinforce the communal

bond between the sick person and his clan. The success of tribal healers derives from their ability to bring the awesome power of community
into the therapeutic arena.[1] Only recently has modern science recognized the compelling influence of social support on recovery from disease and maintenance of health (see Chapter Five).

Ayurveda, the ancient healing system of India, perceives health as a
reflection of the proper balance of life forces within each person. The
three *doshas*, or forces of life, are fire, wind, and water. These determine each individual's constitution and cause disease when they are
out of balance. Although *doshas* are recognized as forces of life, the
word *dosha* literally means "that which causes decay." Their excess is
the source of all disease. Ayurvedic philosophy embraces a concept that
modern medicine still struggles to comprehend: Disease results from
the body's own efforts to preserve itself. The task of the ayurvedic physician is to understand the pattern of *dosha* disharmony in each patient
and prescribe remedies to pacify the forces of decay. *Ayurveda*, which
means "wisdom of long life," has always emphasized the promotion of
health and prevention of sickness, an endeavor that Western clinical
medicine willfully cast aside at the beginning of the nineteenth century, much to its detriment.

In traditional Chinese medicine, the fundamental relationships are
expressed through the concepts of *yin* and *yang. Yang* is that aspect of
being that is warm, expansive, bright, or unfolding. *Yin* is that aspect of
being that is cool, receding, dark, or infolding. The cosmic dance of *yin*
and *yang* is never-ending, creating and permeating all existence. The
rhythms of the dance that play through the organs of the human body
determine the state of health. From a modern perspective, *yin* and *yang*
represent a binary system for storing and transmitting information,
much like a computer's. The activity of this system in the cells of the
human body is my focus in Chapter Six.

For the ancient Greeks, human physiology was described by the balance of the four humors: blood, phlegm, black bile, and yellow bile.
The humors were not abstractions. They were visibly discharged from
the bodies of the sick, who bled, coughed, or excreted their humors.
Different qualities of temperature and moisture attributed to each
humor explained the effect of environmental change and unsound
habits in causing disease. Although Greek physicians were able to distinguish among different types of sickness in vague and broad terms,

they saw, in effect, only one universal disease—an imbalance of the humors—the effects of which varied among different individuals, depending upon the unique circumstances of each case.

Most of what we know about ancient Greek medicine derives from the teachings attributed to Hippocrates, compiled by Greek scholars in the Egyptian city of Alexandria in the third century B.C. Although they are undoubtedly the work of many authors and different schools, the Hippocratic texts are pervaded by an ideal that constitutes the Hippocratic tradition: detailed clinical observation, an aversion to superstition and dogma, and an attempt to cultivate techniques of healing that work in concert with the forces of nature, restoring to the body its natural harmony of function. The Hippocratic physician cared not about disease but about the patient as a whole, striving "to know what man is in relation to food, drink, occupation, and which effect each of these has on the other." He relied on careful observation of the patient's symptoms, habits, and environment, from which he formulated practical advice about diet and activity, never forgetting that a disturbance in any organ was unlikely to be localized in that organ but instead corresponded to a disturbance in the whole person.

Dietetics was the cornerstone of Hippocratic therapy. The Greek concept of diet (*díaita*) included much more than nutrition. It incorporated a person's entire mode of living: the relationship between rest and exercise, sleep and waking, the choice and quantity of food, cleanliness, and patterns of excretion. Hippocratic researchers paid exacting attention to the effects of innumerable foods, solid and liquid, raw and cooked, on the human body in health and disease. They also observed the location of a patient's dwelling place, the winds to which it was exposed, the nearness of the sea, rivers, and swamps, and the quality of his water supply.

The Hippocratic approach dominated Western medicine for almost two thousand years, at first expanded by Galen during the golden age of Rome, and later by Ibn Sina (Avicenna) during Islam's golden age. Ibn Sina's *Canon* became the medical bible of medieval Europe and still guides traditional healers in the Middle East, who "cure diseases that Western medicine cannot name, comfort their patients with satisfying explanations of their conditions, and care for patients who do not accept and cannot afford modern psychiatric methods."[2]

Throughout the Middle Ages and the Renaissance, the healing profession in Europe was not called *medicine;* it was called *physic* (from the Greek word *physis,* meaning nature). Physicians were professors of physic and, consequently, were trained to be philosophers of nature. *Medicine* (from the Latin verb *medico,* literally translated, "I drug") meant the treatment of disease with drugs; it was only a small part of the physician's work, and the least highly regarded.

The preservation of health and prevention of sickness were the main goals of physic. They required that the physician be able to understand each person's unique constitution, matching therapy to the patient's individual requirements, prescribing diet and habits of elimination that were most likely to balance the humors, and herbal remedies that would strengthen weak parts of the body. These general principles guide many types of alternative health practices today.

THE GREAT PLAGUES DESCEND

The replacement of physic by medicine occurred slowly, the result of a growing disparity between ancient precepts and the conditions of life in a changing world. The population of Europe increased substantially during the Middle Ages, trade with Asia and Africa expanded, and cities grew like mushrooms, filth and congestion growing with them. Devastating new diseases made their appearance that were ultimately shown to result from *infection,* a concept foreign to all traditional healing systems.

The Black Death, which decimated Europe and North Africa during the winter of 1347–48, killing one quarter to one half of the entire population, defied explanation on the basis of humors. Giovanni Boccaccio, who contracted plague and survived it, mocked the humoral approach to understanding plague in introducing his masterpiece, the *Decameron,* set against the background of plague-ridden Florence: "How many gallant gentlemen, fair ladies, and sprightly youths, who would have been judged hale and hearty by Galen, Hippocrates and Aesculapius (to say nothing of others), having breakfasted in the morning with their kinsfolk, acquaintances and friends, supped that same evening with their ancestors in the next world!"[3]

The plague's devastation altered every aspect of life in fourteenth-century Europe. Petrarch, who lost his beloved Laura to plague, believed that future generations would never comprehend the magnitude of the disaster. This was, it seemed, a preview of the Apocalypse, filled with suffering, desolation, and madness. Florence had become a city of corpses, overwhelmed by the stench of rotting flesh. Funeral rites were abandoned and bodies were dumped into large trenches. The rules of society, civil and moral authority, all disintegrated. The healthy refused to aid the sick. Husbands abandoned wives, parents abandoned their children. Those that did not quarantine themselves in solitude turned to debauchery and drink. When an Easter pilgrimage to Rome from the papal palace in Avignon failed to halt the pestilence, Pope Clement VI retreated to his inner sanctum, shutting himself up between two protective fires and refusing to see anyone.

Medieval medical authorities were convinced that a catastrophic new disease had been unleashed on the world and struggled to understand it in the light of Hippocratic doctrine. A major deficiency in the Hippocratic texts was their failure to address the concept of contagion. An epidemic was not understood as a contagious infection spreading from person to person, but rather as an event that occurred at a particular place under particular conditions, nothing more: "There was unseasonably wintry weather in Thasos early in autumn, and rainstorms suddenly burst to the accompaniment of northerly and southerly winds. . . . Many people had small styes break out which gave them trouble. . . . there was vomiting of phlegm, bile and undigested food. Sweating occurred and the patients became flaccid all over."[4]

Today we believe that plague results from epidemic infection with a species of bacteria, *Yersinia pestis*, which was isolated in Hong Kong in 1894 during the last pandemic of plague. We also know that the distinctive characteristics of plague, which galvanized medical theorists on the eve of the Renaissance, derive from two factors: the ecology of *Yersinia* and the immune response of infected people.

The usual home for *Y. pestis* is in the tissues of burrowing rodents like field mice and ground squirrels; these are the source of occasional human exposures. Wild rodents transmit plague bacteria to the black rat, *Rattus rattus*, which became the reservoir responsible for the worst human epidemics. Medieval peasants learned to predict the next wave of human pestilence. When armies of moles and marmots came out from their burrows, acting as if they were drunk and then falling down dead, human deaths would inevitably follow. Medieval physicians blamed the plague on noxious vapors, called *miasmata*, generated within the bowels of the earth, first affecting underground animals and then humans. The source of these vapors was hotly debated. The medical faculty of the University of Paris issued a report to Pope Clement attributing the Black Death to the conjunction of Mars, Jupiter, and Saturn in the house of Aquarius that occurred on March 20, 1345. This august diagnosis was the basis for much future discussion. Some argued that astral forces had attracted poisonous gases to the earth's surface, others that the planets had worked directly on the corporeal humors of those who became sick. The pope's surgeon, Guy de Chauliac, confessed that physicians felt useless and ashamed because the plague resisted all conventional therapies. When traditional attempts at helping patients equilibrate their humors failed to prevent or reverse disease, influential physicians became more concerned with classifying outbreaks, attaching names to them, and attempting to help people avoid exposure.

Recognition that plague was contagious led to Europe's first quarantine laws. These failed to halt the spread of disease because the complexity of transmission was not understood. A severely infected person, developing small abscesses filled with plague bacteria in his lungs, can fill the air with hordes of *Yersinia* merely by coughing. Spread of infection through the air produces deadly *pneumonic* plague, marked by sudden onset of chest pain, cough, and fever, rapidly proceeding to hemorrhage. The victim of pneumonic plague bleeds into his skin, becoming a collage of purple bruises (hence the name, Black Death). He coughs blood and vomits blood and, choking on his own bloody sputum, suffocates within one to three days of contracting the infection.

Most plague does not spread by the pneumonic route, however, which explains why quarantine measures failed to stop its spread and why dedicated doctors and nurses (apparently there were a few) could minister to the sick without getting sick themselves. The usual mode of transmission for plague bacteria is from rats to humans via the bite of an infected rat flea. The human victim is known as the *host*, who provides shelter for an unwelcome guest. The rat is the *reservoir* of infection and the flea is known as the *vector*. The black rat's flea, *Xenophylla cheopsis*, has been the most diabolically efficient vector for transmitting the common *bubonic* form of plague. When plague bacteria enter the human body from a flea bite, they provoke an immediate fever, followed by swelling of the lymph nodes—buboes—in areas near the bites.

Fever and formation of buboes are part of the body's immune response to the bacteria, an attempt to limit infection. Medieval physicians observed that the best prognosis was found among those patients who developed large buboes that drained copious amounts of pus. When trapping of *Yersinia* by the lymph nodes is inadequate, the bacteria spread to the lungs and the nervous system, causing shortness of breath, chest pain, cough, headache, anxiety, mental confusion, and hallucinations.

If epidemics of plague during the fourteenth and fifteenth centuries were difficult to fit into the classical model of Hippocrates and Galen, the appearance and spread of syphilis in 1495 demonstrated clearly that contagion, not humoral imbalance, was the cause of epidemics. In 1494, the king of France, Charles VIII, employed fifty thousand mercenaries to besiege the city of Naples. The men were serviced by a small army of prostitutes. Naples's fall was followed by an orgy of looting and sexual debauchery, after which the soldiers and their camp followers scattered and returned to their homes in various parts of Europe. The epidemic had begun.

The earliest symptom was a painless ulcer on the genitals, followed within a few weeks by a skin rash that covered the entire body before turning into hideous scabbing sores that might ulcerate and eat through skin, cartilage, and bone. Fever, swollen lymph nodes, patchy bald spots, and agonizing pain in bones and muscles would occur within weeks or months. Years later, the disease would spread to the brain and spinal cord, producing paralysis and madness. In August of 1495, Maximilian I, the Holy Roman Emperor, motivated by his political dispute with the French king, signed an edict proclaiming that this new pestilence was God's punishment for blasphemy and had never before been seen on earth. Italians called it the French Disease; in Paris it was the Neapolitan Disease. Elsewhere it was known as the great pox, to distinguish it from smallpox. Almost everyone recognized that it was spread through sexual contact.

Girolamo Fracastoro, an Italian physician and scientist, studied the spread of great pox throughout Europe during the sixteenth century and reasoned that the disease must result from sexual transmission of microorganisms, "invisible seeds [germs]" with the power to multiply within the human body.[5] Fracastoro's germ theory found few adherents; the concept of a microorganism as the cause of contagion violated all traditional thinking, but the presence of this new scourge meant the time was ripe for a retreat from Hippocratic concepts of balance.

THE RISE OF "THE NEW MEDICINE"

Ironically, the harbinger of change was an astute and charismatic physician of the seventeenth century, Thomas Sydenham, who was hailed as "the English Hippocrates." A cavalry officer in Oliver Cromwell's Parliamentary Army, Sydenham came to medicine later in life and with far less formal education than most of his peers, receiving his bachelor of medicine from Oxford at the age of thirty-nine. Like Hippocrates, Sydenham believed that it was the physician's task to assist the body's natural healing processes, avoid heroic remedies, observe patients closely, and let common sense guide a practical approach to treatment. Horseback riding was one of his favorite therapies for mental or physical disorders. Sydenham is reported to have sent one of his difficult patients on horseback from London to Inverness to consult a brilliant Scottish physician, who did not exist. The patient's anger at being tricked was mitigated by the incontestable cure of his infirmities, which had disappeared during the long and arduous journey to the Highlands of Scotland.

Sydenham's greatest impact in changing the shape of medical care came from his masterful studies on the use of quinine for the treatment of malaria. Although the devastation wrought by epidemics of plague and smallpox has been more dramatic, the unrelenting toll of death exacted by malaria, century after century, makes it the greatest killer that humankind has ever known. In the seventeenth century, malaria's debilitating fevers, racking chills, and drenching sweats tormented countless citizens of European river cities, like London and Paris. Mosquitoes thrived in the marshy floodplains adjoining zones of commerce and spread disease by injecting malarial parasites into the bloodstreams of rich and poor alike. Not only was the parasite that causes malaria unknown, but transmission by mosquito bites was unsuspected.

Malaria, as its name implies, was thought to be spread by bad air, hence its association with swamps and marshland.

Cinchona bark, a natural source of quinine and a traditional Incan remedy for fever, was brought to Europe from Peru by Jesuit priests who had seen its wonderful effects in relieving the symptoms of dreaded tertian malaria. Demand for this remarkable New World remedy drove its price higher and higher. So many worthless or dangerous imitations were placed on the market that public confidence in cinchona bark plummeted. Overcoming his distaste for the Jesuits, who controlled the world's cinchona supply, Sydenham, a Puritan, carefully demonstrated the efficacy and the safety of quinine, when properly used. Completely ineffective against any of the fevers that were not malaria, quinine was the first great proof for a new theory of medicine: a specific treatment for a specific disease.

Sydenham proposed that diseases existed as real and distinct entities, independent of the individual patients whose minds and bodies they attacked, and as clearly separable one from another as if they were different species of plants. His religious beliefs committed him to classifying diseases by their outward phenomena, the patient's symptoms, which he called "the outer husk of things," because God had given man the ability to see the surface of the body but not its inner workings. He opposed chemical and pathological analysis in favor of detailed attention to the medical history. "Nature," he wrote, "in the production of disease, is uniform and consistent; so much so, that for the same disease in different persons the symptoms are for the most part the same."[6] He separated patients' symptoms into two groups. *Pathognomonic* ("disease-knowing") symptoms were those shared by most patients with the same disease; they indicate which disease is present. *Idiosyncratic* symptoms were unique to particular patients and not useful in identifying the disease. Sydenham's concept is still employed today.

Despite the great esteem in which Sydenham was held, his dream of a comprehensive, consistent typology of diseases was not realized until the end of the nineteenth century, perhaps because Sydenham was wrong. His theory of disease entities could not be built from the "outer husk of things." By its very nature, it needed to be built upon knowledge of the inner workings of the body, and that required the use of the one procedure that Sydenham most abhorred: the autopsy.

Human dissection had thrived in Renaissance Italy and revolution-ized Western notions concerning the nature of the body. A Belgian anatomist, Andreas Vesalius, brought glory to the University of Padua, where he taught, with the publication of his classic treatise, *On the Fab-ric of the Human Body* (1543), regarded as the first advance in anatomy since the time of Galen. A judge in Padua's criminal court was so en-thralled by Vesalius's research that he scheduled executions according to the anatomist's need for fresh bodies. In the eighteenth century, an-other professor at the University of Padua, Giovanni Battista Morgagni, extended the work of Vesalius by attempting to find correlations be-tween clinical symptoms and postmortem pathology. Detailed record-ing of the patient's symptoms followed by meticulous dissection led Morgagni to describe disease as the result of pathological changes found in different organs of the body.

Morgagni's concept of pathological anatomy as the basis of disease, developed during the eighteenth century, received its greatest impetus from research conducted in the charity hospitals of Paris at the start of the nineteenth century. This is the place where modern clinical medi-cine was born and the eclipse of the patient commenced.

Bursting at their seams in the aftermath of the French Revolution, Parisian hospitals were museums of end-stage pathology, the last refuge for the sick, the poor, and the incurable. Infectious diseases—"hospital fevers"—spread like brushfires through their overcrowded, unsanitary wards, killing 15 to 25 percent of the patients and afflicting over half of the medical students who attended them and assisted in their autopsies. The bright and narrow beam of pathology, powered by the dissection of corpses, became the guiding light of the New Medicine, as its fathers called it.

In fact, the New Medicine was poorly named, because its propo-nents held the treatment of disease in disdain. One of its founding fa-thers, Philippe Pinel, vehemently attacked as quackery the notion that the physician's task was to support the body's natural healing processes. According to Pinel, "charlatanism . . . pretends to cure all diseases and does not see in the violence and order of . . . symptoms anything but a sort of harmony and gathering of preservative efforts."[7] Pinel's mean-ing was clear and erroneous. He believed that the signs of sickness were manifestations of the disease, not—as we now know them to be—manifestations of the body's attempt to heal itself.

Pinel's colleagues cultivated their therapeutic pessimism, preferring to act like scientists and observe the "natural history" of diseases. Jean Corvisart, physician to Napoléon I and a leader of the Paris School, warned the French people to stop expecting "health from the healing art."[8] Medicine was about disease, not about health or longevity, and the physician's task was to discover, in life, through physical signs, what organic lesions were present in the patient's body. To explain this concept, Corvisart coined the term "internal medicine," which is still in use. The result was a new way of looking at patients.[9] The inventor of the stethoscope, René-Théophile-Hyacinthe Laënnec, divided diseases into two classes: *organic* (those accompanied by obvious pathological changes in various organs) and *nervous* (those lacking such changes). For the first time in the history of medicine, a formal distinction had been made between physical disease, which could be seen in the tissues of the body, and mental disease, which could not.

From its inception, the New Medicine was troubled by limitations. Although its proponents believed that their attention to detailed clinical observation made them the modern disciples of Hippocrates, they mistrusted and denigrated the information communicated by their patients. They warned their students that the Parisian lower classes, who filled their hospitals, deliberately falsified or exaggerated complaints, were too stupid or too incoherent to provide reliable histories, and were highly influenced by ideas and jargon contained in popular medical books.[10] Pathology, argued Laënnec, was more important than the stories of patients.

FROM MICROSCOPE TO MICROBIOLOGY

The greatest impediment to the full application of Laënnec's viewpoint was the failure of dissectors to find pathology where pathology was expected. To begin with, autopsies seldom disclosed the immediate cause of death and rarely gave information about the underlying causes of disease. A more troubling flaw was that for many patients who had died of fever, no organic lesions were apparent at autopsy. The remedy for this last limitation would require physicians to enter the world of the microscope.

The microscope had been invented about the year 1600, an accidental occurrence in the craft of making spectacles. Fascination with the new device spread quickly, and the seventeenth century witnessed an explosion of information about the fine structure of plants and insects and the discovery of "little animals" in pond water and in feces. Marcello Malpighi, a professor at the University of Pisa, used the microscope to discover the tiny air sacs that comprise the lungs, called alveoli, and the smallest divisions of blood vessels, the capillaries.

Antoni van Leeuwenhoek, a linen draper in Delft, was the most famous and controversial of the early microscopists. At his death, over four hundred microscopes were found in his home, with different types of lenses, used for different purposes. Unprejudiced by medical dogma, Leeuwenhoek allowed his insatiable curiosity to drive his investigations. He examined with his lenses everything he could find, from plants and insects to crystals and rocks, scrapings from his teeth, samples of saliva and semen. He identified sperm in the semen of healthy men and numerous types of animals and concluded that these tiny animals were the basis for new life, rejecting the prevailing view that vapors in seminal fluid were the cause of conception. After his death, the art of microscopy made little progress until the middle of the nineteenth century, when improvements in the structure of lenses and new staining techniques made detailed study of the solid tissues of the body possible.

Rudolf Virchow, Germany's "Pope of Pathology," established the cell as the ultimate unit of structure and function in the body and initiated the movement that traced sickness to cellular dysfunction. He resisted, however, the temptation to localize disease within the cell. As an ardent political activist, Virchow held the social conditions under which patients lived to be more important determinants of health than the tissue changes he saw through the microscope. "Medicine," he wrote, "is a social science. Don't we see that epidemics everywhere point to deficiencies of society?" In 1847, at the age of twenty-six, he founded the *Archives of Pathological Anatomy*. In the journal's first issue, he challenged his readers with the question, Where in the body's cells is disease to be found? His answer: "Diseases have no independent or isolated existence; they are not autonomous organisms, not beings invading a body, nor parasites growing on it; they are only the manifestations of life processes under altered conditions. . . . Therapy is confronted not by diseases but by conditions; everywhere we deal only with the alterations in the life circumstances."[11] For years, Virchow resisted the germ theory of disease, warning his colleagues that the simplistic attribution of contagious disease to bacteria "hinders further research and lulls the conscience to sleep."

Despite Virchow's objections, it was the field of bacteriology that gave medicine its most dramatic advances and supplied the foundation for modern medical practice. Although Leeuwenhoek had identified living microbes in 1667, most physicians and scientists considered them to be harmless by-products of putrefaction, the result of disease, not its cause. That microbes were elemental life forms, far older than any organism visible to the unaided eye, and that they permeated all habitable space on the earth's surface, was incomprehensible.

No group suffered more grievously from medical resistance to the concept of infection than did pregnant women. Childbed fever was a dreaded complication of pregnancy with a high rate of fatality. A careful reading of ancient texts suggests that it was uncommon before the Renaissance. The replacement of home births with hospital deliveries and of midwives by obstetricians created epidemics of childbed fever in the major cities of Europe and the United States throughout the eighteenth and nineteenth centuries. In 1843, Oliver Wendell Holmes, the American physician and poet, studied the pattern of childbed fever in a Boston hospital and concluded that the disease was spread from patient to patient, with the obstetrician acting as the vector. He was angrily denounced for maligning the honor of the medical profession.

I. P. Semmelweiss, a Hungarian obstetrician working in Vienna, observed that the death rate from childbed fever sometimes reached 50 percent in wards where medical students examined patients, and was less than 3 percent on wards attended only by midwives. He attributed the difference to the participation of the students in autopsies of women who had died and concluded correctly that infected material was transmitted from the autopsy room to mothers in labor, despite the cosmetic hand-washing required of students and physicians. He brooded over the agonizing conclusion that he, too, had been a vector, unwittingly killing many of the women he had delivered because of the numerous autopsies he had performed in searching for the fever's cause. In 1847, Semmelweiss proposed that all students and physicians wash their hands in a solution of chlorinated lime before examining patients. Wherever Semmelweiss introduced his system of antisepsis, the maternal mortality rate fell dramatically. His supporters, unfortunately, misunderstood his doctrine and blamed "cadaveric matter," not microorganisms, for the spread of childbed fever. Because some hospitals that did not routinely perform autopsies suffered from high maternal mortality rates, Semmelweiss was dismissed as "the Fool from Budapest" and his ideas rejected. Deepening depression and feelings of guilt slowly drove him mad. He entered a mental asylum in 1865 and died of infection soon after. A decade later the famous French chemist Louis Pasteur isolated bacteria from the blood of victims of childbed fever. The medical profession still refused to yield. One outraged physician challenged Pasteur to a duel for suggesting that hospital personnel carried the deadly germs from infected women to healthy women.

Resistance to the concepts of microbiology was soon swept away by a deluge of useful new discoveries. Inspired by Pasteur's early work, Lord Joseph Lister, a prominent English surgeon, had been publishing studies of antiseptic techniques in surgery since 1867. Lister's techniques were so effective at reducing the postoperative death rate that, by 1880, they were widely used throughout Europe, not only for surgery, but also for obstetrics, a posthumous victory for Semmelweiss. Guided by the discoveries of microbiologists, surgeons soon replaced antisepsis (an attempt to kill bacteria) with asepsis (an attempt to prevent bacteria from contaminating a sterile surgical field). Aseptic technique made the great advances of modern surgery possible and dramatically elevated the status of surgeons.

In the decades after 1880, the dreaded ancient epidemic diseases yielded their secrets to science, one by one. Malaria. Leprosy. Typhoid. Tuberculosis. Cholera. Diphtheria. Plague. Dysentery. The microbes causing each of these were isolated and identified in the laboratories of France and Germany. For the first time in history, the actual causes of disease could be identified with certainty. The specificity of diseases had been proved. Soon, it seemed, the scalpel of laboratory science would dissect every clinical disorder, isolating each as a distinct entity with a unique cause. The Hippocratic notion of disease as disharmony seemed quaint and irrelevant.

THE FALSE TRIUMPH OVER TUBERCULOSIS

No disease more clearly illustrates the triumph of this new vision than tuberculosis. Its old name was "consumption," and it was defined by its symptoms, which had been lucidly described in the Hippocratic texts:

> It began during the winter. . . . By early spring, most of those who had taken to their beds had died. . . . In most cases, the illness started with sudden deterioration. The symptoms were: frequent shivering attacks, often high continued fever, much untimely sweating although the patients remained cold throughout, and much chilling so that it was difficult to get them warm again. . . . Weight loss was pernicious. Coughing continued throughout the illness, and it was common for patients to bring up large amounts of ripe moist sputum without excessive pain. . . . These patients . . . suffered by far the greatest harm from their loss of appetite. They would not even take fluid nourishment, but remained without thirst. As death approached, they showed heaviness of the body, swelling, shivering and delirium.[12]

A disease of cities, consumption flourished in ancient Rome and almost disappeared during the pastoral conditions of the early Middle Ages, returning in fury with the urban squalor of the sixteenth century. By the middle of the seventeenth century it had become "the captain of the men of death," killing one person out of five in the capitals of western Europe.

The name "tuberculosis" supplanted "consumption" during the nineteenth century, because of the characteristic pathology consistently found in the tissues of consumptives. Lungs, livers, and lymph nodes were filled with tiny nodules called tubercles, each composed of a palisade of white blood cells surrounding a core of pus. Rod-shaped bacteria were sometimes discerned growing within the cells. These elusive and mysterious microbes were called "tubercle bacilli."

Robert Koch, a general practitioner in rural Germany, had begun his efforts to identify the tubercle bacillus in secret, working at a makeshift laboratory that adjoined his consultation room. From the lungs of people who had died with tuberculosis, Koch succeeded in isolating a species of large, slow-growing bacteria which was named *Mycobacterium tuberculosis*. When he transferred these bacteria to guinea pigs, the animals died of tuberculosis. At autopsy, Koch was able to culture the mycobacterium from the organs of the dead animals. This, he believed, proved that the bacteria he had cultured were the cause of the human disease and not mere bystanders.

On March 24, 1882, Koch nervously presented his findings to the Physiological Society in Berlin. A young physician in attendance, Paul Ehrlich, a future Nobel laureate himself,[13] described Koch's presentation as a masterpiece of scientific research and a deeply moving experience, "the most important experience of my scientific life."

Overnight Koch became the world's most celebrated scientist. Not only had he discovered the cause of the greatest killer in the industrialized world, he had set a new standard of proof for the cause of disease. Tuberculosis was soon dubbed "T.B.," which stands for "tubercle bacillus." The illness was no longer named by its effect on the individual, which could be quite variable, but by the organism that was its cause.

The irony of Koch's famous presentation is that almost certainly every person in the meeting room that day was infected with *Mycobacterium tuberculosis*, yet none of them had the disease and few would ever develop it. Paul Ehrlich used Koch's method to discover his own asymptomatic tubercular infection and "cured" himself by taking a long vacation. But Ehrlich may never have been sick from TB and was certainly never cured of the bacteria. People who harbor *M. tuberculosis* in their lungs are infected for life. Live tubercle bacilli persist within the tubercles, imprisoned by the white blood cells. The tubercle is not a product of the bacteria, but a defense thrown up by the host. When immunity falters, the bacteria escape. Healthy people who carry the germ for tuberculosis rarely become sick with TB. Impairment of immunity, on the other hand, is known to activate the sleeping infection. Impairment of the host's immunity is as important for the development of tuberculosis as is the microbe itself.[14]

Paradoxically, it was Louis Pasteur, the father of microbiology, who demonstrated the truth of Virchow's contention that the conditions of life, not the microbe, are the cause of disease. Crippled by a stroke, but still active in his work, Pasteur brought two caged chickens to a meeting of the French Academy in 1878. Both birds had been injected with deadly anthrax bacteria. One bird, exposed to cold temperature before infection, was blackened and dead. The other, kept at a warm temperature, was alive and clucking. Limping to the front of the room, the renowned scientist stared intently at his astonished audience as an assistant held the chickens up before their eyes. "You see," he proclaimed defiantly, "a microbe is nothing; the *terrain* is everything!"[15]

MEDICINE IN AMERICA

Most mainstream American physicians believed that the traditions of Europe were not vigorous enough to flourish in the New World. Benjamin Rush, a medical doctor and a signer of the Declaration of Independence, held that American doctors should beware of placing "undue reliance upon the healing powers of nature in curing disease."[16] Influenced by the philosophy of the Enlightenment and the mentality of the frontier, Americans have always embraced new technologies and believed that it was better to do more rather than less. Vigorous bloodletting and strong purgation were standard therapy for many diseases in the early years of the Republic. Physicians in general were less interested in theory than in results and would engage patients in an ongoing process of treatment by trial-and-error. They prescribed prodigious quantities of mercury, rhubarb, opium, and medicinal spirits, along with tonics and stimulants.

The excesses of mainstream American medicine during the nineteenth century stimulated the growth of numerous alternative therapeutic systems based upon personal hygiene, nutrition, water therapy, and herbal folk remedies. Chiropractic and osteopathy originated in the Midwest during the late nineteenth century, and homeopathy, which had been developed in Germany during the early years of the century, was readily transplanted to the United States. By 1900 there were twenty-two colleges of homeopathic medicine and fifteen thousand homeopathic practitioners in the United States, one-sixth of the U.S. medical profession. (The AMA at this time had only eight thousand members.) A major medical center in Philadelphia is still named after the founder of homeopathy, Samuel Hahnemann.

As much as they differed among themselves, all the alternative sects shared the traditional notion that diseases are not distinct entities with unique causes but manifestations of disharmony and imbalance. The influence of the alternative sects was substantial. The dean of medicine at Tulane University complained in 1897 that "quacks [are] the greatest foe to the medical profession . . . [an] obstacle to the financial success of the reputable medical practitioner."[17]

During the first decade of the twentieth century, the leaders of organized medicine concluded that the time had come to change the outlook and the social composition of the American medical profession, increasing at the same time its commitment to science, its income and its social status, and separating its practitioners more obviously from the quacks. The United States, they believed, had a surfeit of bad medical schools and incompetent doctors, many of whom had been recruited from the working and lower middle classes. Their membership in the profession swelled its ranks, creating a physician surplus that reduced professional incomes. In his presidential address to the AMA in 1903, Dr. F. Billings talked with disdain of medical night schools, "sundown institutions [which] . . . enable the clerk, the street-car conductor, the janitor and others employed during the day to earn a degree."[18] The presence of women in the profession was also thought to diminish income and prestige. In 1900, there were more than seven thousand women physicians in the United States, compared to fewer than three hundred in England. In Boston and Minneapolis, almost 20 percent of the practicing physicians were women.

Limiting the numbers of physicians by reforming medical education was the key to progress. Medical students would first study the basic sciences. Clinical instruction would follow, confined to the wards of teaching hospitals, where the teachers would be men of research, not local practitioners. Specialized postgraduate training would be encouraged.

THE FLEXNER REPORT

Between 1906 and 1910, the AMA joined forces with the Carnegie Foundation in an effort to define the future shape of medical education. Their goal was to reduce the number of medical schools from 160 to 31, with the survivors being dominated by the values and standards of academic specialists. Their tool was *Bulletin Number Four*, prepared for them by a young educator, Abraham Flexner. The Flexner Report, as it has been called, directed medical attention *away* from the training of general practitioners, those physicians who took care of the common, everyday ills that make up the bulk of medical work. The great medical centers of this country, most of them affiliated with private universities and built with private funds, owe their very existence to the Flexner Report. For them, *Bulletin Number Four* is as sacred as the Bible.[19]

Flexner's stated goals were never fully met. Because he had no interest in assuring an equitable distribution of physicians or in allowing any but the upper classes to have access to a medical education, his plan called for twenty states to be left without any medical school. State legislatures, however, had to deal with reality. Their commitment to ensuring a supply of general practitioners for their constituencies led to a marked expansion of public, state-supported schools, which have trained most of the nation's generalists over the past eighty years. Only in the 1960s did the number of specialists finally surpass the number of primary physicians.

The reform of medical education embodied in the Flexner Report rapidly fulfilled its purpose in a number of ways. It succeeded in increasing the social and intellectual homogeneity of the medical profession, driving out the lower classes and the immigrants, reducing the number of blacks and women, and, initially, of Jews. It succeeded in creating a shortage of physicians in poor communities and in rural areas.

There is no evidence that implementation of the Flexner Report did anything to improve the care of patients. In 1937, when Lewis Thomas, scientist and author, completed his internship, he discovered that hospitals were "simply custodial. . . . Whether you survived or not depended on the natural history of the disease itself. Medicine made little or no difference."[20] Thomas's simple statement is more than a critique of medical therapy. It describes with uncanny clarity the change in perception that attended the growth of modern medicine. Thomas acknowledges two factors—and only two—that determine recovery from sickness. One is "the natural history of the disease" and the other is medication, which was quite ineffective in the years before antibiotics. The *person* who is sick, within this perspective, plays no active role.

IN THE SHADOW OF MEDICINE

The eclipse of the patient, seen dimly in Thomas's memoir, is the most profound, lasting, and unfortunate effect of the Flexner Report: its insidious and destructive success in altering the relationship between physicians and patients. For the doctor in training, the patient was to become an object of study, stripped of personal identity, plucked from the context of his life and placed in a hospital bed. Here, the process of diagnosis and treatment would be increasingly directed by the wonders of technology as manifested in the laboratory or the X-ray department.

As decades passed, the depersonalization of health care and the dependence of physicians on laboratory testing intensified. In 1944, Tinsley Harrison, the editor of a renowned textbook of medicine, sharply criticized "the present-day tendency towards a five-minute history followed by a five-day barrage of special tests in the hope that the diagnostic rabbit may suddenly emerge from the laboratory hat."[21]

The addiction of American physicians to laboratory testing has not diminished since Harrison's critique. One of the sharpest memories of my internship at Bellevue Hospital is the maniacal look on the face of a junior medical resident as he prepared a case for the hospital's chief of medicine at grand rounds. His obsession was the laboratory results; he had to make absolutely certain they were thorough and complete.

"Oh, my God!" he suddenly moaned. "There's no uric acid result here. The chief will have my ass! I am dead!" He promptly made up a value and filled in the empty box. Measurement of uric acid levels had no particular significance to the case he was presenting, but their absence would, he thought, be a sign of his incompetence.

The entry of insurance companies into the health care market, during the years after World War II, actually increased the reliance on the laboratory and decreased the involvement of physicians with their patients. This effect seems paradoxical, because the profligate use of technology is the single greatest factor in raising the cost of medical care. A brief history of health insurance explains the paradox.

Blue Cross and Blue Shield, originating in the 1930s, were designed to give middle-class patients better access to doctors and to hospitals, and to guarantee hospitals access to the middle class. They were *provider-controlled* plans, developed by the hospitals themselves. Blue Cross was inflationary by intent. Hospitals were paid according to their total operating costs; the higher their operating costs, the higher the reimbursement rate. Blue Cross inexorably encouraged hospital growth, turning large hospitals into huge corporations controlling tremendous financial resources and wielding considerable political influence. The expansion of the health care industry that followed World War II, supported largely by federal grants, had as its primary goal an increase in the number of hospital beds and the affiliation of those beds with research institutions. Other approaches to health care expansion (e.g., development of community-based clinics or preventive health care programs) were passed over.

The growth of expensive, hospital-based medical care attracted commercial indemnity insurance companies. By the mid-1950s, commercial insurers had more clients than the Blues; by 1980, 80 percent of Americans had private commercial health insurance. Initially, the commercial insurers ran a high profit margin. As costs increased they simply passed them on to their clients by increasing the premiums. As long as they could raise their rates, commercial insurers had no incentive to control health care costs. Money obtained from clients was invested at a profit which offset the cost of indemnification. In the economic inflation that characterized the 1960s and 1970s, merely delaying the payment of benefits resulted in substantial profit.

Medicare was the third horseman of the medical cost apocalypse. Although Medicare and Medicaid initially increased access to health care for the poor and the elderly, publicly funded insurance played right into the hands of the private insurers and the Blues. To begin with, the government followed corporate rules: hospitals were reimbursed according to their total costs and physicians were reimbursed more for services performed in hospitals than for services rendered outside hospitals. The fee structure provided financial incentives for physicians to perform procedures on patients and disincentives for them to spend time talking to patients. Today, doctors treating elderly patients covered by Medicare cannot make ends meet unless they perform lots of procedures.

The administrative rules that confound and demoralize physicians are all based on the theory of diseases. It is now possible for a panel of doctors and administrators to know what the appropriate diagnostic evaluation and treatment are for almost any disease without consideration of the person who is sick or the circumstances within which the sickness occurred. These judgments are codified so rigidly that they can be performed on a daily basis by clerical workers servicing HMOs. Even scientific studies that attempt to evaluate the impact of medical care on patients' quality of life rarely ask the opinion of patients. They use measures for quality of life determined by the scientist. The beliefs of patients, it seems, lack scientific validity.[22]

Medicine as an institution now seems to deify technology even as it depersonalizes the patient. My own medical training was a vivid illustration of how doctors as individuals have absorbed that same attitude.

2

MEDICAL ODYSSEY

"Iron Man" was the highest praise possible at Bellevue Hospital, where I trained as a physician. Its meaning depended upon context. On the wards, an Iron Man was an intern who needed no sleep and no help. In the emergency room, an Iron Man was a resident who admitted no one after midnight, protecting the sleep of his fellow interns and residents by guarding the frontier between the hospital's wards and the outside world. The opposite of Iron Man, in the ER context, was "sieve," the most insulting epithet one resident could hurl at another. To be a sieve was to lack clinical judgment, courage, and group loyalty all at once.

The old Bellevue was a beehive of large open wards and dark, winding hallways sprawling across four New York City blocks, a world of its own, connected to the city outside only by the never-ending deluge of the sick and the poor that flowed, unhappily and often unwillingly, through its emergency room and into its overcrowded wards. Most patients entered Bellevue bereft of identity; they had left it somewhere outside the walls. For those of us who worked there, it was safer that way. So many of them died. As interns, we worked a hundred hours a week with little supervision or technical support. We barely had time to think about ourselves—let alone our patients—as persons. Sometimes, however, the identity of a patient thrust itself upon us, even in death. I remember the agonizing thirty-six hours in which I lost three people to heart attacks.

THREE FUNERALS

Elsie Buell, sixty-two years of age, a cashier at a midtown market, felt a crushing weight on her chest as she walked from the subway to her job. She had never been very sick before, but she knew the meaning of that pain. It chilled her to the bone, robbed her of breath, dimmed her vision. She barely managed to hail a cab and whisper, "Hospital!"

I was about to start my rounds when I heard the voice page: "DR. GALLAND TO EMERGENCY, *STAT!* DR. GALLAND TO EMERGENCY, *STAT!*"

All hospitals have emergency rooms, frontiers that separate the world outside from the world inside. Only Bellevue had an emergency ward, or "EW," an intensive care unit adjacent to the emergency room where the sickest patients could receive immediate attention, whatever their problem. Hit by a bus, overdosed on heroin, collapsed with a heart attack—Bellevue's EW was ready and waiting.

When I arrived there, Elsie Buell was being lifted from a stretcher to a bed. Her lips were blue, her forehead covered with beads of sweat.

"Cardiogenic shock!" said the ER resident emphatically. "Crushing chest pain, started about thirty minutes ago. Blood pressure is sixty by palpation. Rhythm is okay." He flashed a cardiogram before my eyes. "Anterior wall myocardial infarction. Looks like a big one. Good luck." He was gone.

I turned to Elsie, who lay trembling on the bed. "You've had a heart attack," I told her. "We're going to do some things to make you more comfortable." That was not exactly true. The oxygen mask may have helped to ease her breathing. But the catheter in her bladder, the IV line in her left arm, and the heart monitor were there for our use, not for her comfort.

In 1969, in fact, there was little we could do for a patient like Elsie. Bed rest, oxygen, morphine for pain, and a drug called isuprel, which stimulated the heart to beat with greater force, were about all we had to offer. We came to learn that isuprel was the worst drug you could give for cardiogenic shock. Using isuprel was like whipping a horse that could no longer walk. Elsie's failing heart needed rest, not a chemical beating. By 1975, isuprel had been abandoned. The physics of cardiogenic shock had been unraveled and new drugs had emerged, smart drugs. Yet the mortality rate from cardiogenic shock remained the same: three out of four died. By the late 1980s, emergency surgical techniques and mechanical wizardry like balloon counterpulsation had been added; yet still, four out of five died.[1]

I examined Elsie and ordered the isuprel drip. Over the next hour, her pulse became weaker and weaker. Then it stopped—a cardiac arrest—and her eyes rolled back in her head.

"Code Blue!" I called, and three nurses rushed over with the resuscitation equipment. I began pressing rhythmically on Elsie's breastbone, so that the pressure of my hand, transmitting the weight of my body, substituted for the beating of her heart. The response was amazing. She awoke and tried talking to me.

"You're getting a good femoral pulse," said a nurse, feeling the pulse in her leg.

"Blood pressure is ninety over fifty," said another. "That's better than she was doing on her own."

False alarm, I thought. No need for resuscitation. As soon as I stopped the chest massage, her pulse disappeared and she lapsed into coma, only to awaken when I resumed pressing.

So it went, for six hours. Elsie stayed conscious through it all, as we took turns massaging her heart. It was backbreaking labor, and one person could only keep it up for ten to fifteen minutes at a time. Exhausted to the bone, we couldn't abandon the resuscitation of this patient, even when the futility of our efforts became clear. I wondered what it must be like for Elsie, being awake for her own resuscitation, feeling the weight of a stranger pushing on her chest sixty times a minute, knowing that his thumping was the only thing keeping her alive. She slowly became less and less responsive. However hard we worked, there was no way that the pressure we supplied could really compensate for a heart unable to pump. When the line on the cardiac monitor became flat, we finally stopped.

We were all veterans of many resuscitation attempts, most of them unsuccessful. This one was different. Almost always, the object of a "Code Blue" was unconscious, a body lying naked on the bed, plastic tubing emerging from the mouth, the arm, the genitals. The person within was unseen and often unknown. But as I leaned over Elsie Buell, her sad brown eyes were open, looking into mine, entreating. We mourned her death, numbly and in silence. The nurses had to clean and wrap her body before their shift ended. I had to return to my ward and complete my rounds for the day.

The next morning, as I prepared to eat breakfast, the dreaded page sounded again: "DR. GALLAND TO EMERGENCY, *STAT!* DR. GALLAND TO EMERGENCY, *STAT!*"

Dora Borelli was only forty, but had suffered from high blood pressure for several years. Chest pain and difficulty breathing had awakened her at 6:00 A.M. Unable to afford a cab, not realizing she needed an ambulance, she took a three-mile bus ride to Bellevue from her apartment on the Lower East Side, accompanied by her ten-year-old son. I caught a glimpse of the boy sitting alone and stone-faced in the dingy waiting room as I rushed into the emergency ward.

Dora was already slipping into shock and soon had no measurable pulse or blood pressure. We spent four hours attempting resuscitation. I went out to speak to her son, Rickie, twice during that time. He never said a word. Haunted by the empty stare in Rickie's face, I refused to stop trying to save his mother, until the heart monitor showed—once again—nothing more than a straight line. Worn down from the physical work and the futility of cardiac massage, and dreading what I had to do next, I walked slowly into the waiting room. The boy stared silently ahead, refusing even to acknowledge my presence.

"I'm very, very sorry," I said. "We did everything we could to save your mother. I'm afraid she's dead." I waited expectantly. There was not a flicker of response. "I'll take you home," I added.

I knew from Dora's clinic record that her husband had a brain tumor and was receiving radiation therapy, and that her mother, who lived with the family, had severe rheumatoid arthritis. They had no phone. I would have to bring them the news in person.

During the past nine months I had not stepped outside of Bellevue once during daylight, except to go home to bed on Saturday mornings. The brightness of the afternoon sun and the bustle of cars and pedestrians on First Avenue startled me. I had been seeing so much of death, I didn't quite remember what ordinary life was like.

The taxi ride felt bizarre. We cruised down FDR Drive, the East River dancing in the sun beneath the graceful arch of the Manhattan Bridge. The world outside seemed vibrant. Inside was a stony silence hiding the agony of a boy who refused to speak.

His home was in a housing project, a stark brick building covered with graffiti. A confusion of smells filled the hallway—chicken soup drifting from a doorway, the acrid smell of urine from the stairwell. Rickie opened the door to his apartment and let me in. I stared at two people more crippled than I had expected. His father was missing half the top of his skull, removed for brain surgery and replaced with a flat metal plate. His legs were too weak to support him; he hobbled forward on crutches. Grandma's hands and legs were as twisted and gnarled as branches of mountain laurel. She needed a four-legged walker merely to stand. The enormity of this tragedy was unbearable. They had lost more than a wife and daughter. Dora had been their only link to the world of sunlight we had just left behind. A crushing weight lay on the shoulders of the boy. As his father and grandma sobbed and moaned, Rickie never once surrendered his silence or his blank stare.

I returned to the hospital at 5:00 P.M., haunted by the faces of Dora's family, as tired as if I had spent the entire night working in the emergency room. I hoped to grab a quick nap before my next admission and slipped away to my room. The coolness of the bedsheets and the softness of the mattress felt delicious. I had never wanted to sleep more.

The phone rang. The panicked voice of a medical student shouted hoarsely on the other end. "Come quickly! There's a visitor vomiting blood on the balcony."

I bolted from the bed, threw on my clothes and ran down the hallway, not knowing what to expect.

The man on the balcony was Carlos Morales, about thirty-five, the husband of my patient Lydia. He had climbed a flight of stairs to visit his wife, felt short of breath and walked to the small balcony, clutching his chest.

He was *not* vomiting blood. A torrent of pink frothy liquid gushed from his mouth. Pulmonary edema—fluid in the lungs—most likely due to acute heart failure. I had seen it many times before, but never so fulminant. He stood by the doorway, sweat pouring from his face, a look of terror in his eyes. We helped him to a vacant bed, and the nurses threw up screens to shield this scene from his wife, who stood in the hallway, her face in her hands. The man was transferred to the intensive care unit, where he died that night. His wife's shadow, outlined by the late afternoon sun against the gray wall of the hallway, frozen with grief and horror, is etched indelibly into my brain.

STAYING HUMAN

When pushed beyond the limits of endurance, as Bellevue interns were, the emotional response of doctors often turns from compassion to anger. Sometimes the anger is explosive. One medical intern dumped a jug of urine on the desk of an assistant hospital administrator because he could not get its contents analyzed before his patient died. We all supported the intern, and no charges were brought.

Sometimes the anger turns inward. One resident used Dexedrine and morphine to numb his pain. To the rest of us, he looked amazingly energetic. We envied his even temper, his ready smile, his ability to work without sleep or food. He was found dead one morning in his on-call room. A suicide note addressed to his wife lay on the desk.

Sometimes the anger simmers, brewing cynicism and hostility directed toward the patients. For some doctors, patients become the enemy, hated for their self-destructive habits, their foul smells, their incurable diseases, their relentless interference with a night's sleep. The phrase "veterinary medicine" was jokingly bandied on the wards of Bellevue. Rumors spread of a clandestine classification used by residents in the emergency room. Patients were being rated "POS" or "SHPOS": Piece of Shit or Sub-Human Piece of Shit. At first, I refused to believe them. I took it for part of the dark mythology that surrounded the hospital like the pestilent fog of a Gothic novel. In one apocryphal story, a previous chief medical resident would make his morning rounds on the streets surrounding Bellevue before coming to the hospital itself. There he would look for derelicts who had died after being discharged from the emergency room and would turn them around, to make it look as if they had died on their way to the hospital instead of on their way out. The stories were just gallows humor—or so I thought until I saw the letters "SHPOS" written on ER records.

As I recall that year of struggling to stay human, I remember with amazement the praise heaped upon Bellevue's training program by its chief of medicine, Dr. Saul Farber. Farber has been one of this country's leading medical educators, president of the American Board of Internal Medicine, a master of the American College of Physicians, provost of New York University. He always believed that Bellevue was a superb place for training new physicians. "When you've worked on city hospital patients with multiple diseases and multiorgan failure," he explained during my application interview, "then the University Hospital patients, who only have one thing wrong with them, are a piece of cake."

To Farber's critics, his attitude embraced the teaching hospital's exploitation of the destitute, a tradition deeply rooted in the soil of the New Medicine. Defenders of the medical school argued that the blame lay with society, not the school, if the disenfranchised were used for training. The teaching program, after all, brought a quality of medical care to the poor of lower Manhattan that was otherwise unavailable to them.

It took me several years to understand that Farber's attitude was not based on social class or race. It was the vision of the biomedical mechanic. The physician's job was to "work on" patients, the way we worked on dogs in the physiology lab. The dimension of healing had been completely abandoned. In 1991, one of Dr. Farber's favorite aphorisms was respectfully quoted by *New York* magazine in its report on the best hospitals in New York: "The best way to learn medicine is to teach it."[2] This statement appears innocent, until you attend to its actual content. When professors of medicine teach, they stand at the foot of the patient's bed, reviewing the chart, talking primarily with the residents. They have no relationship with the *patient*, only with the *data*. For the professor of medicine, the patient is just a footnote to the disease.[3]

As I look past the failures and frustrations of my time at Bellevue to remember my clinical triumphs—the patients that I "worked on" successfully—I am struck by the poverty of insight that Dr. Farber's vision supplies.

MEDICAL MECHANIC OR HEALER?

The first time I saw Miguel Benitez, he was a silhouette on a stretcher at the end of a dark hallway. It was two in the morning, and I was checking my ward before going to bed. The sight of the stretcher was startling.

"What's that patient doing there?" I asked the nurse on duty, hoping to be told he was not a new admission.

"That's your new admission," she replied. It felt like a slap in the face.

"There's a mistake," I insisted. "Check with Admitting. I just admitted a patient to the Intensive Care Unit. This patient must belong to the other side."

"Sorry. The rotation's gone around and you're up for this one."

I grabbed the ER record and read it quickly: "Miguel Benitez, 28-year-old Puerto Rican. Fever, chills, weakness — 36 hours. Sore throat, headache, cough, sneezing for 5 days. Temperature 102, pulse 112, blood pressure 110/70. Lungs clear. Grade 2 systolic cardiac murmur. Abdomen negative. Rule out endocarditis. Ronald Fishbein, M.D."

This description matched the flu far better than endocarditis, which is an infection of a heart valve. I was angry at Fishbein. When had he become such a sieve? If he didn't know what to do with this patient, why didn't he just hold him overnight, instead of admitting him to a medical floor?

My only recourse was to be quick. I could still get to bed by three. I walked over to Miguel's stretcher. His appearance was frightening. He moaned softly and constantly, staring into space. His skin was pale but mottled, looking more like marble than like flesh. I had never seen anything like it, but I remembered the description from textbooks: "*livido reticularis,*" a network of slate blue lines, suggesting a disorder of the circulation. I reached down to feel his pulse. It was weak and threadlike. He looked at me and continued moaning.

"Miguel, I'm Dr. Galland. Can you tell me what's wrong?" He shook his head and moaned. "Miguel, *¿Qué pasa?*" The response was the same.

All thoughts of sleep vanished, along with my anger at Fishbein. This man was very sick. Maybe he was dying. He belonged in the hospital, but not up here, on a floor with so little staff. I walked back to the nurses' station.

"This patient should have been admitted to the EW," I said. "Call the head nurse and tell her I'm bringing down a patient who was admitted to the floor by mistake."

"You're not supposed to do that," cautioned the nurse. "You'd better take this with you." She handed me a sheaf of papers eight inches thick. "It's the old chart, from the Chest Service."

I walked back to the stretcher and told Miguel that I was moving him to another part of the hospital. His old chart looked daunting. As we waited for the elevator, I skimmed the last discharge summary. At the age of twenty-three he had been hospitalized four times for a condition called constrictive pericarditis, an inflammation of the sac that surrounds the heart, an organ called the pericardium. On each admission his pericardium had became so taut with fluid that the heart could not effectively pump blood. The pressure exerted by its sac constricted its movement. After draining the fluid with needles, only to have it return each time, the surgeons finally operated, peeling away the pericardium and removing most of it. Although the organ was dissected, cultured, and examined, the cause of its inflammation was not found. Knowing that tuberculosis can cause constrictive pericarditis, and having no other diagnosis, his doctors prescribed drugs for tuberculosis, which he had taken for about a year.

Miguel scared me. I had completed fourteen weeks of internship, and I knew that whatever was wrong with him was way beyond my experience. I was glad to have Barry Zaret on call that night as the senior resident. He had a reputation for brilliance that was well deserved. By the age of thirty-eight, he was to become the chief of cardiology at Yale University, a dazzling accomplishment.

The emergency ward was organized chaos, as usual. As I stood over Miguel, searching for a vein, I heard his moaning abruptly stop. I felt for his pulse. There was practically none. My own pulse was booming like a drum, but I knew I had to keep my head. I called to the surgeon at the next bed.

"Kenny, this guy's going into shock. Can you slip in a subclavian line for me?" I had done the procedure half a dozen times, but I knew that his hand would be much quicker than mine.

"Sure." He smiled. His surgical gloves were already on, because he was about to perform a "cut down" on his own patient. He stepped over, took a needle from the nurse and punctured Miguel's skin, just below the right collarbone. Using the bottom edge of the bone as his guide, he thrust the needle into the large subclavian vein and threaded a plastic cannula through it, then handed the free end of the cannula to me. I attached a syringe to the plastic tubing and drew out as much blood as I thought I would need, removed the syringe and attached a bottle of salt water, which ran into Miguel's veins as fast as gravity would carry it. He received two quarts of salt water within thirty minutes and his pulse came back. Shock, in Miguel's case, was caused not by heart failure, but by lack of blood volume.

"What's the story?" Zaret asked me, as he approached the bed, the clothes looking rumpled on his lanky frame. He passed his fingers through the wiry black hair that was still plastered to the side of his head. He was obviously surprised at being called out of bed. The date was October 11. On October 1, a new rule had gone into effect: interns were no longer required to consult residents about patients who were admitted after midnight. The assumption was that we had enough experience by now to handle any patient until 7:30 A.M., when the junior resident in charge of the ward came in for rounds.

I told him what I knew about Miguel. "I'm glad you called me," he said. "First, do a spinal tap. Then go up to the lab and check the specimens while I go over the patient and review the old chart."

"I haven't examined him myself, yet," I protested. I was the intern. I was supposed to examine the patient first, before anyone else.

Zaret shook his head. "There's not much time," he said.

I knew he was right. Medical interns had a small laboratory of our own for nocturnal use. There I processed all the specimens myself, the old way, by hand. I placed samples of blood and spinal fluid into sterile tubes of nutrient broth designed to grow bacteria, if they were present. I placed a drop of blood on a slide and deftly smeared it with the edge of another slide, producing a thin film of blood to be stained and examined under the microscope. I filled a pipette with blood and set it upright in a rack to determine the sedimentation rate, the distance that the column of blood cells would settle in one hour. This is an old, simple, and useful test, based on an observation first recorded by ancient Greek physicians—not a test for a specific disease, but rather an index of sickness and inflammation. The normal sedimentation rate is about ten to twenty millimeters per hour. In a patient with bacterial infection, it tends to be much faster. I prepared cultures of blood, urine, and spinal fluid and placed them in an incubator. Then I sat down at the microscope for the part of lab work that I enjoyed the most.

To peer through the microscope is to enter a silent and mysterious world, hidden to the naked eye. Microscopy fills me with the same excitement and sense of discovery as scuba diving or gliding in a small plane. I scanned the cells of Miguel's blood, searching for some secret clue that would reveal his diagnosis. Unexpectedly, I found it. The cells were all torn apart, as if they had been run through a leaf mulcher. I phoned downstairs to Zaret and asked him to come up to the lab.

He held the slides up to the light and examined them. "The blood smears are nicely feathered," he said, approvingly. "We have to assume that the fragmentation of blood cells is real, not the result of poor technique. So, what does it tell us?"

I didn't want him to be Socratic. I wanted him to have the answers. "Maybe it has something to do with his weird sed rate," I responded. "I would have expected a very fast sed rate, at least fifty. His is barely one millimeter."

He studied the pipette and then stared at me intensely. "Did you notice all the bruises on his legs and lower abdomen?"

"No," I answered. "I didn't have the opportunity to complete my examination."

"He's also bleeding around the site of the subclavian line," he mused. "Let's put this all together. What determines the sedimentation rate?"

The answer to that one was easy. "Acute-phase reactants," I said, "fibrinogen in particular." Fibrinogen is a protein made by the body to initiate the clotting of blood. Its production is increased during infection and states of inflammation.

"Exactly!" snapped Zaret. I felt like Watson, being grilled by Sherlock Holmes. "If all the fibrinogen in the blood were depleted, we might expect a sed rate of zero, and we might also expect that the patient would bleed abnormally. Now, what consumes fibrinogen?"

"Clotting of blood," I said.

"Very good. This patient has a disease that makes his blood clot inappropriately, consuming all his fibrinogen and leaving him to bleed into the skin. It also hacks his red cells to pieces, making him anemic, and causes shock and a high fever. It sounds like disseminated intravascular coagulation."

The term was barely familiar to me. I had seen it once, in the small print of a textbook. DIC was considered rare, so exotic, in fact, that Michael Crichton, a doctor turned novelist, employed it as the means by which a virus from outer space destroyed its victims in *The Andromeda Strain*. Today, DIC is a well-known disorder, recognized as a common complication of severe infection and of certain drug treatments. DIC is one mechanism by which the greatly feared Ebola virus kills its prey. With DIC, a person's blood clots spontaneously inside blood vessels all over the body. At the same time that vital organs are deprived of blood flow, all the blood's clotting factors are consumed, so that the patient bleeds internally and externally.

Zaret outlined a strategy for treatment, based on the likelihood that Miguel had DIC, that it was caused by an infection somewhere in his body, that there was no relationship between this illness and the disease he had suffered five years before, and that the possibility of other complicating conditions should be considered. Then he returned to bed and left me to implement the plan. It was now four o'clock in the morning. I had no trace of fatigue, no thought that did not relate to the treatment of Miguel Benitez. I knew that I would spend the next twelve hours in the emergency ward, postponing all my other commitments for the day. Until he died, or turned the corner toward recovery, all my attention and all my energy would belong to this patient.

I wrote the orders as instructed: Large volumes of intravenous fluid to maintain the maximum possible flow of blood through his tissues. Fresh plasma and whole blood and as much fibrinogen as we could get from the blood bank to replace what he was losing. The strongest antibiotics available, combined to cover as many types of bacterial infection as we could imagine. Heparin, a potent inhibitor of blood coagulation, in a desperate attempt to slow the consumption of clotting factors in his blood vessels. A quarter century later, with all that's been learned about DIC, the treatment is much the same. There are new antibiotics, of course, and heparin is rarely used, because no one has managed to show that it really helps. When explosive, as it was with Miguel, DIC is still usually fatal. In 1990, it claimed the life of Jim Henson, creator of the Muppets, shortly after his admission to New York Hospital for pneumonia.

I returned to complete my examination of the patient. He was still moaning incoherently and appeared to be unconscious. His pulse was still threadlike, his skin a collage of purple bruises. Blood oozed from around his teeth, his IV line, and every needle puncture on his body. We were losing the battle. A great weariness seized me. I wanted to cry.

The specialists in hematology and infectious disease arrived, heard the story, took more samples of blood, and did a biopsy of the bone marrow—one more site from which he bled. They had nothing to add to Zaret's plan. I presented the case to the junior resident in charge of my ward and to the faculty physician responsible for teaching. All the options had been taken. There was nothing left to do but wait. Miguel's fate lay in the hands of time.

At three in the afternoon, I sat at the counter of the nursing station, which was on a raised platform overlooking the emergency ward, writing up my summary of the case. The head nurse of the day shift placed a slip of paper before my eyes.

"Bacteriology called," she said. "They've got four positive blood cultures on your patient. This is what they're growing."

I stared at the paper: *Pneumococcus, type 18*.

Pneumococcus, the bacteria that causes lobar pneumonia. So, the infection entered his body through the lungs, in the wake of a simple cold. A sudden exhilaration lifted my spirits. The enemy was known and penicillin could destroy it. Following Zaret's instructions, I had ordered penicillin at 3 A.M. This time we would win! Shivering with exhaustion and exultation, I could barely write. Looking down the ward, I saw Ron Fishbein, the emergency resident, standing at the foot of Miguel's bed. He walked to the nurses' station and looked up at me, grinning broadly.

"Good admission, wasn't he?" he said with pride.

By the next day, Miguel was awake and feeding himself. His bleeding had stopped, his fever was gone. This was a rare and coveted triumph, a reward for quick thinking and knowing how to "work on" patients. Few had been snatched so efficiently from the brink of death. Our handling of Miguel's case was celebrated throughout the department.

Three months later, I sat talking to Miguel in the outpatient clinic. He was a nervous wreck; he couldn't sleep; he was losing time from his job and had lost all desire for sex with his wife. The reason was no mystery. He was afraid the sickness would return. Twice in five years he had almost died. Why should he believe it wouldn't happen again? Could I help him?

Nothing in my training had prepared me for that request. Once a patient was cured, he was supposed to be . . . cured. I understood Miguel's anxiety. Had I been him, I probably would have felt the same way. But I couldn't tell him that. I did not know how to help him, and there was no one I could turn to for advice. I explained to him, as simply and clearly as I could, the nature of the disease that had almost killed him, and tried to convince him that it would not come back. He listened. He was not convinced. I urged him to return for regular follow-up visits, which he did, every few months, for another five years. The dreaded disease did not recur. His anxiety slowly dissipated, while mine increased.

My attempt at reassuring Miguel had left me with considerable self-doubt. I really understood very little about him and the circumstances that had created his illness. Why had he experienced two apparently unrelated nearly fatal diseases by the age of twenty-eight? Why had he gone from a common cold to DIC? How sure could I really be that it would never happen again? Was there any means of prevention? I realized that the content of my education and the conditions of my training had been designed to make me a good medical mechanic, not a healer. I had spent half a decade learning how to analyze data, but I had been taught almost nothing about patients.

FRESH CURRENTS

By the time I left Bellevue in 1973, fresh currents seemed to be changing the course of medicine. They came from all directions. The social unrest of the 1960s had created a rights-conscious environment. People had a right to health care. Communities had a right to administrative influence over the health centers that served them. Patients had a right to privacy, to informed consent, to refuse treatment, to see their medical records, to participate in therapeutic decisions. The growth of powerful, life-prolonging technology, like artificial respiration and kidney dialysis, had created new ethical dilemmas in health care that could not be resolved by physicians alone. The women's movement challenged paternalism in medical care and the bias that ignored or denigrated women's health concerns. A resurgence of research on the epidemiology of chronic diseases suggested that cancer and heart disease were not the inevitable outcome of an increase in average life expectancy; they were preventable disorders, caused by patients' environments, diets, and personal habits. Ethicists, educators, statisticians, psychologists, and anthropologists analyzed the health care industry from novel points of view, drawn from expertise intrinsic to their own disciplines. They chastised the medical profession for training too many specialists and for failing to recognize that patients are not just the bearers of diseases, but individuals who become sick within a social, cultural, and demographic context.

Stronger currents opposed and virtually nullified the changes. Alarmed at the soaring cost of maintaining Medicare and Medicaid, federal and state governments unleashed an army of bureaucrats to regulate the distribution of services; private insurers followed. Bureaucrats and businessmen trampled the individuality and autonomy of patients, erecting a rigid system of medical payments based on ossified concepts of disease. Physicians fought threats to their professional authority and to their incomes by deserting primary care in record numbers, seeking refuge in specialization.

In response to these conflicts, a small group of general internists and family practitioners sought to revitalize personal health care by absorbing the insights of psychologists and social scientists, by analyzing the most common and understudied health problems, and by seeking alternatives to the uncontrolled growth of invasive technologies, enhancing the stature of primary physicians. Hoping to bring their wisdom into medical education, I joined the faculty of a new medical school founded by the State University of New York at Stony Brook. The medical school was so new that there was no university hospital.

For the first time, I had to deal with the kinds of chronic health problems that don't end up in the ER. My patients complained of common ailments like fatigue, headache, dizziness, back pain, chronic sinusitis, recurrent bladder infections. I was skilled in crisis management and the differential diagnosis of uncommon diseases, but I knew very little about the causes or the treatment of the common disorders that bring misery to so many people. I began to study what was known about these conditions and discovered how severely neglected their investigation had been.

One afternoon, I examined a graduate student who suffered from recurrent urinary infections.

"I think I brought this infection on myself," she confided. "I noticed that whenever I get so involved or stressed out by my work that I don't empty my bladder when I feel the urge, an infection will occur. I've discussed this with other women, and most of them agree."

I told her that I had been reviewing research on recurrent bladder infections. Little had been written, and most of the material published had been of poor scientific quality. I had decided to organize my own research and enlisted her help. With no funding, but with the active, voluntary participation of students at the university, we conducted a study of behaviors that might contribute to recurrent urinary infections. Our results were eventually published. We found that most women with recurrent infection (but very few women without recurrent infection) habitually deferred urinating for extended periods of time. Furthermore, regular and complete bladder emptying was effective in preventing reinfection.[4] I wrote proposals for grants to conduct similar behavioral research on other common health problems. It was an exercise in frustration; there was no funding. I realized that the longer I remained at the medical school, the better I would become at the mastery of institutional politics and the more time I would waste in my quest to broaden the clinical investigation of chronic or recurrent disease.

In 1977, I resigned my academic position and moved my family to northwestern Connecticut to start a general medical practice in a small town in Litchfield County. By immersing myself in the primal encounter between physician and patient, which has always been the foundation for healing, I hoped to better understand the real origins of sickness and the requirements for restoration of health.

At the end of my first year in practice, I began making phone calls to patients whom I had not seen for several months, to find out how they were feeling. I was constantly impressed by the differences among individuals. The same disease and the same treatments appeared to affect different people in very different ways. "Classic cases" were the exception, not the rule. With regard to drugs, there were no "classic" responders, just as there were no "average" patients. I also found that a patient's short-term response to treatment was a poor predictor of how she would be faring six months later. The "natural history of the disease" simply failed to explain the high degree of individual variability. I searched for patients' characteristics that might explain the variability of response, and settled upon three that seemed worthy of further study: nutritional status, physical conditioning, and psychological distress.

I spent the next four years studying nutrition, psychology, and therapeutic exercise and attempted to apply them in a general medical practice. I hired an artist who prepared sketches of specific exercises for relieving pain and spasm in different parts of the body. I taught patients relaxation techniques for control of anxiety and published these methods in a journal called *Patient Care*,[5] intended for primary physicians. I reviewed psychological techniques for helping patients cope with the stress of surgery and published these in *Connecticut Medicine*, the journal of the state medical society.[6] I read about the work of Chandra Patel, a general practitioner working in the British National Health Service who taught yoga and meditation to patients with high blood pressure.[7] For Patel's patients, these practices lowered blood pressure as effectively as drug therapy. During a trip to England, I visited Dr. Patel at her one-room office in a suburb of London. I felt certain that the strength of Patel's personality was as much a part of the treatment as any of the procedures she taught. She was unhurried, completely focused, dynamic but quiet, almost serene. The doctor herself presented a model of behavior more important than any technique. Other researchers, attempting to replicate her findings, have usually failed. Perhaps they missed the point.

My local community hospital was so small and informal, I felt, that any innovation would be welcome if it originated with a member of the medical staff. I was able to establish a cardiac rehabilitation program, a stress reduction workshop, and a nutritional support service long before these were available at most larger, more technically sophisticated medical centers. Among all these therapeutic innovations, the benefits produced by nutritional support of hospitalized patients were the most dramatic.

Anna Caprio was an elderly woman who had been admitted for removal of a small cancer in the large intestine. Her hospital stay had been prolonged by an infection of the surgical wound, which quickly came under control with antibiotics. After ten days in the hospital, she suddenly went crazy, screaming gibberish and striking the nurses. Her surgeon ordered her restrained in bed and asked me to see her as soon as possible.

The scene in her room was like a flashback to Bellevue. A painfully thin, disheveled, gray-haired woman lay tied to her bed with a soft waist restraint called a posey. She struggled incessantly against the restraint, emitting a stream of nonsensical sounds and half-formed words in an eerie, high-pitched monotone. Her daughter, Nina, walked in right behind me and almost went berserk herself when she saw her mother.

I released the restraint and sat Anna on the bed, between her daughter and me. Nina tried to soothe Anna by stroking her head. She stopped struggling, but was still visibly agitated. The incantation of nonsense continued.

"I don't know why this happened to your mother," I said to Nina. "I'm going to examine her. But first I'd like you to tell me how she's been the past week."

"She hasn't seemed right since the operation," said Nina, tearfully. "She's been like . . . distant. And forgetful. And she has no appetite. I don't think she's had anything but a little bit of Jell-O since she's been in the hospital. Look at how thin she is!"

"What was she like before the operation?" I asked. "Was she nervous about surgery? Did she know she had cancer?"

"She was great! She had a great sense of humor and deep faith in God."

"How was her appetite?"

"That's been terrible. Her teeth are really bad. She won't get them taken care of. . . . She can be really stubborn. She just eats custard or Cream of Wheat. No meat, no vegetables. She won't listen to me."

"Does she take any vitamins?"

"The doctor gave her iron when he found she was anemic."

My initial impression had been that Anna had suffered an unusual stroke, because of the suddenness of her attack. From Nina's story, I surmised that the abrupt change had actually been preceded by a slow deterioration. Her poor diet led me to suspect that the stress of surgery and infection had unmasked an underlying deficiency of B-vitamins. To confirm my theory, I ordered a blood test for thiamine (vitamin B$_1$). Immediately after the blood was drawn, I administered an injection of thiamine and B-vitamin complex. Within less than an hour, Anna was calm and talking coherently. She left the hospital two days later, after nutritional counseling and arrangements for dental care had been made. The test result came back a week later, confirming thiamine deficiency.

Stephan Bruner, a man in his seventies, almost lost his life to hospital malnutrition. He had been in the intensive care unit for three weeks before his case came to the attention of our nutritional support service. Stephan had entered the hospital a month earlier for removal of his gallbladder. After surgery he developed pneumonia so severe that he needed a breathing tube inserted into his trachea. The tube had been connected to a respirator, which delivered oxygen at high concentration to his lungs. Oxygen and antibiotics were not enough to cure this infection. They were merely prolonging the agony of death, as pneumonia spread slowly and the function of his lungs deteriorated.

The hospital's dietitian noticed that Stephan had received little more than intravenous sugar, water, and vitamins since his admission. She asked Stephan's doctors to request nutritional consultation, which allowed me to examine his record and make recommendations. The poor man's nutritional problems were glaring. He had been fed so little protein that the protein level in his blood had dropped by 50 percent and he could not mount an effective immune response. When I presented this fact, as tactfully as I could, to Stephan's doctors, they looked at me as if to say, "Come on, Galland. You don't really think that *feeding* him is going to make a difference!"

It felt as if the gauntlet had been slapped across my cheek. If the model of health care I embraced was to mean anything, nutritional support should do something for Stephan Bruner, even as his death approached. I ordered the regular administration of a predigested high-protein food supplement through a feeding tube and personally checked twice a day to make sure it had been given and retained. An amazing change occurred within one week. Stephan's pneumonia receded, his lung function improved, and he was able to breathe without a respirator. After ten days of supplementary feeding, Stephan was able to leave the intensive care unit. His doctors said nothing, but consultations to the nutritional support service began to increase.

If protein could bring an old man with pneumonia back from the brink of death, it seemed that proper nutritional support might also help nonsurgical patients inside or outside the hospital. I began looking for vitamin and mineral deficiencies in chronically ill patients who were not responding as expected to conventional treatment. Deficiencies of folic acid, vitamin A, vitamin B_6, iron, magnesium, and selenium were quite common. When I reviewed data from studies of nutrient intake among U.S. adults, I realized that a large fraction of the population fail to consume the recommended daily allowances of these nutrients.

The most important nutritional deficiency I encountered was not readily measured in the laboratory. It was a deficiency of essential fatty acids, or EFAs. I surmised this deficiency from the dramatic improvement in dry skin or brittle nails that occurred about a month after patients added fish oil to their diets. Often, their medical problems would improve in parallel with changes in the skin. I first observed this phenomenon in 1979, when treating Ruth Quinn, the sixty-year-old grandmother of one of my patients.

Ruth had been admitted to the hospital five times in eighteen months, complaining of chest pain. Each time, the evaluation showed no evidence of heart disease and she was discharged within seventy-two hours. When I first saw her, the pain was mild, but from her story and the physical examination, I concluded that the source of pain was inflammation of the cartilage that attaches the ribs to the breastbone (the costochondral junction). I prescribed anti-inflammatory drugs, which are the usual treatment for this condition, but she could not take more than two or three doses without experiencing severe stomach pain. After I exhausted the drugs available at that time, I begin searching for an alternative treatment approach. I had read about the use of cod liver oil as a folk remedy for arthritis, so I prescribed one tablespoon a day plus four hundred units of vitamin E. Within two weeks, Ruth became virtually pain-free. Along with relief of chest pain, she experienced dramatic improvement in the dry skin and eczema that had troubled her since adolescence. Research concerning the anti-inflammatory attributes of fish oils was not yet well known, but the biochemistry of cod liver oil suggested that its effects on inflammation and on skin quality must result from its high content of an EFA called EPA (eicosapentaenoic acid). EPA alters the way in which the body produces a group of chemicals called *prostanoids*, which play a critical role in the development of pain and inflammation.[8] The quantity of EPA in a tablespoon of cod liver oil is not enough to give it the potency of an anti-inflammatory drug. I reasoned that Ruth may actually have been deficient in EPA and that dry skin, eczema, and susceptibility to inflammation were not separate diseases, but rather signs of her EFA deficiency.

Investigating further, I uncovered research that determined that dietary intake of EPA and related EFAs had declined substantially in Western nations over the past hundred years. I began to suspect that alterations in dietary fat consumption during the twentieth century might play a role in many different disorders. Understanding the relationship between dietary EFAs and patterns of disease began to alter my understanding of disease in general. During the next decade I wrote and lectured extensively on the therapeutic applications of EFAs and was delighted to find other clinical researchers and nutritionists following the same track. (The profound effect of dietary EFAs on body chemistry—and the keys to establishing optimal EFA balance—form the core of Chapter Six.)

THE BIRTH OF BEHAVIORAL MEDICINE

During my years in general practice, I maintained a faculty position at the University of Connecticut, supervising residents at the University Hospital and teaching medical students in my private office. The director of general medicine, Dr. Frank Davidoff, who is now editor of the esteemed *Annals of Internal Medicine*, was as troubled as I was by the narrow vision of contemporary medical practice and knew of my interest in alternative treatment strategies. One day he called to tell me of an unusual learning opportunity. One of the university's teaching hospitals had been awarded a grant to establish a fellowship in the new field of behavioral medicine. The grant for the first year was mine, if I wanted it.

Behavioral medicine is a field created by the broad intersection of behavioral psychology with clinical and preventive medicine. Most research in this field has been very practical in its orientation: how to help people overcome self-destructive habits, such as smoking, drinking, and compulsive eating, and embrace self-enhancing habits such as regular exercise; how to improve patients' compliance with prescribed medical treatments; and how to help patients control their chronic pain with a minimum of functional disability.

I hoped the fellowship would give me tools to increase my effectiveness as a physician. Helping patients change seemed to me to be the greatest challenge facing modern medicine, because the major causes of disease and disability spring directly from our behaviors—the choices we are free to make and change: cigarette smoking, alcohol and drug abuse, poor diet and hygiene, sexual promiscuity, lack of physical fitness, reckless driving. The fellowship year led me back onto the wards of a teaching hospital. There I was struck once again by how much physicians had abrogated their responsibility to help patients change, because they had withdrawn from personal interaction with patients. They were so enmeshed in the technical aspects of examination and treatment that they had lost touch with the the power of empathic communication. They failed to listen carefully to patients because they distrusted them. They only trusted the results of tests.

One of the tasks of my fellowship year was to establish a consultation service for patients suffering from addiction or from chronic pain. My first consultation concerned Charles Wright, a middle-aged engineer with unremitting, severe back pain of six months' duration.

"Extensive investigation reveals no evidence of organic pathology," read the consultation request form. "He appears depressed and has lost 30 lbs. Please evaluate for psychogenic pain."

I invited Charles into the consultation room, reviewed the data in his chart, and asked him about himself. He was married with teenage children, had a few close friends and no hobbies except trout fishing. He loved his work. In fact, he spent most of his time working and had recently received a promotion. He drank wine before dinner, had never smoked, and rarely thought about his health. He had endured six months of increasing pain that had become constant and severe, like a drill boring into his spine. He had lost his appetite for food, for work, for sex, even for fishing. He had become withdrawn and depressed. His wife finally brought him to the hospital, pleading for pain relief. He had been extensively "worked up." His blood tests and X rays were all normal. A CAT scan (a computer-directed series of X rays) had failed to reveal any abnormalities. Pain relievers containing codeine had provided no relief. He was getting scared.

As I listened to Charles speak, I gave his words my full attention. I wanted to experience the person who was speaking, to develop a feeling for who he was. Without this connection, I would be no closer to understanding Charles's pain than the medical resident, who, unfortunately, had found nothing to guide him but the negative results of X rays and blood tests.

I strongly suspected that Charles had cancer, originating in the pancreas and eroding into his spine. This man was not accustomed to seeking solace from doctors or drugs. An engineer, he tended to view his body as a machine that should run, whatever ailed it, until it would run no more. His profound depression was a response to the loss of autonomy created by his disabling pain. He needed exploratory surgery, but before that he needed morphine, in frequent high doses. I asked the resident on the medical service to prescribe it and to maintain it for the duration of his hospital stay.

"Well . . . ," drawled the resident, reluctantly, "he does complain a lot. But there are no objective findings to support his symptoms. He seems pretty depressed."

I was furious! What made this doctor believe that what an X ray or a blood test said was more "objective" than what the patient said? Only the prejudice instilled by his training. Two days later Charles underwent exploratory abdominal surgery. The cancer was found, in the exact spot where the pain occurred. Six months later he was dead.

Charles Wright spent two weeks in the hospital, denied effective pain relief because X rays failed to find the cause of his pain, even though his story screamed "pancreatic cancer" to any physician willing to listen. But X-ray vision is no sharper than clinical vision. An X ray is just a shadow cast on a piece of radiation-sensitive film, not by light, but by gamma rays that pass unabsorbed through most tissues of the body. The pictures produced are not true representations of the body; the transformation of an X-ray image into a picture of the body requires the *imagination* of the person reading the films. The reading and interpretation of an X ray is a subjective experience, readily influenced by what the physician already believes to be true about the patient.

Newer imaging techniques utilize computer-generated images produced by mathematical algorithms. For CAT scans (which also failed to detect Charles's cancer) the electronic input is multiple X-ray projections of a cross section of the body from which the computer reconstructs the internal structures being scanned. Magnetic resonance imaging (MRI) creates a visual image of radio signals emitted by molecules within the body when their atomic nuclei are exposed to an external magnetic field. Positron emission tomography (PET scanning) is a visual rendering of chemical changes in tissue related to blood flow and metabolism. The digital data produced by these new technologies are manipulated to produce images with features desired by the observer. They are not real pictures but fabrications; their accuracy in representing the body's interior structures depends at many levels upon subjective decisions that determine the sharpness given to edges, the degree of contrast enhancement achieved, and the perception of the artificial picture by a human being.[9]

Far from constituting "objective evidence," medical tests mean absolutely nothing in and of themselves. Their only significance derives from their interpretation, which in turn depends upon the subjectivity of the patient's physician.[10] A doctor's decision about whether a given test result is normal or abnormal often depends upon her concept of what is good for the patient and how much ambiguity she is willing to tolerate.[11] Despite the best efforts of science and technology, physicians and patients remain, inherently, partners in subjectivity, and empathic listening is still the physician's most important diagnostic tool.

I became aware of my own need for empathic listening from other practicing physicians, and began a search for doctors who were actively challenging conventional medical practices, hoping we could learn from one another. I soon found that I was not alone. A surgeon at Yale named Bernie Siegel had just established a support group for patients with cancer, organized around the premise that healing the mind could heal the body. Bernard Raxlen, a psychiatrist trained in family therapy, had made a different type of discovery: children with learning disabilities and hyperactivity were not being driven to distraction by their families. They often suffered from dietary deficits and food allergies. For most of them, nutritional therapy proved more effective than psychotherapy. From these men I learned that the distinction between physical and mental diseases was as artificial as the distinction between subjective and objective.

In September 1979, a small group of medical mavericks began a series of quarterly meetings at an inn in the Berkshire Hills. The group was originally called together by Stephan Rechtstaffen, a family practitioner and director of the Omega Institute for Holistic Studies in Rhinebeck, New York. As the size of the meetings grew, we organized ourselves into a society, the Academy of Integrated Medical Studies (AIMS). We invited guest speakers, who were given a full day, sometimes more, to present their work. We brought the charts of difficult cases for deliberation. We conducted in-depth discussions of selected topics in nutrition, environmental health, and alternative healing strategies.

These meetings intensified my friendship with Sid Baker, a pediatrician from Yale, whom I had first met through Bernard and Bernie. Sid had recently been named director of the renowned Gesell Institute of Human Development in New Haven. The mission of the institute had been shaped by the work of Arnold Gesell, whose research at Yale's Child Study Center laid the foundation for the modern study of childhood development. In accepting the directorship, Sid asked the institute's trustees to create a medical department in which he could treat sick children and adults with nutritional and environmental therapies. All of the patients who came to the institute had complex, chronic health problems, had undergone previous medical or psychiatric evaluations, and had found them wanting.

In 1982, I joined the staff at Gesell as director of medical research. My goal was to look with the broadest perspective possible into the origins of chronic illness and develop a systematic alternative to standard medical diagnosis that would serve as a guide to new therapeutic strategies. The patients coming to Gesell were eager partners in this endeavor, knowing through personal experience the limitations of conventional medicine. Sid called our work "resort medicine," because so many of our patients opened their initial interview by saying, "Doctor, you're my last resort."

THE PATIENT AS TEACHER

Our first step was to evaluate each patient anew, considering aspects of the patient that had previously been ignored. We were interested in the effects of the common components of life: a patient's thoughts and beliefs, home or work environment, exposure to potential toxins and allergens, food and drink, stressful life events, social interactions, patterns of physical activity. Instead of identifying the *disease* by looking for its symptoms, we would attempt to learn something about the *patient* by understanding her idiosyncratic symptoms, those complaints and physical findings that would reveal information about her independent of the disease diagnosis.

Research at Gesell was barely beginning when it came to an end. By the mid-1980s, high administrative costs had doomed the medical department, and the institute was about to be absorbed by Yale University. I left New Haven for New York City, returning to the place where my medical education had commenced. I was determined to create a diagnostic structure within which patients could be assessed as individuals. This structure would have to shed light on both the patient and her sickness and unify biological and psychosocial domains within the same analysis. I recognized that diagnosis is not an abstract activity. It is goal-oriented and related to treatment. So, I worked backward. I examined what I did that was most helpful to my patients and asked myself, What questions about the patient were being answered by these treatments?

In the spring of 1990, in the hills outside Florence, I first presented my new model for diagnosis to a small international gathering of physicians who were prominent in the development of nutritional medicine. We met in the gallery of the Castello di Montegufoni, a seventeenth-century castle that served as the hiding place for the masterpieces of Florence's Uffizi collection during the German occupation in World War II. It was an extraordinary place for a medical symposium. The gallery's thirty-foot-high painted ceilings are brightly festooned with floral and feral images in the baroque style. Eighty feet of glass-paneled doors open onto a formal garden that overlooks a rolling landscape of vineyards and olive groves. That we spent three full days in intense discussion with drapes drawn was a tribute to our passion for our work, as well as to the damp chill and driving rain of April in Tuscany.

I have since presented this model to several different groups of physicians and have worked to refine its components. I called it *patient-centered diagnosis,* and it forms the core of this book. The response has been so consistently favorable and enthusiastic that I believe it truly addresses our need to renew the art of medicine with the vigor of science.

3

PATIENT–CENTERED DIAGNOSIS

THE BIOMEDICAL MODEL

Contemporary medicine approaches illness with a set of concepts and procedures referred to as the *biomedical model*. Practically, it is supposed to work like this: A patient brings one or more problems to a physician, who uses the nature of the problems, the general medical history, and the physical examination to generate the *differential diagnosis*, a menu of competing possibilities that attempts to answer the question, "What disease does this patient have?" Laboratory tests, techniques for imaging body organs, and invasive procedures, when needed, help to confirm the answer. The diagnosis guides the treatment; a positive response to treatment helps to further substantiate the correctness of the diagnosis.

The problem with the biomedical model is that it doesn't work.

The biomedical model fails to accurately describe either the form or the substance of modern medical practice. The form is shaped by social forces. Physicians have been valued for the procedures they perform and not for the time they spend talking with patients; they practice defensively, afraid of lawsuits by disaffected patients who equate bad results with malpractice, or constrained by bureaucratic rules that penalize them for straying from a predetermined protocol. Laboratory testing is frequently performed on a "rule-out" basis, not to confirm a suspected disease but to rule out other diseases. When I review the records of a patient who has consulted many different specialists, I sometimes get the impression that the main reason for taking the medical history is to decide which procedures to order. Headache? An MRI of the brain. Diarrhea? A colonoscopy.

I first realized how bad this situation generally is when a senior faculty member at the University of Connecticut startled me by confiding, "You know, Leo, I've discovered that patients are much happier if you give them thirty seconds of undivided attention during each consultation. We have to teach that to the residents!"

On a substantive level, the most obvious failures of the biomedical model occur because most people who consult physicians do not have the kinds of diseases that physicians are trained to identify. In one large published study, 74 percent of patients seen by general internists for various common symptoms were left with no medical or psychiatric diagnosis to explain the cause of their problems.[1] When a disease *is* diagnosed, it is often not the real source of symptoms. I have seen dozens of patients who had their gallbladders removed because they had abdominal pain and an X ray showing gallstones, but who were no better after surgery than before.

ILLNESS AND DISEASE ARE NOT THE SAME

The slippery nature of medical diagnosis is quite clearly revealed in the relationship between chronic knee pain and a condition called osteoarthritis, which results from degeneration of cartilage lining the inside of the knee. Evidence of osteoarthritis is readily seen on X rays of the knees of people who have made it past middle age. When an elderly person complains of knee pain, a diagnostic charade is often enacted. The doctor orders X rays of the knees, which frequently show evidence of osteoarthritis. The diagnosis is made: "osteoarthritis," a disease that is conventionally treated with rest and anti-inflammatory drugs. When the condition is very severe, the preferred treatment is surgery to remove the diseased knees and attach artificial ones.

Numerous studies, however, have shown that the degree of pain and disability the patient experiences bears little relationship to the amount of osteoarthritis demonstrated by an X ray. Pain and disability are more strongly correlated with the patient's age, weight, general fitness, degree of anxiety or depression, and especially with the strength of the quadriceps muscles in the thighs. In most cases of chronic knee pain, the *illness* experienced by the patient is not directly caused by the *disease* identified by the doctor. The knee pain and its associated disability result from personal characteristics of the patient that determine the function of the knee joint, such as weakness of the thigh muscles. The most effective long-term treatment for knee pain is not rest and medication, but regular physical exercise.[2]

Discrepancies between what the doctor *sees* and what the patient *feels* occur in most diseases, because sickness is not caused by disease, but by disturbed function, and function involves a complex set of phenomena with physiological, psychological, and cultural dimensions. Most people who are chronically ill have more than one species of disease. This condition, called *co-morbidity*, is the rule, not the exception, in clinical medicine. Co-morbidity suggests that functional disturbances make individuals susceptible to many diseases at the same time. Functional disturbances are the basis of sickness. They can be identified at all levels of personal organization, from cellular to social.

MEDIATORS, TRIGGERS, AND ANTECEDENTS

Patient-centered diagnosis builds upon the foundation of the biological and behavioral sciences to identify the *mediators, triggers,* and *antecedents* of disease in individual patients. A *mediator* is anything that produces symptoms, damage to tissues of the body, or the types of behaviors associated with being sick. A *trigger* is anything that activates a quiescent mediator in an individual. *Antecedents* are the risk factors that predispose a person to acute or chronic illness.

Knowledge of these three components of illness is the major contribution that modern science has made to the understanding of health. The foremost scientific advance of the nineteenth century was the discovery of bacterial triggers for the devastating epidemic diseases. Unraveling cellular damage to reveal its chemical mediators has been the most productive field of biomedical research over the past thirty years.

Recognition of antecedents has provided a rational structure for the organization of preventive medicine and public health. In patient-centered diagnosis, the mediators, triggers, and antecedents for each person's illness form the focus of clinical investigation. Because mediators, triggers, and antecedents are useful concepts not only in biology but also in psychology, patient-centered diagnosis allows for a seamless welding of the biological and psychosocial dimensions of illness.

Mediators and the Formation of Sickness

The first step is understanding that what appears to be "a disease" is, in fact, nothing more than a pattern of signs, symptoms, behaviors, and tissue pathology occurring in individual human beings. Examining the disease is like watching shadow theater. What you see is an illusion created by the activity of something substantial that you don't see.

The shadow of disease, in all cases, is produced by the activity of a varied group of disease mediators. Mediators contribute to the formation of sickness because their activity is the main determinant of function. They are not the *causes* of disease but its *intermediaries*.

Mediators vary in size and substance, from subatomic to societal. In some patients, for example, abnormal electrical gradients can be measured across the membranes of particular cells: the ions or electrons producing this gradient are the mediators.[3] Some patients are rewarded for remaining ill; they receive attention from family members or relief from the performance of unpleasant tasks. For them, social reinforcement is a mediator. A given illness in any single person usually has more than one mediator.

Cognitive Mediators

Dr. Eric Cassell insightfully argues that the worst part of sickness is the suffering it entails, and that suffering, as distinct from other symptoms, results from fear of loss — loss of life, identity, independence, valued relationships, hopes for the future.[4] The suffering of sickness, then, is mediated by fear, and by the associated thoughts and beliefs, personal and communal, with which we label, explain, and evaluate the experience of being sick. These *cognitive mediators* determine how we appraise our symptoms and what actions we take in response to that appraisal.[5] They may even modulate the symptoms themselves. People in pain, for example, tend to experience more pain when they fear that their pain control will be inadequate than when they believe that ample pain management is within their reach.[6]

When I was in general practice, a woman burst into my office, extremely agitated, complaining of severe headache.

"I have *unbearable* pain in my head," she cried. "It started three days ago and it's getting worse. Nothing relieves it. I took aspirin, Tylenol, my husband's Percodan. You have to do something for me right away, Doctor!"

I tried to get a clear description of the exact location and quality of the pain. The woman felt as if a steel band were wrapped tightly around her head. The muscles on the side of her head, her jaw and the back of her neck were taut and very tender to the touch. She denied any injuries or activities that might have caused strain in these areas.

"Were you upset or tense about anything before this headache started?" I asked.

"Oh, indeed I was!" she moaned. "My husband's business lost a lot of money. He was cheated badly!"

"I think this headache results from muscle tension," I said. "Your emotional upset is probably at the root of it."

"Is that all?" she exclaimed, joyfully. "Oh, thank God. I thought it was a brain tumor!"

"There are several things you can do to get relief," I suggested.

"I already have relief!" she snapped back. "I don't need anything else." She left the office looking like a completely different person from the one who had walked in. Her sickness was in large part mediated by her fear that headache was a sign of terrible disease.

If the cultural conditions are right, fear can actually kill. A California research team examined the death records of twenty-eight thousand Chinese Americans and compared them with four hundred thousand death records of people who were described as "white." Their goal was to examine the effect of expectation of death on actual mortality, and they devised a clever method for discerning it. Chinese astrology predicts that the association between certain birth years and certain types of sickness dooms the victim to an early death. The researchers examined astrological data to ascertain whether people of Chinese ancestry who bore these unfortunate concordances died younger of the same causes than people whose birth years and diagnoses were not star-crossed. The control group was people with no knowledge of or attachment to Chinese astrological doctrine. Their findings: "Chinese-Americans, but not whites, die significantly earlier than normal (1.3 to 4.9 years) if they have a combination of disease and birthyear which Chinese astrology and medicine consider ill-fated. The more strongly a group is attached to Chinese traditions, the more years of life are lost. Our results hold for nearly all the major causes of death studied. The reduction in survival cannot be completely explained by a change in the behavior of the Chinese patient, doctor or death-registrar. . . ."[7]

The same investigators found the opposite effect when they examined the relationship between the Chinese festival of the Harvest Moon and mortality. Every year, the death rate among Chinese Americans with cancer, strokes, and heart disease dips by over one third during the week before this important event, no matter what its date in the calendar year. For other groups of Americans, there is no change in death rate during that week.[8]

Self-esteem is less dramatic than fear, but it is another cognitive mediator that molds the shape of illness. The component of self-esteem that has been most studied in relation to illness is called "perceived self-efficacy." It is the belief in one's ability to cope successfully with specific problems. People with a high degree of self-efficacy usually adapt better to chronic disease. They maintain higher levels of activity, require lower doses of pain medication, are more likely to adopt health-promoting lifestyles, and are more compliant with prescribed therapies than are people with low self-efficacy.[9] A patient's low self-efficacy contributes to the formation of sickness, increasing disability and decreasing the effectiveness of treatment. Fortunately, it responds to treatment. Patients can be taught to improve their capacity for self-care and enhance their self-efficacy, which has been proved to benefit patients with several types of chronic disease, including asthma,[10] arthritis,[11] and diabetes.[12]

Biochemical Mediators

The *biochemical* mediators of disease, best known by their ability to promote cellular damage, are not intrinsically "bad." Like the *doshas* of Indian medicine, they are agents of health that can create sickness through excess or imbalance. They include *hormones* like adrenaline and cortisone, secreted by the adrenal glands in response to stress;

prostanoids, which are made by every type of living cell in response to signals from every other type of living cell; and *free radicals*, a by-product of our use of oxygen, which play a critical role in the production of energy and destruction of toxins. At present, a group of small proteins called *cytokines* is receiving vast attention because of their importance in regulating inflammation and the body's response to infection.

The most striking characteristic of chemical mediators is their *lack of disease specificity*. Each mediator has been implicated in many different, apparently unrelated diseases, and each disease usually involves multiple chemical mediators in its formation. The mediator most often responsible for producing fever, for example, is a cytokine called interleukin-1 (IL-1). It is produced by cells in the connective tissues of the body and by a group of white blood cells called monocytes, usually in response to infection or injury. IL-1 induces many of the symptoms other than fever that we associate with infection or injury, such as pain, loss of appetite, lethargy, and depression. Through its actions on different organs, IL-1 stimulates both the immune system and the adrenal glands; it also causes hypoglycemia, bone loss, and decreased thyroid function. A sudden burst of IL-1 activity can cause intravascular coagulation (remember the story of Miguel Benitez in Chapter Two). Prolonged overproduction of IL-1 has been demonstrated in many chronic diseases, especially those involving inflammation, like arthritis, colitis, and asthma. IL-1 may speed the development of AIDS in people infected with the human immunodeficiency virus (HIV). Recent research suggests that IL-1 plays a role in promoting arteriosclerosis (hardening of the arteries), endometriosis (a cause of pelvic pain and infertility among women), and osteoporosis (thinning of the bones).[13]

Mediators never work alone. All mediators are organized into complex cascades and circuits that work to maintain health and stability in response to external danger and internal malfunction.

Several years ago I was asked to see a fourteen-year-old boy named Gary, who had missed most of eighth grade with one symptom or another: headaches, stomachaches, stuffed nose, sneezing, joint pains, and fatigue. When his mother brought him in for the initial evaluation, she told me that he had been cured. Two weeks before he had developed the flu. For the first time in his life, she let him run a high fever and did not feed him aspirin. When he recovered from the flu, all his previous symptoms were gone. He remained perfectly well for about eight months, at which time the headaches, joint pains, and sneezing began to return. His problems were primarily caused by allergies and were easily controlled with a series of allergy shots.

Why did a high fever cause remission of Gary's allergies? Probably for the same reason that high fevers sometimes induce remission of cancer. Fever is part of a protective response; it can stimulate the production of mediators. The cascade of mediators activated during fever include not only IL-1, but also prostaglandin E (PGE), a prostanoid that can inhibit allergy,[14] and Tumor Necrosis Factor, a cytokine that can kill cancer cells. By allowing this cascade of mediators to flow freely, Gary's mother bought him eight months of good health. (This is not to say that fever should always be allowed to run its course. High fevers can be very dangerous, particularly in children.)

Although hundreds of different chemical mediators have been discovered, they work so closely together that it seems possible to describe a handful of mediator families that together promote or hinder most of the common diseases.

Cytokines like IL-1 and prostanoids like PGE are part of a family of signals used by adjacent cells to communicate with one another and to talk back to themselves. They couple a cell to its immediate environment.[15] Because they regulate the growth and activity of many types of cells, they are mediators of the normal healing response to injury and infection. When their activity is not properly regulated, the cell growth and activity they induce can contribute to cancer, arteriosclerosis, and states of chronic inflammation, like arthritis.

Neurotransmitters and stress hormones are another extended family of chemical mediators. They include the adrenal hormones adrenaline and cortisone; the neurotransmitter serotonin, best known for its effects on mood, sleep, and appetite; and neuropeptides like beta-endorphin and substance P, which are known for their effects on pain. These substances modulate the body's response to stressors in the external environment and help to set the biological clocks that govern the daily cycles of sleep and waking. When their activity is improperly regulated, they can promote fatigue, depression, and anxiety, and even make heart attacks more likely.[16]

These two giant families of chemical mediators are not really separate. Like the residents of a small town in Italy, where everyone talks to everyone, neurotransmitters and hormones endlessly interact with cytokines and prostaglandins, so that disturbances in the regulation of stress hormone production affect immune function, contributing to heart disease, cancer, and allergy, and disturbances in cytokine production affect mood and sleep.[17]

The investigation of novel chemical mediators continues at a dizzying pace. The most intriguing new substance is the simplest one yet, a gas called nitric oxide, voted "molecule of the year" by the editors of *Science* in 1992. Ten years ago, nitric oxide was best known as a noxious pollutant found in auto exhaust, contributing to acid rain and destroying the ozone layer. A series of discoveries has drastically changed its profile. The first hint that nitric oxide might be more than just a pollutant was the finding that nitroglycerine in the body is broken down to produce nitric oxide. Nitroglycerine has been used for the treatment of cardiac chest pain (angina) since 1867. It is still the best drug for relieving angina, and does so by dilating the arteries that carry blood to the muscle of the heart.

Nitric oxide is made by the cells that line blood vessels. Its effect is to relax the muscles in the vessel wall, dilating arteries and increasing blood flow. Too little nitric oxide may contribute to high blood pressure, arteriosclerosis, and male sexual impotence. Nitric oxide has been found in the brain, where it serves as a neurotransmitter and appears to be important for the storage of memory. In the stomach, nitric oxide protects the lining from the effects of acid; in the pancreas it stimulates the release of insulin. White blood cells synthesize nitric oxide and use it to kill microbes and tumor cells. Although a modest production of nitric oxide is important for normal cell function, high levels may be extremely toxic, killing the body's own cells and causing shock. Recent evidence suggests that destruction of the pancreas by nitric oxide is an early event in the genesis of juvenile diabetes.[18]

Nitric oxide is a classic mediator: it is multifunctional; it participates in the formation of numerous different, unrelated "diseases"; it does nothing by itself, acting only in conjunction with other mediators that inhibit, mimic, or stimulate its effects; its baseline activity is modulated by diet. Most of the body's nitric oxide is directly synthesized from a dietary amino acid (a building block of protein) called *arginine*, found in nuts, beans, and numerous vegetables. Vegetarian diets may be beneficial in part because they stimulate the production of nitric oxide.

The most basic elements of life—diet, exercise, sunlight, recreation, social interaction, thoughts and mental images—affect your levels of chemical mediators. Age, sex, phase of the menstrual cycle, the season, or the time of day may also affect the activity of mediators. Breast cancer grows most rapidly in spring and most slowly in the fall. The cure of breast cancer by surgery is far more likely if the operation is performed between two and three weeks following the first day of a woman's menstrual period than at other times in her cycle. Asthma attacks frequently occur during the night, when levels of adrenaline are naturally low. Fatal heart attacks are more likely to occur just after dawn.[19] This well-known phenomenon was first recorded on a tombstone in the village of Sevenoaks, England: "Grimm death took me without warning / I was well at night and dead at nine in the morning."

It is in the early morning that blood has the greatest tendency to clot. Tiny particles called platelets, which are made in the bone marrow and travel through the bloodstream, initiate the clot by clumping together and attracting a heavy coating of fibrous protein that stems the flow of blood. When platelets clump, they release chemical mediators into the circulation. Platelet-derived mediators make blood vessels constrict and increase the tendency of other platelets to clump. This is called a "feed-forward" cascade, and it plays a critical role in protecting the body from blood loss when injury occurs. It also contributes to the cellular events that initiate a heart attack.

The tendency of platelets to clump together varies with the time of day and with exposure of platelets to a variety of chemical mediators that either increase or decrease platelet aggregability (stickiness), counterbalancing one another in a physiological tug-of-war. The stickiness of platelets is naturally greatest in the early morning.[20] It increases when you eat a meal high in saturated fat, smoke a cigarette, or feel fear or anger, which causes the adrenal glands to flood your tissues with adrenaline. Platelet stickiness is decreased by eating fish, vegetables, or garlic, drinking red wine, and exercising regularly. Platelets may in fact be the link between emotions, habits, and heart attacks.[21] Platelet stickiness may also explain why fatal heart attacks occur more frequently on Monday mornings than on any other day of the week.[22]

Social Mediators

Social stress has clearly been shown to increase the rate at which people develop heart attacks. A person's degree of social isolation,[23]

COMMON MEDIATORS OF ILLNESS

Biochemical
    stress hormones (e.g., adrenaline and cortisone)
    neurotransmitters (e.g., serotonin)
    neuropeptides (e.g., beta-endorphin and substance P)
    prostanoids
    cytokines
    free radicals
    nitric oxide

Cognitive/Emotional
    fear of pain
    fear of loss (life, identity, independence, relationships)
    beliefs about sickness, including cultural beliefs
    feelings about sickness (anxiety, depression)
    poor self-esteem, low perceived self-efficacy

Social
    rewards for being ill
    behavioral conditioning
    lack of resources (poverty, social isolation)

Subatomic
    ions
    electrons
    electrical and magnetic energy fields

---

poverty, depression, or anxiety[24] predicts the likelihood that he will die from heart disease, if he already has hardening of the arteries. Unexpectedly, people who minimize their symptoms and deny the presence of serious heart disease appear to have a better prognosis than those who worry. Emotional distress increases the release of chemical mediators, which increase platelet clumping.[25]

The modulation of mediator activity by social interaction and habitual patterns of living—what the ancient Greeks called *díaita*—can be a matter of life and death for people with arteriosclerosis. A team of California scientists, led by Dr. Dean Ornish, recognized this when they devised a program that offered social support, group meditation, low-intensity exercise, and vegetarian, very-low-fat meals for people with heart disease. The program not only decreased the participants' rate of heart attacks, it actually improved blood flow to the heart muscle by reversing their arteriosclerosis.[26]

Unfortunately, most practicing physicians haven't learned how to recognize, understand, and respond to the impact of interpersonal relationships and *díaita* on illness. In fact, many doctors fail to meet "essential core competence" in clinical nutrition.[27] A new discipline within health care, called *functional medicine*, is presently emerging. Its mainstay is an understanding of the way in which all components of *díaita* affect human biochemical, physical, psychological, and social function. Its main tenets are described in the next chapter.

Triggers and the Provocation of Illness

It is often possible to identify the *triggers* that activate quiescent mediators in individual patients. They are easiest to find in acute infection, injury, or allergy, but probably occur in all ailments. Common triggers include trauma, exercise, microbes, drugs, toxins, allergens, foods, thoughts, images, memories, repetitive activities, and social interactions. For some diseases, the trigger is such an integral part of our concept of the disease that it is called the *cause*. Concussion, for example, is, by definition, caused by head trauma. "Strep throat," by definition, is caused by infection with the bacterium *Streptococcus pyogenes*.

Triggers are often not disease-specific, however; they tend to be specific to the individual. Many chronic ailments have multiple interacting triggers. People with asthma, for example, may experience attacks that are triggered by air pollution, passive smoking, thunderstorms, exposure to dust, cats, or cockroaches, viral respiratory infection, feelings of anxiety, cold temperature, and strenuous exercise.[28] Sensitivity to each trigger often varies among persons with similar ailments. A prime task of the doctor as medical detective is to help patients identify important triggers for their ailments and develop strategies for eliminating them or diminishing their virulence.

Most triggers are not so easy to track down or eliminate, but it's well worth the time and effort required by both doctor and patient. I once had a patient, Laura, who had been admitted to the hospital three times complaining of severe abdominal pain in her lower right quadrant. Each time the surgeon prepared to do an appendectomy, Laura's pain mysteriously disappeared. The trigger could have been many things—job stress, worries about running the household—but it turned out to be an allergic reaction to the tuna salad sandwiches she ate on the job.

Looking for triggers in the lives of several thousand patients has taught me some rules:

(a) The list of possibilities is endless; listen carefully to the patient's story and seek her opinion.

(b) In chronic conditions there are usually multiple triggers that reinforce one another; be comprehensive.

(c) It's easy to make mistakes and identify the wrong trigger, especially in a condition that fluctuates spontaneously. Be skeptical; challenge each theory.

(d) The same symptom in two different people (e.g., joint pain) may have different triggers; conversely, the same trigger may induce different symptoms in two other people (e.g., headache in one, diarrhea in the other); be flexible.

Such competing demands on the seeker of triggers may explain why so many physicians avoid the search. In one study, practicing physicians were asked how they would treat a new patient with abdominal pain who had a recent diagnosis of gastritis (inflammation of the stomach) made by a specialist in another town. Almost half were ready to put the patient on a drug to lower stomach acid without asking about the patient's use of aspirin, alcohol, or tobacco, all of which are potential triggers for gastritis. The authors of the study concluded, "In actual practice, ignoring these aspects of the patient may well have reduced or even negated the efficacy of other therapeutic plans implemented."[29]

It is not always possible to eliminate the triggers of illness, but understanding them may clarify the mediators that these triggers activate.

In the spring of 1994, I was invited to present my blueprint for patient-centered diagnosis at a medical school in the Midwest. After my lecture, the department chairman asked me to join "teaching rounds" in the university hospital. At teaching rounds, a team composed of an intern, resident, and medical student present to a faculty member the cases admitted the previous day. When I arrived on the hospital floor, rounds were already in progress, in a small conference room behind the nurses' station. The resident promptly apologized for missing my lecture. There had been four admissions the night before and the team was *very busy*. The tone of his voice warned that I was an unwelcome interloper. There was work to be done and not much time for a luxury like patient-centered diagnosis.

"Well, which patient should we present to Dr. Galland?" asked the faculty member.

"How about Mrs. Borovic?" replied the resident, with a hint of malice in his voice.

The medical student began by presenting the patient's history. Mrs. Borovic was seventy-one and suffered from diabetes, high blood pressure, and poor circulation. In the past she had undergone operations on her heart and the blood vessels of her legs, because of blocked vessels. Her husband also had high blood pressure and poor circulation. Both of them had had numerous admissions to different hospitals for one reason or another. For the past few days, Mrs. Borovic had been awakened at night by severe pain in the lower right quadrant of the abdomen, which would last most of the night and clear up during the day. Her gastroenterologist had sent her to the hospital for admission, ordered a CAT scan of her abdomen, and requested that she be started on intravenous antibiotics. The admitting diagnosis was "diverticulitis," which is the formation of an abscess in the large intestine. The medical student was puzzled because this patient had experienced pains in the same place since the age of sixteen. When she was twenty-four, her appendix had been removed, but the pains continued. About a year ago, her gastroenterologist had prescribed a drug that relieves spasm of the intestine; the pain had improved for many months.

The intern spoke next. He was unshaven and looked haggard, having borne the brunt of the previous night's workload. He had examined the patient on her arrival at the hospital, but at that time she had no pain and his examination had been unrewarding. Her white blood cell count and sedimentation rate were normal. He left orders that he was to be called, so that he could reexamine her if and when the pain returned, which it did at 3:00 A.M. The second examination was also unrewarding because she had so much pain that she would not allow him to examine her very thoroughly. I understood his frustration. He had generously given up sleep—an intern's dearest possession—to reexamine this patient in the middle of the night, only to find her not fully cooperative.

"She doesn't have diverticulitis," interjected the resident, with a tone of disgust. "She has irritable bowel syndrome. We're only doing the CAT scan to appease the gastroenterologist. If it's negative, she'll be discharged."

"Well, well," added the faculty member. "The plan is to await the results of the CAT scan. What comes next?" He looked my way and all eyes followed.

"I don't think we should wait for the CAT scan," I said. "I wouldn't even do one. I'd like to know more about this patient. What was she like before this present episode of pain? What was she doing? How active was she? Did she change her diet? Was anything new going on in her life?"

No one had the information with which to answer these questions, so we decided to take them directly to Mrs. Borovic. She was in the hallway when we approached her room, looking quite fresh and cheerful. Her snow-white hair was combed and sprayed, her face was made up, and she had changed from a hospital gown into her own bed clothes, which were still neatly pressed. She looked much better than the intern did, in fact, and she was absolutely delighted to see us.

After being introduced as a visiting professor, I asked her, "How were you feeling last week, *before* this bout of pain started?"

"Oh, I was very fatigued." She sighed. "Whenever I get fatigued, I get sick."

"Why were you fatigued?"

"My husband was in the hospital. Whenever he goes into the hospital, I get so fatigued. I have to drive and visit him every day. I have to walk the dogs by myself. I get so worn out. When he comes home, I get sick. It happens every time. In December he had surgery, and I wound up at another hospital, only that was different. Then, I was vomiting."

A hospital admission was the last thing this woman needed! Without hesitation, she had disclosed the trigger for this hospitalization: her

---

COMMON TRIGGERS OF ILLNESS

Physical injury (e.g., concussion)
Repetitive activities (e.g., overuse syndromes)
Physical exercise (may trigger heart attacks)
Microbes (triggers of infectious disease)
    bacteria
    viruses
    parasites
    fungi
Drugs
    therapeutic (e.g., aspirin)
    "recreational" (e.g., alcohol or caffeine)
    illicit (e.g., cocaine)
Toxins
    air pollution
    heavy metals (e.g., lead or mercury)
    cigarette smoke
    microbial (e.g., botulism)
Temperature extremes (may trigger asthma)
Adverse social interactions (e.g., fights or arguments)
Memories of previous sickness or distress
Feelings of anxiety (may trigger asthma, heart attacks)
Stressful life events (e.g., family illness)

---

husband's previous hospital admission. From her own description, the principal mediator of her illness was the need to rest and be relieved of the responsibility of caring for him at home. During the course of many hospital admissions over many years, she had learned on an unconscious level that being sick was the best way to get relief. Each hospital admission reinforced this pattern of behavior by providing her with the respite she wanted. Psychologists call this *operant conditioning*. For some people with chronic or recurrent illness, it is a powerful and *involuntary* mediator of sickness and disability. Two features of Mrs. Borovic's case reveal the involuntary nature of her symptoms. First, the pain would wake her from sleep at night; it was rarely present during the day. Second, she was clearly not malingering. She made no effort to conceal her motivation and was happy to discuss it when the right question was asked. The woman needed a new strategy for coping with the stress she experienced each time her husband became ill, not a new series of diagnostic tests.

For me, the most rewarding outcome of this interview was the change in attitude of the intern and resident. By the time we returned to the conference room, their hostility toward the patient had evaporated. She was no longer just a "crock" with irritable bowel syndrome, she was a person whose proper care challenged the model of medical practice to which they were accustomed.

The Precipitating Event

For many patients there is a trigger so important that it deserves a separate status; it acts like a boundary in time. Before it occurred, the patient considered himself to be a reasonably healthy individual. Since crossing it, he has become a "patient," someone who sees doctors regularly. I call it the *precipitating event*. The commonest events that cluster around such a boundary, in the patients I have evaluated, are a period of extreme emotional distress, an acute infection, or exposure to some toxic substance. To locate the precipitating event, it is not enough for me to ask a patient, "How long have you been ill?" or, "How long have you had this symptom?" I frequently have to ask, "When is the last time you felt completely well?" Then the patient may laugh or groan and say, "Oh, I haven't felt well for ten years!" or, "Oh, that was before the birth of my last child," or, "Not since I moved to New York." I start my investigation of the causes of the present illness with inquiries about the six-month period prior to that boundary, because often the answer lies there.

Edward Ruiz was a thirty-one-year-old computer technician who had been ill for eighteen months with fatigue, headaches, blurred vision, and inability to exercise. He used to lift weights, but now his muscles hurt and felt weak if he tried to do anything. He saw an internist and an orthopedist who each suspected Lyme disease but didn't find it. He saw a neurologist; the office examination was normal, so the neurologist ordered a brain wave study (an EEG), which was normal, and an MRI (magnetic resonance image) of the brain, which showed many small abnormal patches. The neurologist suspected multiple sclerosis. Edward saw a second neurologist, who agreed. More electrical studies of the brain were done; the results were normal. The second neurologist wanted to do a spinal tap and Edward refused. At that point, a friend referred him to me.

Sitting across from me in the consultation room, Edward shifted his weight from side to side as he told his story. He stared first at the ceiling, then at the floor, anxiously awaiting a verdict. My heart reached out to him. Multiple sclerosis was a dreaded diagnosis that would change his life forever. I wanted to reassure him. More important, I wanted to help him give me the information I needed to find the real source of his problem.

"There are many possible causes for your symptoms," I explained. "The only support for a diagnosis of multiple sclerosis comes from the MRI. Now, the MRI is a very sensitive tool for seeing certain types of physical disturbances in the brain. But it can be misleading.[30] Because there has been no other explanation to account for your symptoms, the assumption has been made that the minor abnormalities on your MRI are the 'cause.' Maybe there are other explanations. What was your health like before these symptoms started . . . say, two to three years ago?"

"I was always healthy as a horse," he answered earnestly. "I never missed a day of work, I never even thought about being sick . . . until I got pneumonia."

"Oh, when was that?" I asked, in a casual tone intended to veil the intensity of my interest in that information. I wanted Edward to lead me; I didn't want to be leading him.

"Almost three years ago, maybe a little less."

"What happened when you had pneumonia?"

"I had the flu. I couldn't shake it. I kept coughing, running a fever. My doctor did a chest X ray and told me I had pneumonia."

"How were you treated?"

"Some kind of antibiotic."

"What happened next? How was your recovery?"

"I got over it pretty quickly. Yeah, I was fine. But, boy, was my stomach a wreck!"

"What do you mean?"

"I could hardly eat anything. It would swell up and rumble. I got diarrhea. I had some pizza and beer after bowling one day . . . forget it! I got so sick I even missed work the next day."

"Did you see a doctor about that problem?"

"No. It would come and go. It slowly got better. I just had to be careful about what I ate."

"Is your stomach back to normal now?"

"No, not really. In fact, I was sick again just last week. But I don't care about that. It's this being so weak that has me worried."

Edward's precipitating event was clearly an acute illness, pneumonia. I suspected that the culprit was not the infection itself, but an effect of the antibiotic he had taken. One of the patterns that my colleagues and I repeatedly encountered during our investigations at the Gesell Institute was the development of chronic illness following the use of antibiotics. We thought that antibiotics might precipitate chronic disease by altering the body's ecology. Each person is colonized by over a hundred trillion bacteria, which crowd themselves onto the surfaces of the digestive, respiratory, and genital tracts and cover the skin. These organisms, called the "indigenous flora," perform some useful functions, so that our relationship with them is normally one of mutual benefit. Destruction of these bacteria by antibiotics may be injurious, allowing the overgrowth of unfriendly organisms, which proliferate when their control by the normal flora is broken. Yeasts are known to take advantage of this situation; in women they cause vaginitis, in infants diaper rash, in men jock itch. Yeasts overgrowing the lower intestine can cause diarrhea and bloating. The evidence that intestinal yeasts can trigger diarrhea has been reported in several studies dating back to the 1950s, a time when antibiotics were first generally available.

The evidence has been widely ignored, which is unfortunate, because yeast-induced bowel disorders are quite common.[31]

I ordered a stool examination for Edward. When an extract of stool was examined under the microscope, large quantities of yeast were seen. I advised Edward to avoid the foods that aggravated his digestive symptoms, suggested that he supplement his diet with a preparation of *Lactobacillus acidophilus*, which are friendly intestinal bacteria, and treated him with nystatin, a drug that is highly effective at killing yeast. Over a period of several weeks, all his symptoms disappeared. He has remained perfectly well for the past five years.

The notion that yeast colonizing the intestinal tract can cause symptoms such as fatigue or headache has generated heated controversy within the medical profession over the past few years. The terms of the debate have been misguided. Detractors of the yeast theory have discussed the problem as if yeast overgrowth were supposed to be a new disease. It's nothing of the kind. It is a toxic reaction of a type that can occur with any infection, aggravated by the ability of yeasts to generate strong allergic reactions in people they infect.[32]

Often, the effects of a precipitating event cannot be readily reversed. A high level of emotional distress may predispose people to conditions that persist after the stress subsides. Childhood diabetes, hyperthyroidism, appendicitis, and chronic headache are all associated with preceding stressors.[33] In pregnancy, an increase in life stress in the third trimester more than doubles the rate of serious complications affecting the newborn infant. Marital disruption due to death or divorce is one of the greatest stresses a person can undergo, and recent or pending marital separation is associated with suppression of several measures of immune function.[34] It's often difficult to discover the truth about a patient's life stressors; sometimes it's impossible.

One evening, when I was still teaching at SUNY Stony Brook, I was about to go home for dinner when a graduate student named Carla, whom I did not know, appeared at my office door asking if I could see her. She had a severe sore throat and fever; her doctor had prescribed penicillin, but she was getting worse, not better. I led her into an exam room and looked at her throat. My blood froze. She had a large ulcer on her left tonsil filled with shaggy gray pus. Her gums bled at the

COMMON PRECIPITATING EVENTS FOR CHRONIC ILLNESS

Severe emotional distress (e.g., loss of a spouse, being
   fired from a job)
Severe infection (viral, bacterial, parasitic, fungal)
Exposure to toxins, drugs, or allergens

Precipitating events appear to increase a person's
   sensitivity to the triggers that act to maintain
   illness.

touch, her skin was pale, and there were bruises on her arms and legs. I feared that she had acute leukemia, so I admitted her directly to the nearest hospital. A blood count confirmed the diagnosis. I started intravenous antibiotics and consulted a hematologist, who began chemotherapy.

Carla told me how determined she was to fight this disease; she had a wonderful husband, Russ, and was about to finish her thesis. The prognosis for acute leukemia in adults is grave, however, and she lost ground quickly. We talked about her life and family. I asked her if she had experienced any major loss or disappointment prior to her diagnosis. No, she said, her life had been wonderful.

About a month after I first saw Carla, I had another visit from a graduate student, a young woman whose name was Lauren. She couldn't sleep. She had daily migraines. She was an emotional wreck. I would understand the cause, she said.

"It's Carla Harmon," confided Lauren. "I've been having an affair with Russ. We're in love. He wants to divorce her and marry me. He told her a few weeks ago. He's only staying with her now because she's sick. I know she's going to die soon. I feel awful."

Carla died a month later, denying that she had any problem in the world except her disease. I have no way of knowing what relationship the disintegration of Carla's marriage, or her denial of it, had to the rapid onset of her leukemia and the speed with which it killed her. No one can know that. I can only wonder.

ANTECEDENTS AND THE PREDISPOSITION TO ILLNESS

Looking through the disease to search for the mediators and triggers of illness is just the first step of patient-centered diagnosis. No expert in art restoration would feel confident restoring an important work without knowing as much as possible about its history and background: When and where was it painted? Who was the artist? Who were his masters? What other works did he create? What was this painting like when originally completed? Similar information must be gathered about patients, because patient-centered diagnosis must preserve and clarify the identity of each person.

Diathesis

To reach this goal, a physician must seek to know those features of the patient that created the setting in which illness occurred. These characteristics are known collectively by the Greek word *diathesis*, which means "predisposition." When interviewing patients with multiple symptoms and complicated medical histories, I invariably find that knowledge of diathesis is essential for forming a coherent picture of the present illness.

A complete diathesis includes a search for all those factors that existed before you fell sick that contributed to the evolution of your illness. These factors can be congenital (those with which you were born) and developmental (those you acquired after birth). The most important congenital factor is sex: women and men differ in their susceptibility to many disorders. The most important developmental factor is age: what ails children is rarely the same as what ails the elderly. These two are obvious. Beyond them lie factors as diverse as our genetic differences and the very life experiences that distinguish one person from another. In a brilliant and, unfortunately, neglected essay, Dr. Jeffrey Fessel, a professor of medicine at Stanford University, explains,

> In most circumstances, disease is not an inevitable outcome of a single event occurring at a point in time but generally a probabilistic result of many events, each impinging on the organism at separate times and each producing its own sequence of biological reactions. The sum total of these events produces sufficient discomfort to the

person to be recognized as illness. . . . Although the [body's] ultimate
. . . reaction . . . may be the same in different persons, suggesting a
uniform illness and, by extension, a disease entity in its own right,
each person nevertheless probably has a unique and separate illness
by virtue of the probability that no one else has the same combination and permutation of antecedents and their time relations. In this
sense, every disease consists of multiple diseases; in this sense, too,
there are no diseases but only sick people.[35]

The identity of the patient, in all relevant dimensions—genetic, environmental, psychosocial, structural, nutritional—is as critically important to the diagnostic process as is the identity of a painting *in
restauro*. The effort to understand and accept the uniqueness of each
patient defines the art of medicine. To better serve this art, medical science needs to pay more attention to what makes us unique individuals.

Congenital factors, those present at birth, may be genetic (inherited
through the chromosomes) or acquired in the womb. They can most
readily be evaluated from a comprehensive family history, including
the mother's health before and during pregnancy. *Developmental* factors shape an individual's health risks and resilience prior to the illness.
Doctors learn of them by asking about family life, diet, environment,
occupation, drug use, life stress, and sexual behavior, chronologically
since birth. The key developmental factors in illness diathesis appear to
be nutrition, trauma (physical and emotional), learned patterns of behavior, alterations in the body's microbial ecology, and chronic exposure to drugs or environmental toxins.

Understanding diathesis is not merely an intellectual exercise. A
proper diathesis will reveal most of the usual triggers, precipitating
events, and common components of a person's life that modulate the
activity of mediators. Including diathesis in the diagnostic process helps
guide the physician in developing a patient-centered treatment and
bridges the traditional gap between preventive and clinical medicine.
Modern preventive medicine is based on the understanding of individual risk factors, those characteristics of a person that predispose him
toward disease. Risk factors are the flip side of diathesis; they form the
diathesis for an illness the patient does not yet have but which might be
prevented if they were altered.

In subsequent chapters, I will describe some of the developmental factors in greater detail and relate them to various agents of disease. I'll mention some key ones below.

Infections, especially the common infections of childhood, help shape our resistance to disease, for better or for worse. A study done in Copenhagen found that people who had measles in childhood, with the typical rash, were *less* likely to suffer from a wide variety of diseases in adulthood than were people who had suffered an unrecognized measles infection without the rash.[36] In other words, a strong case of measles at a young age was associated with increased hardiness later in life. Other infections may have remote—and negative—effects. Cytomegalovirus (CMV) is an extremely common, often asymptomatic, viral infection. Recent research indicates that a brisk immune response to CMV infection may injure arteries in the heart and contribute to the eventual development of coronary heart disease.

When it closely precedes illness, trauma (either emotional or physical) can be seen as a trigger. The Northridge earthquake, which battered Los Angeles in 1994, quintupled the death rate from heart attacks in Los Angeles County, for one day. The emotional trauma of the quake was the apparent trigger.[37] When repeated trauma has occurred long before the onset of symptoms, it can be viewed as a developmental component of the illness diathesis. Daily exposure to loud noise, for example, may result in high blood pressure (hypertension).[38] Similarly, a single blow to the head may be the precipitating cause of headache. On the other hand, several blows to the head, occurring sporadically over a period of years, may so change the postural alignment of the neck that chronic muscle tension eventually produces headache. The event that finally creates pain may not be an injury; it may be an extended period of emotional distress or prolonged work in an uncomfortable position. The injuries, then, are not part of the precipitating event, they are part of the diathesis. These distinctions are relative, not absolute; they may not even be important in every case. Their purpose is to structure the diagnostic process in such a way that treatment is guided by the characteristics of each patient and not by the anonymity of the disease.

Are Genes Destiny?

When a disorder like heart disease or cancer "runs" in a family, doctors tend to seek its origins in the genes. The prevailing belief is that the pattern of DNA found in a person's genes creates a tendency toward a particular disease that will be expressed if the environment also favors the development of disease. Genetic differences between individuals are invoked to explain the differential susceptibility to disease of two people in similar environments. The greatest impetus for the genetic hypothesis comes from studies that contrast the health of identical and fraternal twins. If a condition occurs in both twins, the two people are said to show *concordance* for it; if a condition appears in one twin but not the other, the twins are said to show *discordance* for it. The finding that a given trait, like high blood pressure, occurs with greater concordance among identical than fraternal twins is usually taken as an indication that the condition is likely to be genetic, rather than environmental.

We have entered an age that places undue reliance on the genetic hypothesis, obscuring the complexity of human development. Numerous early life influences may be shared by identical twins and not by fraternal twins. Identical twins are usually nourished by a common blood supply (placenta) when developing in the womb, whereas fraternal twins are not. Identical twins who share the same placenta are more likely to be concordant for developing hypertension as adults than are identical twins with separate placentas.[39] This shows us that nongenetic factors, at work in the womb, may strongly influence the tendency toward the development of chronic illness in adulthood. Their importance lies in the greatly expanded opportunity for prevention. A low birth weight, for example, strongly increases the risk that a person will develop hypertension, diabetes, or elevated cholesterol and die from a heart attack or chronic lung disease.[40] Birth weight is strongly influenced by the mother's diet and whether she smokes or drinks alcohol when pregnant.

Numerous drugs predispose to physical deformities at birth. A high rate of multiple minor physical anomalies, such as widely spaced eyes, a highly arched palate, and a curved fifth finger, is thought to result from some unidentified injury occurring in the womb; it is associated with hyperactivity and learning disabilities in children and with clum-

---

ANTECEDENTS OF ILLNESS: THE ILLNESS DIATHESIS

Congenital Factors (those with which you are born)
Genetic (sex and inherited traits)
Acquired in the womb (resulting from maternal
        nutrition, toxic exposures; e.g., fetal alcohol
        syndrome)

Developmental Factors (those that develop over time)
Effects of age
Nutrition
Traumatic events (physical or emotional)
Effects of toxins, drugs
Effects of learning and conditioning
Altered microbial ecology (e.g., depletion of normal
        intestinal bacteria)

---

siness, aggressiveness, and high sociability in adults.[41] I have noticed, among my patients, an apparent relationship between the nature of the fingerprint pattern and changes in heart rate and blood pressure that occur when standing up quickly. As the fingerprints and the nervous system develop at the same time, in about month three of pregnancy, it is likely that factors that affect the growing fetus at that time lie behind this association.[42] Congenital factors cannot be changed, but recognizing them may be essential to understanding the varied ways in which patients respond to treatment.

WHEN THE DIAGNOSIS CANNOT BE MADE

There are some patients for whom no disease can be identified, because no diagnosis really fits. For them, patient-centered diagnosis may be the *only* way to reach a rational understanding of the illness. This proved to be the case for a teenage girl I first met in May 1990. Janine and her younger sister, Gail, had been out of school for four months with a vague cluster of symptoms that included fatigue, dizziness, sore

THE ANATOMY OF AN ILLNESS

clinical disease
symptoms, signs, changes in behavior, changes in cells/tissues

mediators
psychosocial, biochemical

diathesis
congenital factors
genetic
acquired in utero

developmental
factors
age–related
environmental
nutritional
drug–induced
disease–related
learned
traumatic

triggers
psychosocial stress
injury, infection
toxins, allergens
thoughts, feelings
drugs

precipitating events
stress, infection
trauma, toxin exposure

The same factors may act as triggers, precipitating events, or elements of the illness diathesis, depending upon the structure of each individual's illness. Illness is dynamic and changing: Mediators act as triggers for the activation of other mediators. Sickness creates the diathesis for further sickness.

throat, and headache. For Janine, this was part of a pattern reaching back six years, to the time she was seven.

One of the benefits of treating children is that I often get to meet the whole family. I set aside a Friday afternoon to spend with the Stephensons, who drove down to Manhattan from their home in upstate New York, and I prepared for them by reviewing the questionnaires they had completed. Something seemed very strange. Two intelligent girls who were good students felt too tired and dizzy to go to school for four months. No particular illness had been identified, yet they just stayed home. Maybe their parents were part of the problem. On the other hand, I knew their doctor to be a competent and thorough physician, well attuned to treating his patients as individuals. He had referred about a dozen of his toughest and most complicated cases to me and he had been very astute in handling each one. He wasn't likely to have missed anything as obvious as mere parental bungling.

When I interviewed the Stephensons, I put as much effort into assessing the dynamics of their family life and the effectiveness of the adults as into defining the illness of the children. Sickness had consumed much of their time and energy. Perhaps it had brought them closer together, but I had *no* feeling that this family needed sickness to be close. On the contrary, they had constantly fought its hold on their lives. This recent capitulation was a terrible defeat that left both parents deeply worried about the future. What kind of life could Janine expect if this disabling pattern of recurrent ill health refused to abate? Janine did not voice her fears. She was just "tired of being sick."

She had known seven years of relatively good health, although her mother recalled that she always lacked the stamina of her playmates. In the fall of 1983, shortly after her seventh birthday, she changed suddenly, looked pale and ghastly, and threw tantrums every day. After three months of medical treatment brought no answers, the Stephensons took Janine to a Connecticut allergist, Dr. Marshall Mandell, known for his work with hyperactive children. Mandell videotaped Janine and obtained handwriting samples while she underwent allergy testing. When injected with extracts of wheat, tomatoes, and airborne molds, Janine turned into a screaming demon unable to write her own name. She was treated with an allergy diet and shots to desensitize her to mold spores.

She did fairly well for two years, until she developed pneumonia. The infection left her with fatigue, chills, dizziness, and joint pain that persisted for so long that her pediatrician rendered a diagnosis of chronic fatigue syndrome. Over a three-year span she slowly improved, and by the summer of 1989 began to feel almost normal. In the fall of that year she lost both her grandfathers. She grieved deeply but found that counseling, which included all members of the family, helped restore her spirits. She had three bouts of "flu" that winter; these were acute episodes of abdominal pain, sore throat, headache, and dizziness. Each left her more exhausted than the one before. She stopped attending school and was tutored at home.

Janine's younger sisters, Gail and Cindy, had been plagued by allergies since infancy. When Janine became ill again in the beginning of 1990, Gail slowly developed the same symptoms and the same degree of disability. Her mom suspected that she was depressed. I asked about the health of other family members. Mom and Dad and aunts and uncles were all healthy, except for mild bouts of hay fever.

As I took the family history, one event stood out like a red flag. The summer before Janine's allergies developed, the entire family had taken a cross-country trip to British Columbia. They camped in state and national parks most of the time and paid little attention to the water source from which they drank. Could a chronic infection acquired from contaminated drinking water, fluctuating in its effects over the years under the influence of other types of stress, explain this whole illness? A test for parasites, done promptly in my office, revealed that Janine was infected with the parasite *Giardia lamblia*; the other family members were not.

My physical examination quickly revealed that there was more to be reckoned with than infection alone. When lying at rest, Janine's pulse seemed normal, 84 and regular. As soon as she stood up her pulse rate zoomed to 132, and after three minutes of standing it was still very fast, 124. Ordinarily it takes strenuous exercise to raise a child's pulse rate that much. For Janine, the simple act of standing was enough. Extended bedrest might do this to an otherwise healthy person, but I suspected that Janine had been born with this problem and that it explained her susceptibility to severe fatigue. Perhaps her sisters shared the same abnormality. I studied Janine's fingertips with a magnifying glass. The fingerprint, technically called the *epidermal ridge pattern*, ordinarily consists of whorls, loops, and arches. Whorls are the most tightly coiled and complex, arches the simplest and most open. Janine had only arches. This minor congenital anomaly reflects a disturbance in fetal growth during the third month of pregnancy. There were other signs that Janine may have been troubled during her third month in the womb: an indented breastbone (*pectus excavatum*) and mild scoliosis. The part of the nervous system that regulates heart rate, the autonomic nervous system, also undergoes a critical stage of its development during the third month; so do the valves of the fetal heart. One of Janine's heart valves, the mitral valve, made a clicking sound when I listened. All these associations suggested to me that the speeding of her pulse on standing was not just the result of prolonged rest but represented an inborn disturbance in the function of the autonomic nervous system, a condition called autonomic dysregulation.

I examined Gail, Cindy, and their parents for fingerprint anomalies and signs of autonomic dysregulation. Mom, Dad, and Cindy were normal; Gail was in between on both measures. It seemed no coincidence that the two family members who were ill were the two marked by congenital anomalies.

I had shared each step of the evaluation with Mrs. Stephenson. At the day's end, I sat down with the whole family and drew a blueprint based on patient-centered diagnosis to give structure to Janine's illness. I couldn't be sure of all the mediators, but autonomic dysregulation was a likely cause of fatigue. "When Janine is asked to stand up," I explained, "her body acts as if she's had to run a mile." Fear and despair were also likely mediators. Janine had long ago learned that she could never trust her body to get her through the day. *Giardia* infection was a precipitating event, probably responsible for the sudden onset of allergies at the age of seven. To call her disease giardiasis, however, would be a misleading simplification. The loss of two grandparents may have constituted a second precipitating event. Diathesis included a family history of allergy and her congenital anomalies.

The most reasonable treatment approach would be the most comprehensive. I expected that treatment of *Giardia* infection would improve her energy and decrease the severity of her allergies. The best treatment for autonomic dysregulation is aerobic physical conditioning. I explained to Janine and to Gail that they would both have to start a graduated program of walking for fitness. The school year was almost over. I set goals for them to reach during the summer, and, like most girls their age, they showed less enthusiasm for my plan than I would have liked. I wasn't sure how best to deal with their fear. Psychological counseling might be helpful, but they felt that they had had enough of that last autumn and would rather exercise than start counseling again.

By September, Janine and Gail were both back in school. Cured of giardiasis and walking two miles a day, Janine had no fatigue or dizziness and virtually no allergic problems. She sailed through the fall without illness. When I spoke to Mrs. Stephenson at the start of 1991, it seemed as if the problems were over.

Two weeks later, they began all over again. Complaining of shakiness, dizziness, weakness, and headache, Janine missed five weeks of school. She felt cold all the time. This time there was no abdominal pain, gas, or bloating, and no evidence of recurrent *Giardia* infection. This time, Gail did not share her sister's illness.

Janine and her mother returned for an examination at the end of February. From their story, it seemed to me that a brief flu or cold had put her to bed for a few days. A few days in bed can wreak havoc with the nervous system of some people with autonomic dysregulation, and perhaps Janine was one. I examined her. Her pulse rate response was still abnormal, but it was considerably better than it had been when I first saw her.

"What is it that keeps you from going out of the house?" I asked. "I know you feel pretty awful, but there are people who feel awful and still manage to do things they have to, even if it's difficult." My remark was meant to provoke her; I wanted to gauge her response.

She spoke without emotion. "There's a time every day when I feel so dizzy I can't even stand up. I never know when to expect it, but if I overdo anything, even walking, I can be pretty sure I'll get it." This dizziness was not a true vertigo, which sends the room spinning, but a sensation of being lightheaded. I didn't think Janine was faking her symptoms, but my subjective response to her presentation was that she had given up rather easily. At the first return of symptoms, she had succumbed to disability, almost without a fight. Was it fear, that familiar dread of being deserted by her own body, that had conquered her? Was there an element of depression in this illness? Janine felt somewhat depressed; beyond that she could acknowledge nothing.

Her mother was concerned about the girl's thyroid. Janine's temperature was low. Could this, she asked, be a sign that her thyroid was underactive? It might be, I thought, but blood tests for thyroid hormones were normal, and autonomic dysregulation by itself can lower the body's temperature. On the other hand, I reasoned, thyroid function is in part regulated by the autonomic nervous system. Could dysregulation impair thyroid function by means too subtle for any available test? There were arcane and anecdotal reports asserting that thyroid extracts could help overcome autonomic dysregulation, acting as a spark to the nervous system. Some psychiatrists use thyroid to treat depression, presumably for the same reason. I decided that a short trial of thyroid would do little harm and might do some good. I prescribed the hormone, but made two requests: Janine would again begin a graduated exercise program, and she would resume psychological counseling as soon as possible.

What followed played out like a game of chess between the girl and the specter of her disease. Within three weeks, her coldness and dizziness were improved, but her lethargy continued. A month later she began exercising in earnest despite her fatigue, but was irritable and at times depressed. She acknowledged that she felt better after a brisk walk, but spent most of her time reading. "I can never get too much quiet," she told me. I urged her to step up the pace of exercise and to start psychotherapy, which she had postponed. She surprised me by enrolling at a school for karate. Psychotherapy finally began in midsummer, in the context of family counseling. It was a revelation. Janine was not depressed. She was furious. Illness was a thief that had stolen her childhood and made her a stranger to her friends. Karate, I thought, was an appropriate response.

By September, Janine had regained most of her lost ground, although she still chilled easily. An hour a day at karate class and weekly psychotherapy helped her unload the baggage of seven years of sickness. She went through the winter without a relapse and missed only four days of school all year. Her long-lost sense of humor returned, and she became so busy with after-school activities that by midwinter there was little time for karate. By early spring, her resting pulse rate had dropped to 60 and her standing pulse to 72, a victory of physical conditioning over autonomic dysfunction.

So, what *was* Janine's illness? It was nothing more and nothing less than Janine's own individual unique disease, presenting with symptoms of dizziness and fatigue, mediated by autonomic dysregulation and fear of her body, triggered by infection, grief, and anger, occurring in a girl whose autonomic nervous system was poorly modulated from birth. From this understanding came a plan not only for treating illness, but for preventive maintenance. I explained to Janine that a lifelong commitment to strenuous physical exercise would be her best guarantor of a stable autonomic nervous system and her best insurance against future disease. Janine took this advice to heart, with dramatic results. In February 1993, an unusually cold and snowy month, she fractured her pelvic bone in a sledding accident. Fortunately, the fracture was above her hip in a part of the bone that does not bear weight. After five days in the hospital, she was sent home with crutches. Determined to stay active, she was up and about despite her pain. Five weeks after leaving the hospital she left the country, with her crutches, for a long-awaited archeological tour of Israel. She impressed everyone. Janine had come to see that the director of restoration was not her doctor but herself.

4

THE FOUR PILLARS OF HEALING

Dr. Caroline Bedell Thomas of Johns Hopkins University has developed an eloquent metaphor for understanding disease, which stands in sharp contrast to the biomedical model. She calls it "the kaleidoscope model."

YOUR PERSONAL KALEIDOSCOPE

"The kaleidoscope model, which is rooted in psychobiology, states that *many* genetic and environmental factors enter into the health equation. While some factors are more important than others, it is the overall pattern that determines the outcome. As life goes on, the kaleidoscope turns a little as each new positive or negative factor is added. Thus the pattern is constantly changing, and is susceptible to future change. The persistence of good health, or the development of disease, depends upon the particular configuration of factors in a given individual at a given time."[1]

Patient-centered diagnosis provides a blueprint for analyzing the pattern in each person's kaleidoscope at any point in time. Drawing upon the interview, the physical examination, and relevant laboratory tests, we attempt to understand the mediators of disease that operate in each case, identify their triggers, determine the precipitating event(s), and dissect the varied, tangled threads of diathesis. The application of this blueprint requires knowledge of the patient, common sense, and a wealth of factual information that is not part of conventional medical training. Difficulty in acquiring this information is a major impediment for physicians and other health professionals who are trying to expand the scope and improve the efficacy of their practices.

Despite a plethora of medical organizations that offer educational symposia, I felt frustrated in attempting to disseminate information about patient-centered diagnosis. Existing groups of conventional or alternative physicians are generally organized around commitment to treating a cluster of diseases, providing a defined array of therapeutic techniques, or looking at the clinical encounter between physician and patient with a lens I judged to be too narrow in focus. So I welcomed the opportunity, which presented itself in the spring of 1993, to participate in the founding of a new organization, the Institute of Functional Medicine. IFM is dedicated to providing education and fostering research in keeping with the principles of the kaleidoscope model of health, and patient-centered diagnosis is its eyepiece.

The energy for IFM's creation came from Jeffrey Bland, a dynamic biochemist who had participated in the Italian conference at which I first unveiled the blueprint of patient-centered diagnosis. Dismayed at the lack of critical analysis in medical education, Jeff had left medical school in 1967 to pursue a doctoral degree in biochemistry. He had devoted most of his efforts to teaching and research concerning the impact of nutrition on physiological function. After several years of work with Linus Pauling, Jeff had founded his own organization, called HealthComm, to pursue his vision with full independence. Our paths had crossed many times at many symposia. Each time I marveled at his ability to synthesize concepts that extended far beyond the boundaries of his expertise in nutritional biochemistry. IFM gave me the chance to couple my vision with Jeff's and to work closely with the team of physicians, biochemists, and nutritionists that Jeff had brought together.

The goals of functional medicine are the improvement of physiological, emotional, cognitive, and/or physical function of individuals, sick or well. Restoration or enhancement of health, not suppression of disease, is the aim, so that functional health care is *restauro* for sick people. The principles that guide the restoration of health are different from the principles that guide the suppression of disease. Disease-suppressing therapies have a role to play in medical care, but their importance has been exaggerated. The core of this book is formed by the elements of health restoration. I call them the *pillars of healing*. There are four pillars on which each person and each physician must depend for the restoration process to be complete.

THE FIRST PILLAR: RELATIONSHIP

Forty-five years ago, René Dubos, the renowned microbiologist and environmentalist, observed that outbreaks of tuberculosis had been more closely related to wars and other disruptions of the social fabric than to any other factor.[2] A decade later, research demonstrated that widowed men and women were two to four times more likely to die prematurely than those still married.[3] For men over fifty-five, the death rate soared by 40 percent during the six months after the death of a wife.[4] Thirty years ago, a series of studies conducted in different countries revealed that social ties and social support softened the effect of stress, decreased sickness, and prolonged life. Middle-aged men with severe anxiety were half as likely to experience angina (chest pain) if they felt their wives were loving and supportive than if they felt isolated from their wives.[5] A famous study in Alameda County, California, found that marriage, close friendships, and voluntary membership in church or community organizations decreased the death rate from cancer, heart disease, and stroke, as well as the total mortality rate, for both men and women. The most socially isolated women in the community had a death rate almost three times as great as the most socially involved.[6] More recent studies have demonstrated that men or women with heart disease are far more vulnerable to heart attacks and death if they live alone, lack friends or family, or perceive a lack of emotional support from others.[7] Women with early breast cancer have been found to live longer if they receive emotional support from close friends and family.[8] Dr. Leon Eisenberg of Harvard Medical School observed that "inadequate social support is analogous to nutritional deficiency. One cannot write a prescription for spouses and friends, as one can for vitamins or trace elements, because we lack the equivalent of the neighborhood pharmacy. . . ."[9]

An ambitious study at Stanford University showed that social isolation can be overcome. People with cancer often feel alone, even if they were not previously isolated, because those around them are uncomfortable discussing the illness. The Stanford study offered women with widespread (metastatic) breast cancer the opportunity to join a weekly support group led by two therapists, one of whom had been treated for breast cancer. The groups, which met for one year, were structured to encourage members to express their feelings about the illness and its effects on their lives, and to discuss ways of coping with cancer, pain, and the side effects of medical treatment. Group members encouraged one another to be more assertive with their doctors and focused on ways of extracting personal meaning from the tragedy, using their experience of illness to help others. Strong bonds developed among members, which may have persisted after the groups ended. The survival of group members was compared with the survival of other women with metastatic breast cancer who received the same medical therapies but were not offered membership in a support group. Women who participated in the group lived an average of three years after the diagnosis of metastatic cancer; women in the control group lived an average of nineteen months. The near doubling of survival time associated with the support group shows a greater effect in prolonging life than could be offered by any available medical therapy.[10] Similar results were later reported by another California research team among two groups of patients with melanoma, a highly malignant cancer of the skin.[11] The improved survival was associated with an increase in the activity of a group of white blood cells called natural killer cells, an important component of the body's defense against cancer.[12]

Varied mechanisms compose the link between social support, health, and mortality. Satisfying relationships may buffer the impact of stress, actually lowering the levels of chemical mediators, decreasing the strain on mind and body.[13] The rewards of friendship may include an increase in self-esteem and with it a boost to perceived self-efficacy. As I discussed in the previous chapter, a higher level of self-efficacy improves an individual's ability to cope with symptoms, adopt healthful habits, and cooperate with medical treatment.

Relationship as a pillar of healing has two components. First is the network of mutual obligations that leads a person to believe she is cared for, loved, and esteemed.[14] Second is the encounter with givers of health care, which may foster, supplement, and occasionally substitute for her natural support network. "The physician," says Eisenberg, "is one valuable source of social support. Family and friends may respond to medical recommendations for more frequent contacts. The patient can be encouraged to link up with culturally appropriate social and religious organizations. Self-help groups, associations of lay persons who share a common problem and band together for mutual aid, can be of enormous help in sharing knowledge, in enhancing coping skills and in providing affective [emotional] support. . . . whether the physician wills it or no, all medical practice is a set of social and interpersonal transactions. Surely, if the patient is inevitably going to be affected in important ways by the relationship with the doctor, it is an imperative for good clinical care that the doctor increase the knowledge and the skill he or she brings to bear on that relationship, the one invariant in healing encounters, folk and professional, medical and surgical."

The sharing of *information* is an aspect of the doctor-patient relationship that is central to functional medicine. Patients in general want considerably more information about the nature of their problems than doctors think they do. The desire for information is universal and has no relationship to the patient's level of education or social class.[15] The more information the patient receives and the more the patient is actively involved in making decisions about treatment, the higher the level of mutual satisfaction and the better the clinical outcome.[16] The kind of information needed is personal, not statistical. It must answer the question, "What can *I* do?" The answer to that question is *never* "Nothing." Even when the outlook for recovery is bleak, there are powerful personal strategies for reducing the suffering of illness. The many layers of *relationship*, and their relationship to the greatly misunderstood "placebo effect," are discussed in Chapter Five.

THE SECOND PILLAR: *DÍAITA*

The precursor of our word *diet, díaita* is an ancient Greek concept that includes diet and regulation of the daily cycle of rest and exercise. A

Hippocratic physician, observing Americans today, would marvel at the *irregularity* that governs our lives. Convenience foods and electric power have given us a remarkable freedom from the constraints of those natural rhythms that determined the lifestyles of people prior to the industrial revolution. In evaluating the diet of Americans, the Hippocratic physician might be less concerned with *what* we eat than *how* we eat.

In 1984, I was invited to address the French Society for Magnesium Research at their annual meeting in Paris. From that symposium I developed close personal friendships with several French scientists and have returned to France many times for travel and conferences. Those experiences could fill another book. They gave me—among other things—the opportunity to observe firsthand a phenomenon called "The French Paradox." Traditional French cuisine is very high in sugar and fat, yet the French in general are quite lean, especially when compared to North Americans. Despite their high consumption of animal fat, their rate of heart disease is low. Spending time with French families showed me how the French can eat so "badly" without gaining weight. Although their meals are copious and heavily adorned with cheese and creamy sauces, *they don't snack*. They only eat meals at which the whole family sits down together. What a delightful custom!

I recently evaluated a Norwegian boy whose father is a visiting professor at Princeton, to determine the cause of the child's hives. When taking a dietary history, I asked him a routine question: "What do you eat for snacks?"

Although his English was perfect, he gave me a blank stare. His mother responded to his silence in an apologetic tone. "You see, Norwegians don't snack." She then added, "Whenever friends from Norway visit us, they say that people *here* eat all the time. It seems so strange to them."

Snacking is big business in the United States and makes a major contribution to obesity and ill health. In 1994, Americans bought 5.7 billion pounds of salty snack foods, twenty-two pounds for every man, woman, and child, up by one pound per person from the year before.[17] These salty foods are high-fat foods; potato chips and corn chips accounted for half the junk food sales. The statistics do not even include the huge amount of sweet snack foods like candy bars and cookies. Americans obtain about one-third of their total calories from nutrient-poor junk food. The more junk a person eats, the lower the daily intake of vitamins, minerals, and protein.[18] Three-quarters of U.S. adults are overweight, one-third of U.S. adults are frankly obese, and both the prevalence and amount of obesity are on the rise.[19] The rate of obesity among children has doubled in the past generation. Obesity makes a significant contribution to the risk of heart disease, hypertension, diabetes, several types of cancer, arthritis, fatigue, depression, and general ill health.

Eliminating junk food snacks and avoiding foods with added fat and sugar will significantly improve the nutritional quality of what you eat.[20] This has become conventional wisdom. It is an important step in preventive medicine and in healing. One would expect all physicians to advocate and practice its precepts. Attend a medical convention, however, and you'll find that the meals and snacks are no different from those at any other type of convention.

Before attempting to provide patients with individual nutritional guidelines, functional medicine stresses the importance of consuming foods that are high in nutritional quality. There is no mystery in discovering these. They are, to begin with, foods that have not had nutrients removed by processing and that do not contain added sugar or shortening. Vegetables, fruits, nuts, and seeds are an important part of this diet and can be used for snacking, if desired, as well as for meals. The evidence that increased consumption of fruits and vegetables is beneficial for health, offering protection against cancer and heart disease, is overwhelming, yet only 9 percent of Americans eat the five servings of fruits and vegetables each day that are recommended by the National Research Council. That statistic may even be too generous, because "French-fried" potatoes, which are loaded with fat, are included as vegetables. Among children, French fries account for about a quarter of the alleged vegetable consumption.[21] Even well-educated, presumably well-nourished adults taking nutritional supplements frequently do not consume nutritionally adequate diets and, despite their supplement, fall short in their consumption of important minerals like magnesium, iron, zinc, and calcium.[22] The impact of nutrition on physiological function is so vast and extensively researched that a summary of available knowledge is beyond the scope of this book. In Chapter Six I will discuss some of the most exciting and medically relevant current research and use it as the basis for specific dietary guidelines. I will also discuss exercise and rest, the second and third components of *díaita*, which constitute a balanced regime for health.

THE THIRD PILLAR: ENVIRONMENTAL HYGIENE

The bond between health and cleanliness is venerable, but more honored in some cultures than in others. Ancient Egyptians adopted laws for town planning that reflect a sophisticated understanding of the hazards of environment. They forbade building in damp or humid places, employed mosquito nets for preventing malaria, and required that all homes have windows, ventilation, and toilets connected to a sewage system. According to the Book of the Dead, deceased Egyptians had to swear on the Day of Judgment, "I did not pollute any water."[23] A visitor to modern Cairo might think that Egyptian city planning had deteriorated over the past four thousand years.

In the Hippocratic worldview, environment was a major determinant of health and sickness. Throughout the European Middle Ages and the Renaissance, physicians trained in the Hippocratic approach believed that terrible epidemic diseases, like malaria and the Black Death, resulted from environmental toxicity. They called these epidemics *miasmata*. When the microbial agents causing epidemics were discovered in the late nineteenth century, the miasmatic concept fell into disrepute and environmental hygiene focused on control of microbial contamination. Despite our efforts in this area, microbial contamination of food and water continues to be an important cause of sickness in the United States and other developed nations. The problem is addressed in Chapter Eight.

As public health measures were attempting to eradicate microbial pollution, chemical pollution increased, a problem predicted by René Dubos in his memorable work *The Mirage of Health*.[24] The sources of chemical contamination are legion. The modern understanding of *miasmata* began about fifty years ago, with the chemical analysis of outdoor air pollution. On December 5, 1952, a severe temperature inversion occurred over London, with warm air at ground level trapped below a blanket of Arctic air, causing the worst smog in the city's history. The result was four thousand deaths from respiratory disease.[25]

The main culprits were thought to be sulfur dioxide gas and ultrafine particles produced by car exhaust, power plants, and heavy industry.[26] Numerous studies conducted since that time in U.S. cities demonstrate a close correlation between increased daily death rates and fine-particle air pollution, even at levels of pollution that are considered safe by the World Health Organization.[27]

Community-wide pollution has been well established as a cause of respiratory ailments,[28] but its effects extend beyond the respiratory tract. The rate of cancer among suburban women increases with outdoor exposure to airborne dust particles.[29] Nitrogen dioxide, a common component of polluted air, has been shown to increase the spread of cancer in experimental animals.[30] Nitrogen dioxide may have other undesirable effects. Psychiatric admissions increase when the nitrogen dioxide levels in ambient air increase.[31] Among apparently healthy people, air pollution can provoke general symptoms of ill health, including headaches, fatigue, and irritability, which are relieved by breathing pure air.[32]

Silent Spring, Rachel Carson's impassioned manifesto, published in 1962,[33] kindled the first sparks of public interest in the perils of pesticide abuse. Corrective actions have typically occurred *after* a great deal of damage has been done. Over a billion pounds of pesticides are still used every year in the United States alone. Environmentalists, farm workers, federal agencies, and food growers continue to disagree about what constitutes "safe" levels of the twenty thousand registered pesticides. Since many of the most toxic agents remain in the environment for decades, and are most harmful to the young, their full impact has not yet been realized.

Living safely in a polluted world is no easy task. In 1991 my life was thrown into turmoil when I discovered that the health of my patients and my staff was being threatened by mold and bacterial contamination of my medical office. The problem had started slowly: a brown discoloration of ceiling tiles in the reception area and of air vents in the waiting room, and occasional leaking of the roof. Strange odors were noticed intermittently, some drifting up the fire stairs or the elevator shaft, others seeming to emanate from the air vents. I consulted an environmental engineer who removed the ceiling tiles and crawled inside the vents. The look on his face when he emerged shocked me.

"You have a big problem here," he said ominously. "You may not be able to fix it."

What he had seen looked like nothing more than soot, but microscopic examination revealed that the black coating on the primary ceiling and on the tiles, streaking down the walls and through the ductwork, was a forest of mold and bacteria, growing in the dampness created by a leaking roof and a poorly installed air-conditioning system. The Old Testament prescribes the treatment for black stains on the ceiling that grow over time: Eight men must surround the dwelling and destroy it by pushing in the walls, so that the debris does not spread outward. The remains of the building must be hauled to an unclean place and dumped. The occupants of the home must burn their clothes and begin life anew.

My request to the landlord was not as dramatic as the biblical prescription, but it was met with complete denial.

"Clean the vents," shrugged the building manager.

The more I researched my problem, the more desperate it seemed. Five years remained on the lease and the landlord had warned me that he would sue for five years' rent if I broke it and moved out. I moved anyway. As this book goes to press, the trial is about to begin.

I have since become an expert on indoor air pollution, a major factor in promoting ill health. Chapter Seven examines its complexities and offers some straightforward solutions for preventing environmental disasters at home.

THE FOURTH PILLAR: DETOXIFICATION

The supply of environmental toxins, chemical and microbial, appears endless. We simply can't avoid all of them. The human body has many natural defenses against environmental toxicity. These include: (1) the constant shedding of the skin and the lining of the gastrointestinal tract, which slowly dispels environmental toxins from the body; (2) the activity of protective immune responses that limit the attachment of toxins to the surfaces of the lungs or the gastrointestinal tract; (3) enzyme systems in the liver that destroy toxins and prepare them for excretion in the bile or the urine; (4) enzymes that repair damaged cells and promote healing.

Traditional approaches to detoxification employed fasting, purging, and herbal remedies to "cleanse" the intestinal tract. Techniques for intestinal cleansing have been used by every system of health care since the ancient Egyptians bestowed upon the pharaoh's personal physician the august title "Keeper of the Royal Rectum." Although ancient Egyptians had no knowledge of the microscopic world of parasites, they used herbs like thyme and minerals like antimony, which we know today are active against intestinal parasites.[34] Élie Metchnikoff was the first modern scientist to study the notion of intestinal toxicity. A highly respected biologist, Metchnikoff was chosen by Louis Pasteur to succeed him as director of the Institut Pasteur in Paris; he was awarded the Nobel Prize for Medicine in 1908, sharing it with his rival, Paul Ehrlich. At the turn of the century, Metchnikoff advanced the theory that intestinal bacteria cause senility and degenerative disease by producing toxic chemicals called ptomaines, which are absorbed into the body. He advocated yogurt as an antidote, believing that the "friendly" bacteria in yogurt, called *Lactobacilli,* would inhibit the growth of harmful bacteria.[35] Although Metchnikoff's ideas have been largely ignored in the English-speaking world, a substantial body of research supports the basic soundness of his concepts. Intestinal bacteria have important effects on human physiology; they constitute a powerful chemical factory, producing toxins and antitoxins and altering the chemical composition of foods and drugs. They de-methylate methylmercury, decreasing its toxicity. They manufacture half a dozen vitamins, nourish the cells of the small and large intestine, help the immune system to develop normally, and inhibit the growth of disease-producing yeasts and bacteria. I'll discuss these friendly flora in Chapter Eight.

Toxins that enter the body from the intestinal tract are directly transported to the liver, which is the chief site for detoxifying enzymes in the body. The chemical processes of liver detoxification proceed continuously and spontaneously, supported by a nutritious diet. They are extremely complex and barely comprehended by most physicians. This is unfortunate, because the liver not only destroys toxins, it breaks down drugs and hormones. A thorough understanding of liver detoxification can help predict drug interactions and can explain many of the effects of nutrition on the development of disease; it is essential for competence in all fields of medicine. Strategies for supporting and directing liver detoxification will offer great potential as innovative treatments in the coming decades.

The Pillars of Healing naturally and spontaneously sustain the art and the science of medicine. They support every encounter between physician and patient. If they fail, medical care is likely to be ineffectual. Patient-centered diagnosis allows health practitioners to use the tools of science to buttress the Pillars, achieving results beyond the scope of conventional diagnosis and treatment. One of my clearest examples is the case of Michael Finn. His diagnosis was ankylosing spondylitis (AS), a crippling arthritis of the spine that is inherited and starts early in life. In conventional medical thinking, AS is a well-defined disease entity, treated primarily with anti-inflammatory drugs.

Mike's history was classic: minor backaches as early as the age of seven, becoming severe by age eighteen, spreading slowly from low to upper back, neck and jaw, and downward to the hips. His mornings were made of pain and stiffness. Movement helped; as the day wore on, his comfort increased. He accepted the pain without really knowing its cause, drowning it with hard work and alcohol and weekly visits to the chiropractor. At the age of thirty-five he saw a famous orthopedist at New York's Hospital for Special Surgery. Mike's physical exam revealed marked limitation in the movement of his spine. AS was promptly diagnosed and the management of his case was transferred to a rheumatologist in eastern Pennsylvania, where Mike was living. Indocin, an anti-inflammatory drug that is a cousin to aspirin, gave him moderate but incomplete relief of pain. He needed high doses and suspected that the drug clouded his thinking. No, said the rheumatologist, Indocin only causes ulcers; it doesn't cloud thinking. Methotrexate, a relatively toxic drug that suppresses the immune system, was given next. Mike developed chest pain and palpitations. He was hospitalized and taken off methotrexate. Chest pain stopped and palpitations improved. No, said the rheumatologist, methotrexate doesn't cause chest pain, it only causes anemia and hepatitis. He ordered a coronary angiogram (an X-ray study of blood vessels in the heart) to "rule out" coronary heart disease. It was normal. He recommended that methotrexate be continued. When Mike refused to take it again, the rheumatologist chastised him for being uncooperative and warned him that his disease could cause severe disability if not controlled.

As I wrote down the details of Mike's medical history, I burned with an anger I found hard to mask. He had not technically been a victim of malpractice. His treatment, unfortunately, was quite consistent with the standard of care in many communities and would be considered "usual and customary." But it certainly was biomedicine at its worst, trampling roughshod over a patient in its frantic attempt to suppress a disease. In order to help Mike find a path out of his illness, I had to start by learning much more about him than the disease he carried.

Depression had haunted Mike from his earliest memories of childhood. He was cowed by his father's contempt for him, never disbelieving the old man's scornful predictions that he would amount to nothing. His father was an alcoholic, and Mike himself turned to whiskey and marijuana at the age of fourteen, as if trying to prove his father right. A decade and a half later he dropped them both and joined Alcoholics Anonymous. From the age of sixteen to thirty-three, he earned his living maintaining golf courses and was dowsed with pesticides and weed killers many times each season. Sudden bouts of irresistible drowsiness would set upon him during the day; to function at all during each of these took every bit of strength and determination he could muster. His nighttime sleep was broken by nightmares. Muscle spasms in the neck and back were a daily problem, not clearly separated from the pain of arthritis in his spine. New symptoms emerged to plague him. Six years ago came acne of the scalp; about the same time he began grinding his teeth at night. Four years ago, he had been promoted to assistant golf course superintendent, a tribute to his battle against pain and despair. He was no longer exposed to heavy doses of lawn maintenance chemicals. At about that time he married, acquiring two stepchildren, had a baby, attended college during the winter off-season, and developed severe fatigue, frequent headaches, and loss of libido. Two years ago he suffered a urinary infection and inflammation of the prostate gland (prostatitis). He was treated with antibiotics, but still felt discomfort when passing urine. A year ago, canker sores began to inflame his mouth. The palpitations, which had started after he began methotrexate, were not completely gone, and despite four years of psychotherapy, he was still depressed.

On examination, Mike's spine was tender to the touch, with limited flexibility. He had lost an inch of his usual six-foot stature and could not expand his chest fully when breathing. All these are characteristic signs of AS. A thorough physical examination also showed me that his prostate gland was still actively inflamed. When a bacterial culture indicated that his prostatitis was caused by bacteria called *Klebsiella*, I knew that an important trigger had come to light.

The unfolding scientific investigation of ankylosing spondylitis implicates *Klebsiella* as a trigger for arthritis. Ninety-six percent of people with AS produce a protein called HLA-B27, which is prominently displayed on the surfaces of cells that line their joints, as well as on their white blood cells. HLA-B27 is also made by some people without AS; its production is inherited and is controlled by the genes. Exciting research in Great Britain has discovered that *Klebsiella* bacteria produce a protein that is very much like HLA-B27. In fact, patients with AS make antibodies to this *Klebsiella* protein; these antibodies can attack not only *Klebsiella*, but also the cells of their own bodies, which display HLA-B27 on their surfaces. This is called a *cross-reaction*, and the resulting illness is said to involve *autoimmunity*—the body's attack on itself.[36]

Klebsiella that invade an organ of the body, such as the prostate or the lung, cause a local infection, often serious. In a patient with AS, they may trigger autoimmune arthritis. Of course, Mike's arthritis had occurred long before he developed prostatitis, so his prostatic infection was at most a secondary trigger, and another source of exposure to *Klebsiella* had to be sought. Many healthy people harbor species of *Klebsiella* in their large intestines, where they usually do no harm. Australian researchers found from stool cultures that people with AS almost always grow *Klebsiella*. In contrast, people whose blood cells test positive for HLA-B27, but who do not develop AS, almost never grow *Klebsiella* in their stool. They advanced the theory that exposure to *Klebsiella* in the intestinal tract is the usual trigger for autoimmunity in AS.

Mike proved to be a real paradox. Not only did he have one species of *Klebsiella* in his prostate and another species of *Klebsiella* in his intestines, his test for HLA-B27 was, surprisingly, *negative*. I suspected that those few people without HLA-B27 who develop AS may have another protein on their cells, not yet identified, that cross-reacts with

Klebsiella. Ridding the prostate of *Klebsiella* requires strong antibiotics. If it can be fully eliminated from that site, which is not an easy task, it may never grow back. Clearing the stool of *Klebsiella* needs a different approach, because it is never fully eliminated from the bowel, only diminished. Dr. Alan Ebringer, a rheumatologist at Middlesex Medical School in London, has developed such an approach. Its cornerstone is a low-starch diet. Ebringer reasoned that intestinal bacteria have to be well nourished to grow, and their main source of nourishment is their host's undigested dietary starch. He knew of research showing that a low-starch diet markedly decreases the number of bacteria growing in the area where the small intestine joins the large intestine. Ebringer decided that controlling bacterial growth in this area with a low-starch diet would reduce the quantity of *Klebsiella* and might improve the back pain of patients with AS. His studies showed that a diet free of cereal grains, bread, and potatoes (which are the major sources of starch in the Western diet) did indeed help to control the pain of AS; at the same time it decreased the amount of *Klebsiella* in stool and the level of antibodies to *Klebsiella* in blood. When diet alone did not work, he added low doses of antibiotics.

With this information and the blueprint of patient-centered diagnosis, I formulated my concept of Mike's illness. Prostaglandins and inflammatory cytokines were likely to be key chemical mediators. They did not account for symptoms like muscle spasm, palpitation, and insomnia, however. I suspected that Mike might have a secondary magnesium deficiency, resulting from stress, inflammation, and his previous abuse of alcohol.[37] A blood test confirmed my suspicion. Low self-esteem was another mediator, contributing to depression and pain. His advancement at work and the strong bond he seemed to have with his wife must have done a good deal to improve his self-esteem, but his terrible experience with medical care had left him shaken. In a sense, this experience was a trigger for his decision to seek a nonconventional approach to health care. *Klebsiella* was possibly a trigger for inflammation, and prostatitis itself, independent of the germ causing it, was a likely trigger. Localized infection from any cause can aggravate a condition like arthritis, which involves the entire body. Methotrexate and Indocin had been triggers for side effects. Both drugs are also toxic to the intestine. They damage its lining, making it porous and leaky, increasing its permeability to potential toxins. If intestinal bacteria were triggering autoimmunity, the usual drugs for arthritis might actually make the reaction worse. Diathesis overflowed with possibilities: genetic predisposition to alcoholism, AS, and depression; the ability of alcohol and aspirin to increase intestinal permeability. I also wondered about the havoc that heavy doses of pesticides and herbicides had wrought on Mike's immune system.

From my analysis came four treatment strategies intended to remove triggers and bolster the Pillars of Healing. First, I explained my thoughts to Mike and to his wife. They understood the nature of the treatment I was proposing and were eager to cooperate. Next, I recommended a change in diet and exercise. Mike had been injuring himself at work and I advised him to refrain from heavy lifting, which was no longer required by his job. I recommended physical therapy—which he did not pursue—and Ebringer's diet, which he followed assiduously. I modified Ebringer's low-starch regimen to include large quantities of vegetables rich in carotenoids and bioflavinoids. I supplemented the diet with magnesium and with extra doses of vitamins C and E. I advised Mike to keep his exposure to lawn maintenance chemicals to the minimum level permitted by his present job and to stop taking Indocin because of the damage it was doing to his intestine. Finally, I prescribed a strong antibiotic called floxacin to kill bacteria infecting his prostate.

A remarkable thing happened. Within a few days of starting the antibiotic, his joint pain and fatigue improved dramatically. When he stopped floxacin, the pain and fatigue returned. At the time of our first follow-up visit, Mike was in just as much pain and just as tired as before. But when I asked him about his other symptoms, we discovered that a marked change had occurred. His canker sores, scalp acne, palpitations, muscle spasms, and nightmares were completely gone. His depression, headache, low libido, and urinary discomfort were each about 50 percent better. From my experience with other patients, I surmised that correction of magnesium deficiency had improved Mike's muscle spasm, disturbed sleep, headache, and palpitations, and that the change in diet had cleared his canker sores and acne. Improvement in depression and libido may have been attributable to an increase in self-esteem. Mike was enthusiastic about actively taking control of his health care.

As we entered the second month of treatment, I reinforced the initial strategy by prescribing a supplement of fish oil and urging Mike to continue the diet and the other nutritional supplements. Over the next two months, his joint pain and fatigue improved by 90 percent, and his depression, low libido, and headaches disappeared completely. He has needed no medication for pain since that time four years ago. The mobility of his spine and his rib cage have become normal. His disease has not progressed; in fact, it has actually been reversed.

Mike and I both know that the first and most critical therapeutic step was taken by Mike himself, with his wife's support, when he decided to refuse further treatment with methotrexate. He would no longer be a passive victim of his disease and accept dangerous drugs as the only possible solution to pain. In order to take control of his disease, he had to begin by taking control of his medical care.

To maintain or regain your own health, understand and actively support the Four Pillars of Healing:

• Nurture relationships with others. Commit some time each day to give your undivided attention to a friend or family member.
• Involve yourself in a group activity that is meaningful to you and enjoyable.
• Eat regular meals with people you care about. Avoid snacks or meals in front of the television. Especially avoid the salty high-fat snack foods that are an American obsession. Keep them out of your home.
• Engage in regular physical exercise of at least moderate intensity for thirty minutes a day or more. Brisk walking is a good start. Do it with a friend.
• Get enough sleep at night so that you can awaken without an alarm clock.
• Reserve a period of fifteen minutes or more for quiet, focused relaxation every day.
• Become aware of the environmental hazards in your community and your job.
• Keep to a minimum your use of alcohol and drugs, including medical drugs.

• Ask your doctor about the possible side effects of any drug you take, including the effect of the drug on liver detoxification.

• Consume a nutritious diet that is rich in "detox" vegetables like broccoli, carrots, tomatoes, avocado, Brussels sprouts, and cabbage, and in nuts and seeds. Add sea vegetables and green onions as condiments. Further dietary guidelines are found in Chapters Six and Eight.

5

THE FIRST PILLAR: RELATIONSHIP

Love's Alchemy

Roseto, Pennsylvania, was a remarkable community, an Italian hill town sprouting in the Delaware Water Gap. It was first settled in 1882 by immigrants from Roseto Val Fortore, a village in the foothills of the southern Apennines, near Italy's Adriatic coast. Under the leadership of Father Pasquale de Nisco, a Catholic priest, a cohesive spirit of community flourished, based on family ties, church membership, and civic pride. *McClure's Magazine* acclaimed the padre's accomplishments in a 1908 feature story called "One Man and His Town."[1] Marion Carter, who reported the story, was struck by the proliferation of social clubs and of gardens, each with its own grape arbor. The social structure of Roseto maintained a striking stability over the next fifty years. It remained the purest Italian town in America.[2] When a team of medical researchers from Temple University visited Roseto in 1961, they were struck by its distinguishing characteristics:

> The town radiated a kind of joyous team spirit as its inhabitants celebrated religious festivals and family landmarks such as birthdays, graduations and engagements. Their social focus was on the family,

whereas neighboring communities, holding to the traditional American view, were more likely to focus on the individual as the unit of society.

When we interviewed and examined the inhabitants of Roseto and familiarized ourselves with the town and its people, we were surprised at our inability to distinguish by dress, manner, or speech the affluent owners of textile factories from the more impecunious laborers. The well-kept houses of all Rosetans, rich and poor, were clustered close together on streets with colorful Italian names such as Dante, Columbus, and Garibaldi. The lack of display of affluence or even obvious distinction between rich and poor, and the absence of the need to "keep up with the Joneses" appeared to be a central ingredient in the unifying cohesive force of the community.[3]

The scientists were studying Roseto because of a chance encounter with a local physician, Dr. Benjamin Falcone, who had observed that heart attacks were relatively rare among Rosetans. Despite their high-fat diets, being overweight, facing formidable economic stress, and smoking, the people of Roseto experienced a death rate from heart disease that was less than half the rate of residents in neighboring towns who shared the same water supply, hospital, and doctors. Researchers traced the low rate of heart disease to the strong spirit of community that most distinguished Roseto from its neighbors.

Within twenty years, the magic was gone. Roseto's cardiac mortality rate had doubled, matching that in neighboring communities. A decrease in consumption of fatty foods and cigarettes was unable to stop the galloping increase in heart attacks. This unfortunate change had actually been predicted by the investigators in 1961. How had they foreseen it? There was no war, no depression, no major upheaval to rend the social fabric of the town. Yet the researchers had seen something far more subtle, an indication of impending change: many young adults were abandoning the old ways. The spirit of self-sacrifice and loyalty to family traditions that had built the town held no appeal for them.[4] Church attendance was down a bit, the number of extended families living under one roof was declining, wine making had dropped off, the median income had increased. The change was not easily measured, but it could be felt. The spirit of community was dying. Researchers reported a recurrent theme in their interviews of citizens who were disabled with illness: "You don't understand, Doctor; things have changed. People don't care."

THE PLACEBO EFFECT

Rapid social change may cause sickness and death by many mechanisms. The Roseto experience is unique in revealing a face of change not related to major social disruption but just as forceful in its impact: the perceived loss of a caring environment. For health care, a cardinal function has always been the creation of a caring environment to foster healing. Yet there is a remarkable lack of research into the *science of caring*, those aspects of the relationship between healer and patient that enhance health. Studies of medical treatment uniformly attempt to cancel out the effects of that relationship by using placebo controls, without really understanding the nature of placebo effects and their role in healing.

Placebo is a Latin word meaning "I shall please." Our oldest description of the concept comes, naturally, from the Hippocratic texts: ". . . some patients, though conscious that their condition is perilous, recover their health simply through their contentment with the goodness of the physician."[5] In its modern sense, *placebo effect* is used to describe a positive response to treatment that results not from the specific treatment itself but from the patient's psychologically mediated response to undergoing the treatment. The placebo is therefore a pill or injection that contains "inactive" ingredients. Responses to placebo pills are real and reproducible and do not distinguish between "physical" and "psychological" disease entities. Patients with any type of pain, from headache to heart pain to cancer, may benefit from placebo treatment with a pain reduction greater than 50 percent. Placebo analgesia is not imaginary. It results from release of the body's own intrinsic pain relievers, called endorphins, which are biochemically similar to narcotics.[6]

Placebos relieve more than pain. Their administration may reduce symptoms such as nausea, cough, anxiety, and depression; lower cholesterol;[7] and heal peptic ulcers. Placebo healing of ulcers tells a most instructive story. For the past hundred years, the standard treatment for ulcers has been the use of drugs or surgery designed to decrease the production of stomach acid. For most of this time, antacids were the only drugs available. It was obvious to everyone that they were not terribly effective, and surgery for ulcers was common. The development of the drug Tagamet (cimetidine) during the 1970s dramatically reduced the need for ulcer surgery, because Tagamet did not just attempt to neutralize stomach acid; it slowed the production of acid by the cells that line the stomach. When Tagamet was first released, there were many double-blind, placebo-controlled trials to test its efficacy. In these experiments, one group of patients received Tagamet and the other group received an inactive sugar pill. Neither the patients nor the scientists knew which patient was receiving which treatment until the end of the study, hence the label "double-blind." When the results of all studies were pooled, healing of ulcers occurred in 76 percent of patients given Tagamet and in 48 percent of patients taking placebos.[8] Although Tagamet was evidently more effective overall than placebo, in the majority of the individual studies, there was no significant difference between Tagamet and placebo response rates. Most important is the variability of placebo responsiveness in the different experiments. Placebo ulcer healing occurred at rates that ranged from 10 percent in some studies to 90 percent in other studies. In other words, the variation in apparent placebo responsiveness for different studies of the same condition deviated by 900 percent, a far greater difference than one ever finds in the comparison between a placebo and an "active" treatment.[9]

This means that the placebo response is not a fixed entity that remains constant from one doctor-patient encounter to the next. It can change dramatically with the nature of the person, the doctor, and the treatment administered.[10] When the doctor enthusiastically supports a treatment, the placebo response may be greater than 80 percent.[11] When tested against a treatment that the doctor believes to be highly effective, the placebo will have a stronger effect than when it is tested against a treatment that the doctor believes is weakly effective. For example, a placebo that is compared with morphine in an experimental study will provide much greater pain relief than a placebo that is compared with aspirin, because the expectation of benefit is greater with morphine than with aspirin.[12]

The relative difference between "active" treatment and placebo is also not constant. Scientists use a placebo to control for the "real" effect of a drug, assuming that the placebo response and the drug response are separate, independent effects. They believe that the effect of the drug is a property of the drug and the effect of placebo is a property of the person who is being treated. By subtracting the placebo response from the drug response, they expect to determine the "real" effect of the drug itself. This is an illusion. The placebo response may actually determine the drug response.

People who respond well to placebos respond even better to "active" drugs. In contrast, people who respond poorly to placebos show a poor response to "active" treatment, and for them the "active" treatment may work no better than the placebo. In other words, placebo responsiveness actually affects the response to the active drug above and beyond the classic placebo effect.

The conventional viewpoint is based on an equation that reads:

placebo response + active drug response = patient's response

The actual research reveals an equation that reads:

placebo + (placebo response × active drug response) = patient's
response   response

The ability of placebo responsiveness to amplify or diminish responsiveness to "real" drugs appears to derive from something in the relationship between doctors and patients. When patients in a clinical trial are required to give their written informed consent, they respond less well to placebo and there is a decreased difference between placebo and "active" drug. Even when the design of the experiment is kept constant, the difference in response between placebo and active drug varies from clinic to clinic. Drugs and placebos work better when given by a caring physician. When given by a noncaring physician, both drugs and placebos are less effective and the distinction in response between "active" drug and placebo can be wiped out.[13] The effectiveness of a medical treatment, therefore, is not a fixed property of the treatment itself. It is a highly variable quantity that may be more strongly influenced by the relationship between doctor and patient than by any other factor.

Physicians tend to be as confused as researchers about the nature of placebo. Doctors often administer placebos to demanding, anxious, or highly dependent patients, who are the group least likely to respond.[14] They believe that a placebo is a form of ethical deception. Placebo has nothing to do with deception, however. Patients may respond to placebo pills even when they are informed by the doctor that the pill contains no active ingredient, provided the doctor reassures them that it may help them feel better.[15] The placebo lies not in the drug, but in the person of the doctor.

Placebo effects do not even require the administration of a drug or the performance of a procedure. Words will suffice and may even work better than pills. People who are about to undergo surgery suffer less pain, require fewer pain medications, and leave the hospital earlier if the preoperative visit from the anesthesiologist lasts longer and includes information about the nature of pain, advice about simple techniques for coping with pain, and reassurance about the availability of backup medication if their pain is not adequately relieved.[16] For patients with chronic headache, the best predictor of symptom relief has nothing to do with the prescription of a drug. It is the patient's satisfaction with the doctor's discussion of the nature of his problem.[17]

INFORMATION: MORE POWERFUL THAN DRUGS

Doctors in general tend to overestimate the extent to which patients want drugs and to underestimate the extent to which patients want information. In a recent poll, family practitioners estimated that 80 percent of patients visiting them for an acute illness expected to receive a drug as treatment. A poll of their patients disclosed that the doctors had overestimated the patients' demand for drugs by almost 100 percent! The poll's author states, in conclusion: "The placebo effect in general practice is the power of the doctor alone to make the patient feel better, irrespective of medication. It is one of the most important factors in the consultation, yet generally it is neglected."[18]

Research on the placebo effect leads to the inescapable conclusion that placebo is not a pill or a procedure. It is a relationship. The basis of that relationship is a communication that states, "You are not alone. I am on your side." Three hundred years after the Scientific Revolution, placebo is still the strongest force in medicine and, for the majority of patients, the major determinant of the outcome of health care. Strange, that a force so powerful should be treated with such disdain.

Dr. Howard Spiro, professor of medicine at Yale, an internationally renowned gastroenterologist and a teacher in Yale's Humanities in Medicine program, in writing about the placebo effect, stated that physicians rely so heavily on science that most have lost faith in themselves as therapeutic instruments. This belief is shared by many who wish to restore the human face of medical care. Though well intended, it misinterprets the problem in a crucial way. When doctors ignore the importance of the physician-patient relationship in the treatment of disease, they are not relying on science, they are negating it. Medicine is not an abstraction. Medicine is what doctors do. And the single most important thing that all doctors do is to interact with their patients. There simply is no medical treatment response that occurs independent of the person who is sick and the person who administers the treatment. If the science of medicine fails to grasp the importance of this interaction, to embrace it with all its intellectual rigor, to support it by helping physicians and patients understand it better, then what passes for the science of medicine is just the costume of a masquerade, itself little more than the most recent adornment to the powerful placebo effect.

Science and technology do nothing to lessen the importance of placebo. The charismatic role of the physician in healing originates in the power and authority with which society invests physicians. Most Americans share the belief that science and technology can work miracles. The ability of doctors to translate the symptoms that trouble their patients into the abstract and forbidding language of this powerful force and to bring back from its laboratories the newest treatments imbues medical practitioners with an awesome authority that can transform the coldest, most detached clinician into a magnet for the patient's hopes.

Julie Loeb is a high-powered Manhattan attorney who suffers from metastatic breast cancer. Her suffering has not been caused by the cancer itself, but by her fear of death. Her oncologist had quoted statistics to her that indicated she would be dead in less than two years.

"I have to warn you that I hate doctors!" she said at our first meeting.

"Richard Foster may be a great oncologist, but he knows nothing about people. To him, I am basically a statistic. Every time I see him for chemotherapy, I realize that I haven't long to live."

Julie had discovered her own cancer six months earlier, a small irregularity in the contour of her right breast. The tumor was fast-growing and highly invasive. Cancer had already spread from the breast to the lymph nodes beneath her right arm. Soon it appeared in her liver, detected by a scan. Her only symptom was overwhelming fatigue, resulting in part from the chemotherapy she received each week. She had come to me for dietary advice. She had no intention of stopping chemotherapy, despite her feelings about the doctor, but she wanted me to help her strengthen her immunity.

I prescribed a low-fat vegetarian diet and a daily routine of exercise and relaxation. I urged her to discuss her dissatisfaction with the oncologist and to view her chemotherapy in a positive light, as a therapy that would prolong her life, not shorten it. She followed my advice about diet and exercise carefully, but she never confronted Dr. Foster. Outspoken everyplace else, in the oncologist's presence she became silent, and her attitude toward chemotherapy remained the same.

As the weeks passed, a disquieting change occurred. Julie's energy increased, an effect that she attributed to the diet and exercise program. So did her anger. Instead of expressing her feelings to Dr. Foster, she was quarrelsome with everyone else. She returned to work, but was so contentious that her partners asked her to stay home.

Then one day her demeanor suddenly changed. She exuded more confidence and less hostility than I had yet seen.

"There's a new treatment," she said, earnestly. "I'm a candidate for it. There is even a possibility of *cure*." In the new treatment protocol, massive chemotherapy would be followed by bone marrow transplantation, thoroughly destroying the cancer but sparing her own immune system. "Foster explained the whole procedure, reviewed all the statistics. It's still experimental, but I'm ready."

The promise of this technological breakthrough had transformed her relationship with the oncologist and radically altered her attitude toward treatment. I marveled at the tenacity with which Julie's spirit clung to hope and wondered if Dr. Foster had any notion of the magic wrought by the development of this new therapy.

ANTI–PLACEBO EFFECTS

For over a decade, the focus of my medical practice has been on chronically ill patients who have seen many different physicians without much relief. They are usually referred to as "treatment failures," but this label is misleading. It's not the patients who have failed, but the relationship between doctor and patient. Many of these patients, like Julie, have experienced *anti-placebo effects*, which add to the burden of illness. Anti-placebo is a communication that says, "Don't count on me for help." Julie's anti-placebo had been administered along with her initial course of chemotherapy. It said, "The statistics say that you'll be dead in two years, and there's nothing I can do." Even if the statistics were immutable, which they are not, there is still a good deal that a caring physician can do. A caring physician can give advice that helps the patient resist the grasp that sickness holds on her life, controlling pain, improving stamina, and maintaining independence. A caring physician can hold out hope, despite bad news. Despair is the most toxic of emotions, and makes its own independent contribution to sickness and death.[19] If your doctor cannot do this for you, find a new doctor. In the terminal stages of illness, the physician can help the patient find meaning in her life by acknowledging the patient's individuality.

Approaching death in isolation, writer and critic Anatole Broyard believed, ". . . some form of acknowledgment by the physician may be to some extent an antidote. . . . [The doctor] who refuses to acknowledge a patient is in effect abandoning him to his illness. . . . the physician's *presence* may be the assurance that the patient needs."[20] As Eric Cassell admonished, "It should be clearly understood that although there is nothing more that can be done for the body, this does not mean that there is nothing more that can be done for the sick person."[21]

For people who are not dying, the common anti-placebos contain overt or covert messages like, "Your problems are all in your head, don't ask me to fix them," or "This problem is not in my specialty, so I don't care how it relates to the disease for which I am treating you," or "Your ideas are *unscientific* and your concerns are misguided." The last statement is often employed when the patient has shown an interest in alternative medicine. The failure of physicians to acknowledge their patients' concerns accounts for a good deal of consumer dissatisfaction with health care.[22] The enormous growth of alternative medicine in the United States is a reflection of that dissatisfaction. There are presently more visits made to alternative health care providers each year than to all the family practitioners, general practitioners, general internists, and pediatricians combined, and Americans spend more money out of pocket on alternative health services than on conventional care.[23] Mainstream medicine is only now beginning to read the meaning of this trend. It does not result from gullibility, medical ignorance, or psychological dependency. It signifies a demand for personal—cost-effective—thoughtful health care that enlists the active participation of the patient. That demand is not being met within the medical mainstream.

I see residual effects of the anti-placebo response every day—anger, sadness, panic, a sense of betrayal, feelings of inadequacy. Anger and sadness hurt, but they sometimes mobilize patients to seek better solutions for their health problems than those they have been given. The damage wrought by an anti-placebo can be hard to predict. John Gerard and his wife, Edith, found their marriage itself was a victim.

John is a guidance counselor for emotionally disturbed children, a job that requires self-control and an even disposition. Although overweight, he had always enjoyed robust health. In December 1994, he suddenly developed severe cramping abdominal pain and diarrhea. He and his wife believed the problem was food poisoning, traced to a meal eaten at a Chinese restaurant two days earlier. He dosed himself with over-the-counter remedies, Pepto-Bismol, Kaopectate, and Immodium. The diarrhea turned to blood, so he consulted a gastroenterologist who was prominent in his community. After a series of tests, a verdict was rendered: *ulcerative colitis*, an inflammatory disease of the large intestine for which the cause is not known. Ulcerative colitis typically begins in adolescence or young adulthood and lasts for life, although its symptoms may wax and wane. The conventional treatment consists of anti-inflammatory drugs. Occasionally, surgical removal of the entire large intestine is necessary because of uncontrolled bleeding. Prolonged severe ulcerative colitis increases the risk of large bowel cancer, and gastroenterologists often recommend total removal of the large intestine for prevention of cancer.[24]

Ulcerative colitis is considered to be a distinct disease entity, which must be separated from other disease entities, especially infectious colitis. Intestinal infections with amoebic parasites or certain species of bacteria can produce symptoms and signs indistinguishable from those of ulcerative colitis. The main difference is that antibiotics may cure infectious colitis but have a rather inconsistent effect on ulcerative colitis. Actually, the role of infection in ulcerative colitis, although obscure, is not inconsequential. People with a diagnosis of ulcerative colitis have an increased susceptibility to infections of the large intestine, which aggravate their colitis. Many people who develop the disease in adulthood only acquire ulcerative colitis *after* contracting a parasitic or bacterial infection. Antibodies directed against the cells that line the large intestine occur in patients with ulcerative colitis, and may also be found in people with chronic forms of infectious colitis. One theory holds that ulcerative colitis is an autoimmune disease provoked by an allergic reaction to microorganisms in the intestinal tract. Another theory holds that ulcerative colitis may result from toxins produced by intestinal bacteria.[25] Both theories make the boundary between infectious colitis and ulcerative colitis very fuzzy. In addition to the possibility of multiple infectious triggers in ulcerative colitis, the condition may be aggravated by allergic reactions to foods or to the very drugs used to treat mild cases of the disease.[26] Twenty percent of patients with ulcerative colitis improve by eliminating all milk protein from their diets.[27] Low-fat diets may also be useful in decreasing the risk of colon cancer, because there is a direct correlation between the development of cancer in ulcerative colitis and the secretion of bile from the liver; the liver secretes bile in response to eating fatty foods.[28]

Ulcerative colitis is a complex illness that demands a flexible therapeutic approach. Like all chronic diseases, it is far more clearly understood through its mediators, triggers, and antecedents in individual patients than as an abstract disease entity. Conventional drug therapy of ulcerative colitis has as its goal the suppression of the mediators of inflammation.[29] Little attention has been paid to the divergent triggers of different patients. Over the past twenty years, I have found some patients in whom ulcerative colitis was profoundly affected by diet, or the composition of the intestinal bacterial flora, or allergic reactions to intestinal yeast, or emotional distress, or the smoking of cigarettes. Each has responded differently to therapies that included diet change, antibiotics, or the administration of friendly bacteria like *Lactobacilli*, but almost all have responded, sometimes with complete remission of symptoms. There are even some patients who develop colitis when they stop smoking cigarettes and who experience a complete remission of colitis when they resume smoking.[30] I treated one such patient in 1980, and she decided that she would much rather smoke than try to battle the disease using other means.

The specialist whom John Gerard consulted had little to say about diet or infection. He prescribed anti-inflammatory drugs and told John that he would probably develop colon cancer in twenty-five years no matter what he did, but that the drugs would control his symptoms. Since John was forty-seven, he could still lead a full life. John went home despondent. His depression increased when the drugs did very little to control his symptoms. Edith decided to investigate further. A professional writer, she was accustomed to checking her sources of information. To her, it made no sense that John should have developed ulcerative colitis suddenly at the age of forty-seven. John became sullen and accused her of being in denial. Edith recounted her experience to me in a letter. "We had a loving and close marriage of twenty-five years. Deaths in the family, financial setbacks, and armed service separation, and other minor dips in the road had always brought us together. This was different. We were driven apart. Neither of us would admit to one another how scared and frightened we were feeling. Each of us suffered alone and in silence. Our mutual respect, closeness and understanding had suddenly changed on that cold January doctor's visit of '95."

Edith accompanied John to his next appointment with the gastroenterologist, fortified by all the information she could gather about intestinal infection mimicking or aggravating ulcerative colitis and about the role of diet.

"Eat anything you want," replied the gastroenterologist. "Just avoid raw fruits and vegetables."

Edith asked if John's symptoms might be caused by bacteria, parasites, or reactions to food. She mentioned that John had only had one test for parasites and that all the books said at least three specimens should be examined. The doctor became irate and pounded his fist on the desk. "He does not have a parasite! It's not from bacteria! And it is not from the Chinese food he had! He has chronic ulcerative colitis and he'll have it the rest of his life. I have twenty-five years' experience in the field of gastroenterology. Where did you get your license, lady?"

Humiliated by the doctor's tirade, John and Edith decided to seek another opinion. The next gastroenterologist recommended a change in the drug therapy but ordered no further tests. The third gastroenterologist scheduled John for a complete examination of the large intestine—a colonoscopy—during the Easter vacation, and made another change in the drugs. John was still having bloody diarrhea several times a day and had now lost forty pounds. Before the appointment for the colonoscopy, Edith arranged a consultation with me and called this doctor to postpone the procedure. Angered, the doctor fired them as patients. Traumatized by what they described as "eighteen weeks of hell," Edith and John sought the help of a psychiatrist who specializes in helping people cope with chronic illness. "We felt we needed professional help in sorting out and coming to terms with our feelings and to gain back some of our perspective," Edith wrote. "My own physical health has suffered: headaches, dizzy spells, severe anxiety and now, panic attacks. Our children were all affected in one way or another. This stemmed from their father's lack of energy, his obvious pain, his inability to co-play in sports and lowered patience and stamina in assisting with homework and school projects. The children were frightened to look at him because he was so sick. They were sad and sullen and sometimes almost too quiet. It was obvious they were very worried because they kept asking, 'Will Daddy be O.K.?' We would have to lie many times because the truth would only make it worse for them—and we had never lied to the children before."

Once a month an infuriating story like the Gerards' comes my way. They fill me with dread for the future of health care. I often expend half my energy during the first consultation trying to undo the damage of a virulent anti-placebo. The first question I asked the Gerards, after reviewing John's history, was "What can I do that would help?"

Edith answered, "I think he has an amoeba. Can you do more testing?" John gave her a skeptical look.

I agreed with Edith that John needed more testing for parasites. I explained to them that John's symptoms can be caused by many different types of infection. Even if the tests were all negative, I would treat John as if he had an infection, because the sudden onset of bloody diarrhea in a man his age is more likely to have been triggered by infection than by anything else. Negative test results in John's situation are simply not reliable enough to warrant a decision not to treat with antibiotics.

I asked John about the effect of food on his symptoms.

"I feel the best when I don't eat," he said. Almost any regular meal would cause tremendous abdominal pain. I prescribed a diet that would nourish him and help to relieve his diarrhea. It consisted of white rice, bananas, and a powdered drink called Sustain, which is made from rice protein supplemented with individual amino acids, vitamins, minerals, and fructooligosaccharides, a vegetable extract that supports healing in the large intestine.[31] The nutritional therapy decreased his symptoms by about two-thirds, as we awaited the results of the stool tests. Many samples had to be examined before the parasite was found, an amoeba called *Entamoeba histolytica*, exactly the organism that Edith had predicted. Treatment with two antibiotics, metronidazole and diiodoquinol, completely halted John's symptoms.

John was angry at the gastroenterologists for failing to make the right diagnosis. Edith's anger was fired by the first doctor's arrogance as he denigrated her ideas. I was disgusted at the way in which the theory of diseases had been used to falsify a diagnosis. Even if John did have "ulcerative colitis" instead of "amoebic colitis," he deserved a thorough investigation for all the possible triggers and modulators of his illness, not rote treatment with suppressive drugs.

The first step in the *science of caring* is a commitment to understanding as much as can be learned about the person who is sick, *in relation to his sickness*. Patient-centered diagnosis serves as a structure for collecting and analyzing this data. It is the caring physician's task to know the context in which sickness occurs, the physical and social environment, the dietary habits of the person who is sick, her beliefs about the illness, her hopes and fears, the triggers for symptoms, and the likely precipitating events. Unfortunately, medical training and education pay little attention to the science of caring, assuming that it is enough for doctors to know how to recognize and treat diseases. Doctors therefore are adept at ignoring information that is important to patients but seems incidental to treating diseases, even though their ignorance leads to considerable dissatisfaction among patients.[32]

THE QUALITIES OF A CARING DOCTOR

There are several behaviors that distinguish a physician who is skilled at caring.[33] Here are the qualities I believe all competent physicians must possess.

1. Ability to listen. A study done at Wayne State University found that most patients have three reasons for visiting a physician, are interrupted within eighteen seconds of starting to tell their stories, and never get the chance to finish.[34] Although doctors excuse this behavior by citing lack of time, it takes an average of one minute and rarely more than three minutes for a patient to present a complete list of problems. As a patient, you must be allowed to present your major concerns and to tell your own story. Patients who are given the opportunity to present their concerns in their own words are more satisfied with their physicians, cooperate more fully with medical treatment, and show a greater improvement in their health status, losing less time from work and experiencing fewer limitations of function. This is one area in which published research supports common sense: doctors who ignore the patient's concerns are likely to miss important medical information.[35]

2. Willingness to acknowledge. Every patient has his own ideas and feelings about the illness. In most medical consultations, the patient and the doctor are not in full agreement about the nature of the principal problem, and some form of negotiation is needed.[36] A study that carefully analyzed taped transcripts of visits to a medical clinic found that patients attempted to clarify or to challenge what the doctor said in 85 percent of cases. Usually, their requests were ignored or interrupted.[37] Even when physicians are informed of their patients' concerns, they are loath to recognize the patient's perspective.[38] A physician who understands the science of caring will seek to discover your beliefs about your illness by asking questions like "What do you think has caused your problem?" and will address these beliefs rather than dismissing them.

3. The ability to explain. People have an intense need for explanations about the causes of their diseases.[39] Doctors are usually content to name the disease and treat it. Patients want to know *how* they

came to be sick, so that they can attach some meaning to the illness.[40] They want to know what to expect from the illness and what they can do to relieve symptoms or speed recovery. Information can reduce anxiety, increase feelings of personal control, and improve the ability to cope with pain. People change their behaviors more readily when they receive information about the importance and the nature of the changes they need to make, as well as help with setting goals and measuring progress. The amount of information given by physicians consistently correlates with the degree of satisfaction patients express concerning the treatment they have received.[41] Advice and information from physicians plays an important role in helping patients change. And yet, it is rarely given.[42] Doctors consistently underestimate the amount of information patients want and grossly overestimate the amount of information they actually give. In one study in a general practice, doctors spent less than 5 percent of their time informing patients but believed they were spending 45 percent of their time giving information.[43]

4. Willingness to assess family and social support. In the last chapter, I reviewed studies that show that a lack of social support increases the rate of sickness and of death. Conversely, strong family and social bonds alleviate sickness and enhance cooperation with medical treatments. Because illness itself often contributes to isolation, a caring physician must always inquire about a patient's social integration. Helpful questions include "Are there people in whom you can confide?", "How satisfied are you with your marriage/family/friends/social life?", "How much support do you receive in dealing with your health problems?" The caring physician can help patients who are suffering from isolation by calling this isolation to the attention of family members or friends or by attempting to connect the patient with a support group or community agency. Possibly, there is nothing that can be done to relieve the patient's isolation, but the doctor's awareness and acknowledgment of it is important nonetheless.

5. Ability to show empathy. Writing in *The New York Times Magazine*, Anatole Broyard reflected, "A doctor's job would be so much more interesting and satisfying if he would occasionally let himself plunge into the patient, if he could lose his own fear of falling."[44] Empathy is plunging, sharing another person's feelings and understanding them as

if they were one's own. In order to be empathic, the physician must first understand what the patient feels and then communicate this understanding to the patient. A statement like "I understand how you feel" is highly charged when uttered by a physician. It may lead to an angry outburst—"No, you don't understand!"—which allows the real concerns of the patient to come forward. It may strengthen the bond between physician and patient, especially if the communication is correctly focused: "I understand how difficult your daughter's illness has been for you," or "I realize how afraid you are of having a heart attack, because of your father's early death." An empathic bond between physician and patient may encourage the patient to reveal her most difficult problems, enhancing the process of diagnosis. It also allows the doctor to understand why the patient makes the decisions she makes, why she chooses to follow or not to follow the doctor's advice. The doctor then has the option of altering treatment to meet the patient's values and expectations rather than those of the doctor. Empathy enriches the experience of being a doctor. Fortunately, empathy is a skill that can be taught. A halting effort is under way to integrate its teaching into medical education.[45]

6. Willingness to offer encouragement, hope, and reassurance. Our feelings of hopelessness contribute to our sickness and death and inhibit cooperation with medical treatments.[46] Debilitating disease is always accompanied by feelings of guilt or inadequacy. But even if you have a terminal illness, your doctor's offering of hope is not deception. Your doctor can encourage you by praising your determination to get better or your commitment to following the treatment plan. In her landmark work, *On Death and Dying*, Elisabeth Kübler-Ross observed that physicians can share in the hope of their dying patients that remission may occur and that they will outlive the statistics, without deceiving the patient.[47] Patients are most likely to respond positively to reassurance and encouragement if they believe that the doctor has really listened to their major concerns.

HELPING YOUR DOCTOR BECOME MORE CARING

There are several steps that you can take when consulting with your doctor to help him or her become more caring:

1. Describe the effect that illness has had on your life, your daily activities, the way you perform your work, your recreation, your relationships with those close to you. As a rule, physicians ignore or underestimate the degree to which illness impairs their patients' level of function.[48] If your doctor doesn't ask, tell him or her.

2. Express your feelings about the illness—your fears, your frustrations, your anger. If the doctor is not interested, you should be seeing another doctor.

3. Present your goals. What you want from a medical consultation is usually not obvious from the list of your medical complaints. As I mentioned before, doctors tend to assume their patients want drugs, when in fact what their patients want is information. One study of patients in a primary care practice found that 70 percent were hoping for education about their diseases, 43 percent wanted advice about diet and exercise, and 24 percent wanted stress management counseling.[49] A nurse practitioner who studied her own patients found that if she asked, "How did you hope that I might help you this visit?", her patients always had a request and it was usually not one that could have been predicted from the primary medical complaint.[50] If your doctor doesn't ask what you want, tell him or her.

4. Do not wait until the end of your appointment to express your major concerns. People consulting primary care physicians often introduce new problems during the last minute of the office visit, as the doctor is getting ready to leave the room.[51] Not only is it annoying for the doctor to hear, "Oh, by the way . . .", but there is very little chance that your new problem will get the hearing it deserves under those circumstances.

5. Actively participate in developing a therapeutic plan. You are the person who has to implement it, after all, even if it only requires taking pills. The best physicians encourage their patients to take an active stance in their care, so that patients assume a collaborative role. This

improves satisfaction, cooperation, and level of activity for patients with a wide range of chronic diseases.[52] A doctor's refusal to accept your active participation will undermine your treatment and make it difficult for you to cooperate with his or her care.[53] If your doctor dismisses your input, change doctors.

YOUR ACTIVE ROLE

Cooperation with treatment is technically called "adherence" or "compliance." These names are unfortunate, because they emphasize passivity rather than active involvement. Nonetheless, several studies have found that "treatment adherence" has surprising effects on sickness and mortality that cannot be predicted by conventional medical wisdom. The impact of adherence as an independent phenomenon first became evident in some large-scale studies that attempted to assess the effect of drugs in preventing death from heart attacks.

The Coronary Drug Project was a large multicenter study of a cholesterol-lowering drug, clofibrate, which, it was hoped, would decrease the death rate from heart attacks among middle-aged men with high cholesterol levels. Compared to a placebo pill, however, clofibrate had no effect. When adherence to treatment was analyzed, the researchers discovered what they expected to find: among patients given clofibrate, those who took 80 percent or more of their pills had only half the death rate of those who didn't take their pills. Further analysis was startling. Patients who faithfully took the placebo medication also had half the death rate of the nonadherent patients. In other words, the drug had no effect on mortality, but *the act of following directions* was associated with a markedly improved medical outcome.[54]

These findings have been replicated in another drug study that compared placebos with a drug called Inderal (propranolol), which is supposed to prevent heart attacks by decreasing the stress placed on the heart. These results have also been replicated in studies of women, as well as men, and also in patients with cancer. People being treated with anticancer drugs may develop profound immune suppression as a side effect of the drugs. Death often occurs from infection due to immune suppression, rather than from the cancer itself. Immune-suppressed cancer patients who faithfully take antibiotics as prevention against infection have a decreased incidence of infection and fever when compared to patients who do not take their antibiotics. No surprise there. But patients who faithfully take placebo pills *also* have a decreased incidence of infection and fever.[55] Possibly, those people who adhere to research protocols are people who take better care of themselves in numerous ways. We can't be sure, because the data necessary to make such a judgment have not been gathered.

It appears that people who adhere more closely to their prescribed treatment have a greater sense of their ability to accomplish the goals they set for themselves; their "perceived self-efficacy" is high. Individuals with high perceived self-efficacy adopt healthier lifestyles, follow treatment recommendations more closely, recover from illness more rapidly, and live longer.[56] Self-efficacy is not a fixed trait. It is highly responsive to the patient's social environment, including the environment in which he receives his health care. The physician's attentiveness to the patient and willingness to convey information have a measurable impact on self-efficacy. The advice and information about self-care practices that a doctor gives can enhance a patient's perceived self-efficacy and improve his or her medical outcome.[57]

The greatest challenge and the greatest promise in medicine today is not cost control, genetic engineering, or the development of new technologies. From the prevention and treatment of heart disease to cancer to AIDS, it is learning how to motivate people to change their behavior. The relationship between patient and physician is a critical resource for change.

To achieve the greatest support from your relationship with your doctor:

• Present your goals and expectations at the start of each consultation.
• Explain the type of information you need: risks, side effects, nondrug treatment strategies, treatment rationale, results in other patients, treatment statistics.
• Express your feelings about the illness.
• Explain the way in which the illness has affected your life, your daily activities, your work, recreation, and personal relationships.

- Actively participate in developing a therapeutic plan; make your preferences known to your doctor.
- Don't wait until the end of the office visit to voice your major concerns.
- Expect that your doctor will listen to your major concerns without cutting you short, will acknowledge your ideas and your feelings about your condition, will attempt to give you the explanations you seek, will attempt to understand how you feel, and will offer encouragement.

If these goals cannot be achieved, voice your dissatisfaction.

6

THE SECOND PILLAR:
DÍAITA

CELL SIGNALS

Her name was Catherine Fox, age sixteen, and her parents were there to tell me her story. Catherine herself had very little to say. She had been quiet and reserved for most of her life, but no one ever considered her an abnormal child. She did well in school, had several friends, participated in sports.

At the age of fourteen, Catherine had changed dramatically. She'd become increasingly withdrawn, refusing to leave her bedroom for school, or even for meals. Her parents thought she was depressed. When they tried to coax her out of her isolation, Catherine revealed the frightening truth: she had been hearing voices that ordered her to kill other children at school. She begged the voices to leave her alone, but they refused to listen. Fearful that they could compel her to do their bidding, Catherine had withdrawn into a world of solitude where she could be sure she would not kill.

Her distraught parents rushed Catherine to a psychiatrist, who provided a prompt diagnosis, as terrifying as the girl's symptoms: paranoid schizophrenia. The treatment was Thorazine, a potent tranquilizer that does not cure schizophrenia but that may help to control its most obvious symptoms. After taking Thorazine, Catherine found that the voices were silenced. She was far from normal, however. She had no appetite, no interest in anything that took place around her, and, even without the tormenting voices, no desire to leave her bedroom or to speak with anyone. This poverty of speech and will was not a side effect of the drug she was taking. It was the least dramatic but most disabling symptom of schizophrenia, the "negative" or "deficit" symptom complex, which reflects a disengagement from oneself and others.

Meeting Catherine for the first time was an eerie experience. It was not like meeting a girl; it was like meeting the two-dimensional, black-and-white outline of a girl. Her gaze was vacant, her speech vague, her posture limp. There was not a trace of emotion in her face or voice. To her parents, it seemed as if their child were hidden from view in a prison without windows.

Schizophrenia generally strikes people at the threshold of adulthood, making casualties of both parent and child. It usually lasts for life, depriving victims of their identity, independence, and mental capacity. Ten percent of schizophrenics commit suicide.[1] Although medication is usually effective in controlling symptoms like hallucinations and delusions of persecution or grandiosity, the deficit symptoms resist most treatments and prevent most treated schizophrenics from returning to school or work or maintaining ties with other people. Because of its onset at young age, its relentless course, and its destruction of those traits of emotion and intellect that are most prized for being distinctly human—and because it afflicts about one person out of every hundred—schizophrenia has been called "the worst disease affecting mankind, even AIDS not excepted."[2] Between one-third and one-half of homeless people in the United States are schizophrenic.[3]

In 1980, the year in which Catherine Fox became ill, the American Psychiatric Association issued the third edition of its *Diagnostic and Statistical Manual* (DSM-III), which described the exact criteria to be met for a diagnosis of schizophrenia and emphasized the need to separate it from other diseases capable of mimicking its symptoms. Catherine's auditory hallucinations, social withdrawal, extreme emotional flatness, and belief that the voices were capable of controlling her behavior were all characteristic of schizophrenia. The impact of this approach on clinical practice is evident in Catherine's case. Her psychiatrist's role was to determine that the patient met the DSM-III criteria. Once the diagnosis was made, treatment was started with antipsychotic drugs. In a best-case scenario of conventional treatment, psychotropic drugs would be supplemented with counseling designed to help both patient and family cope with this devastating, chronic disease.

But the notion of schizophrenia as a distinct disease, as presented in DSM-III, stumbles over a huge paradox. DSM-III required of schizophrenia that it be "not due to any organic mental disorder." Now, an organic mental disorder is *any* condition in which infection, physical trauma, nutritional deficiency, drug exposure, or medical illness disturbs the function of the brain. *Numerous* organic, metabolic, and infectious lesions have been described among patients with schizophrenia. In the early years of the twentieth century, when the founders of modern psychiatry were defining the common psychiatric diseases, mental hospitals were filled with psychotic patients suffering from vitamin B_3 deficiency (pellagra) or the late stages of syphilis or postencephalitic catatonia (the state of immobile, trancelike withdrawal depicted in the movie *Awakenings*, induced by viral infection of the brain). Until the specific factors that produced psychosis in these patients were understood, many were given a diagnosis of schizophrenia. It is reasonable to assume that today's schizophrenics may also have disorders as diverse and unrelated as those of patients who lived a century ago.

Instead of thinking of schizophrenia as a disease, or even as a group of diseases, it is more useful to think of schizophrenia as an *outcome*, the end result of many types of injury that severely disrupt the processing of information in the brains of individual patients.[4] Furthermore, the *outcome* we call schizophrenia is not even an expression of the injury alone; it also depends upon the nature of the information that has to be processed.[5] The more stressful a person's life, the more schizophrenic behaviors he will display.

Catherine and her parents had come to see me to find an alternative to the conventional clinical approach.

"Don't talk to us about schizophrenia," they insisted. "Talk to us about Catherine. What is it about Catherine that produces *her* schizophrenia?"

I felt that this was a reasonable question, but extremely difficult to answer.

Catherine's illness was quite typical for teenage schizophrenia; consequently, it shed little light on her unique characteristics. Her parents, as far as I could tell from the initial interview, were both supportive and flexible; their family life seemed stable and did not display the kinds of interpersonal tension that can contribute to the stress that schizophrenics endure. Catherine's most distinctive abnormality revealed itself on physical examination. Her skin had the texture of rough sand, visibly peeling from her arms and legs; her hair had the texture of rusty Brillo. She was about the driest teenager I had ever seen.

Having made this observation, I had to decide what meaning I would attach to it. Was dryness really a clue to the mystery of Catherine's illness? Or was the texture of her skin and hair a distraction I would be better off ignoring? I reasoned that dryness, if it had a meaning that was relevant to Catherine's illness, could signify one of two things: either she had an underactive thyroid gland or she lacked the nutrients necessary to give her skin the qualities of luster and oiliness expected in a girl her age. Her thyroid had already tested as functionally normal. Dryness, I thought, might indicate a deficiency of essential fatty acids (EFAs).

Although the body readily makes most of the fat that it needs from dietary starch or sugar, humans lack the ability to make EFAs and must get them in food. EFAs are found in all foods but are most abundant in certain oils. They come in two distinct families, based upon their chemical structure. The two EFA families are not interchangeable and, in fact, tend to compete with each other in the body's metabolic pathways.

The larger family, called *omega-six* EFAs, are abundant in many vegetable seed oils, including corn, sunflower, and safflower. Deficiency of omega-six EFAs causes impairment of growth and fertility, hormonal disturbances, and immunologic abnormalities.[6] An excess of omega-six EFAs may promote the development of cancer.[7] People living in North America and Europe have relatively high levels of omega-six EFAs in their diets, because of the increasing consumption of vegetable oil during the twentieth century.

The smaller family, called *omega-three* EFAs, is most concentrated in fish oils and in flaxseed (linseed) oil. It is also found in green leafy vegetables and in the flesh of animals that feed on grass and leaves. The human brain is rich in omega-three EFAs; their deficiency causes abnormalities in the development and function of the nervous system, as well as immune defects. Omega-three EFAs formed an important part of the diet of Stone Age humans, who relied heavily on wild game and leafy plants for nourishment. Consumption of fish, flaxseed meal, and soybeans supplied omega-threes for our more recent ancestors. The past century has witnessed a systematic depletion of omega-three EFAs from the Western diet because of changes in food choice and in techniques of animal husbandry and food processing. Some theorists have traced the origins of numerous different diseases to a lifetime depletion of omega-three EFAs.[8] One small study, done in Nigeria, found evidence to suggest that some people with schizophrenia metabolized omega-three EFAs very slowly; they might develop signs and symptoms of EFA deficiency more rapidly and more severely than other people.[9]

I explained to Catherine and her parents that Catherine's unusually dry skin might be a sign of EFA deficiency. I asked her to take flaxseed oil, three tablespoons a day, along with a multivitamin, while I awaited the results of laboratory tests for other metabolic or nutritional defects.

When Catherine returned to see me a month later, I felt as if I were meeting her for the first time. She made eye contact, smiled, and had opinions. The outline had been filled in with living color. Incidentally, her skin and hair were far less dry, but still not lustrous. Her main request was that I allow her to stop taking Thorazine.

"It may be a bit too early to stop your medication," I cautioned. "I know you don't like it, but it did help you get rid of those terrible hallucinations."

"The drug didn't do that," protested Catherine. "*I* did! It was very difficult, but *I* made them stop."

"Wait one more month," I asked.

She reluctantly agreed, but in fact never took the medication again. When I saw her a month later, she was attending school every day, doing well in her classwork, engaging in sports, and visiting friends with whom she hadn't spoken for two years. Her skin and hair were normal in texture, and I recommended that she decrease the dose of flax oil to one tablespoon per day.

Catherine made only one more visit to see me. The trip was inconvenient and she had a full schedule. She and her parents believed she was cured and needed no further treatment, so I followed her condition by telephone for two more years. She had no further problems and appeared to be healthy and well adjusted.

I have not personally seen any other schizophrenics cured with flax oil, but Dr. Donald Rudin reported several cases when he did research at the Pennsylvania Psychiatric Institute during the 1970s.[10] Although Rudin's work passed largely unnoticed, the omega-three story, as he predicted, became the leading nutritional breakthrough of the 1980s. Extensive research published since 1985 has demonstrated that flax oil can prevent cancer and birth defects in animals.[11] Fish oils, the other concentrated source of omega-threes, have made front-page news because of their ability to help prevent disorders as apparently unrelated to one another as cancer, heart attacks, migraine headaches, and premature births, and to reverse the effects of conditions as different as psoriasis, ulcerative colitis, rheumatoid arthritis, and cystic fibrosis.[12]

The wide range of clinical benefits that result from omega-three therapy highlights a new way of thinking about the effects of nutrition on the cells of the body. The most obvious role of nutrition lies in supplying fuel for the production of energy. All cells are alike in their need to burn fuel. What each type of cell does with its energy is different, however, and depends upon the special and distinct function of the tissue to which the cell belongs. Muscle cells, for example, use energy to become shorter or longer, which makes muscles either contract or relax. Glandular cells, nerve cells, and cells of the immune system produce chemicals, an immense variety of them, each with its own set of specific effects. The living cells in bone produce a protein matrix on which they deposit crystals of calcium, or else they absorb the matrix and its coating of calcium.

The control and integration of these activities is set by an information network that passes chemical signals from cell to cell, regulating how every cell performs its special function. The signals give each cell two fundamental, opposite sets of commands: "Do less" or "Do more." Although many different chemicals, naturally produced within the body, may act as messengers to carry the signal, the information is transmitted in a binary code that has been called the *yin* and the *yang* of physiology. In Chinese medicine, *yin* is that aspect of function which recedes, withdraws, is cooler or darker, and *yang* is that aspect which advances, expands, is brighter or warmer. The *yin* signal is a "Do less" signal. It instructs each cell to do less of its specific task. The *yang* signal is a "Do more" signal, which accelerates each cell's specific task.

This binary code not only tells every type of muscle whether to constrict or relax and the lining of the stomach whether to secrete more acid or not, it also tells the cells of a tumor whether to keep dividing in two and multiplying their numbers or to stop growing, and it tells nerve cells how to communicate with one another. In this way, each cell functions like a computer. Hormones and other chemical messengers are as varied as the keys on a keyboard, but the information conveyed by striking each key is transduced into a signal that says either "yes" or "no." *Yin/yang* imbalance of the body's binary information network underlies all chronic diseases, from acne to cancer to ulcers. It accompanies the alterations in brain chemistry that cause schizophrenia.

Most of the chronic diseases characteristic of modern industrial societies reflect a response of the body to stress that is imbalanced in the direction of excessive *yang*. The body's cells are *overly* reactive, especially in the earlier stages of disease. The blood clots too readily, cells divide too rapidly, muscles constrict too tightly, hormones and other chemical messengers are released in excess and flood the tissues with signals that amplify the imbalance by evoking further responses from cells that habitually overreact. This *yang* distortion of cellular responsiveness produces the state of cellular frenzy that creates coronary heart disease, high blood pressure, hardening of the arteries, most forms of cancer, all varieties of inflammation, migraine headaches, asthma and other allergic disorders, endometriosis, psoriasis, and acne.

Nutrition and Cell Signals

Nutrition has a profound influence on the body's cellular information network, by affecting the way that cells respond to signals from other cells. Of all nutrients studied, the most direct and dramatic effects are produced by dietary fats and by calcium.

Most of the body's calcium is stored in bone, where it provides density and hardness. Of the calcium that is not stored in bone, 99 percent is bound to protein, which renders it inactive. The remaining fraction of calcium, which is freely dissolved in the cellular fluid, is able to activate or inactivate enzymes, the proteins that catalyze all important biochemical reactions in the body. Regulating the availability of free intracellular calcium is a key function of the binary code.

Most of the fat we eat is simply burned or stored. A special fate awaits dietary EFAs. First, they are incorporated into the membranes that surround cells, giving cell membranes the degree of flexibility needed for each cell to respond properly to signals from other cells. Second, EFAs are plucked from the cell membrane and transformed into chemical messengers called *prostaglandins* and *leukotrienes* (as a group, these substances are known as *prostanoids*). Prostanoids are made by almost every cell in the body; their main function is to alter the cadence at which cells work, speeding it up (*yang*) or slowing it down (*yin*).

Altered production of prostanoids and abnormal regulation of free intracellular calcium levels are universal companions to sickness of any type, from heart disease to cancer, from diseases of the skin, like psoriasis and eczema, to diseases of the mind, like depression and schizophrenia.[13] There are at least fifty different prostanoids active in human physiology. Although they all act on the rhythm of cell function, they may augment or conflict with one another, depending upon the type of cell being studied and the cell's general level of arousal.

When a cell is resting (*yin* predominates) there is usually little prostanoid synthesis and the free calcium level is low. An activation signal coming from another cell elevates the free calcium in the cell, which in turn increases prostanoid production, which further increases the calcium level, turning the cell toward *yang*, increasing its activity. As the cell bustles with action (*yang* predominates), prostanoid synthesis and free calcium levels are high. The prostanoids produced in this state lower the calcium concentration and begin to inhibit further cellular activity, turning the cell toward *yin* once again. This is the neverending rhythm of normal cellular function. Its failure is the ultimate cause of all chronic disease.[14]

A relative deficiency of omega-three EFAs disrupts the rhythm of cell function by distorting prostanoid synthesis. Its net effects are deficient production of prostanoids that favor *yin* and an excess of prostanoids that favor *yang*, the same pattern of altered reactivity found in most chronic disease.[15]

A person's need for omega-three EFAs is not fixed. It varies with the level of other fats in the diet. The higher the consumption of fat in general, the higher the need for omega-three EFAs, because fats tend to compete with one another in their effects on prostanoid synthesis. One of the benefits of a low-fat diet, which has been shown to reduce the risk of heart disease and cancer, is a reduction in omega-three require-ments.

Drugs Versus Nutrition

The world's most commonly used drugs work by inhibiting prostaglandin synthesis. They belong to a pharmaceutical category called nonsteroidal anti-inflammatory drugs (NSAIDs), which includes aspirin and ibuprofen (Motrin/Advil). NSAIDs relieve pain and in-flammation by inhibiting the formation of prostaglandin E-2 (PGE-2). Although high levels of PGE-2 contribute to pain and inflammation, PGE-2 also protects the stomach from the corrosive effects of its own acid, regulates circulation of blood to the kidneys, and modulates the activity of the immune system. NSAID use can have severe side effects, which are a direct result of their inhibition of prostaglandin formation. The side effects of chronic NSAID use include stomach ulcers, intesti-nal bleeding, kidney failure, high blood pressure, and aggravation of immune system disorders like asthma, psoriasis, and colitis.[16]

Some interesting benefits of chronic use of low-dose aspirin under a doctor's supervision have recently been highly publicized. Long-term use of aspirin seems capable of preventing heart attacks, bowel cancer, migraine headaches, and some complications of pregnancy. The opti-mal dose for preventing heart attacks is the equivalent of one baby as-pirin every other day. When used at this level, aspirin does not relieve pain or inflammation and does not block the synthesis of PGE-2. It se-lectively inhibits the synthesis of a prostanoid called thromboxane A-2 (TXA-2), which is a potent stimulus to cellular hyperactivity and possi-bly the most dangerous prostanoid found in the human body. TXA-2 makes blood clot very fast, promoting heart attacks, and makes cells grow very rapidly, promoting cancer. The preventive benefits of chronic ingestion of *small* amounts of aspirin (with your physician's ap-proval) for different, apparently unrelated diseases point once again to the universal importance of prostanoids in regulating cellular respon-siveness, but they leave unanswered the question of low-dose side ef-fects. A recent study from Boston University found that the use of

buffered or enteric-coated aspirin did not decrease the rate of gastrointestinal bleeding among aspirin users, and that even at doses less than
one adult-strength aspirin a day, the risk of major gastrointestinal bleeding increased threefold.[17]

Like NSAIDs, most of the drugs that are used in clinical medicine
behave like chemical straitjackets, restricting the actions of cells that
have gone berserk. They block the response to signals from other cells,
interrupting the flow of information. This role is obvious in the names
doctors give to categories of drugs: antihistamines, H-2 blockers, calcium channel blockers, beta blockers, ACE inhibitors. Although these
drugs may be effective in accomplishing their short-term objectives,
they all have side effects that are a direct extension of their therapeutic
actions. They do not restore the balanced flow of intercellular communication; they merely inhibit cellular hyperactivity. Just as a person
in a straitjacket loses the ability to feed or clean himself, a cell in a straitjacket loses the ability to regulate itself. New drug development needs
to address ways of enhancing the body's regulatory functions, not
merely suppressing them.

Nutritional therapy offers the potential for restoring balance rather
than merely suppressing hyperactive cells. When properly used, nutrients can achieve results that drugs cannot, because nutrients are intrinsic components of the cellular information network. The cure of
Catherine's schizophrenia is an example. There are no drugs effective
at reversing the deficit symptom complex of schizophrenics.[18]

In treating Catherine, I did not rely on flax oil alone; I added a multivitamin and mineral supplement, because the way in which the body
utilizes EFAs is in turn regulated by the availability of vitamins and
minerals that govern EFA metabolism. The important vitamins for
EFA metabolism are E, C, A, and B_3 (niacin), and the important minerals are selenium, zinc, and manganese.

NUTRITIONAL THERAPY: THE FIRST THREE LEVELS

Understanding the effects of nutrients on cellular communication has
allowed me to shape nutritional therapies tailored to the needs of individuals, using data from scientific studies. These therapies are built
around three broad strategies, one level at a time. The steps are not dif-

NUTRIENTS NEEDED FOR EFA UTILIZATION

Nutrient	Adult RDA	Best Food Sources
Vitamin E	10 mg	Nuts, seeds, legumes, whole grains, and dark green leafy vegetables, especially raw sunflower seeds, raw hazelnuts, raw almonds, kale, oatmeal. (I recommend that most adults supplement their diets with 400 mg of vitamin E/day)
Vitamin A	5,000 IU	Liver, crabmeat, egg yolk, and fruits and vegetables with high carotene content like carrots, tomatoes, broccoli, cantaloupe, apricots
Vitamin C	60 mg	Citrus fruit, strawberries, papaya, red and green pepper, tomatoes, collard greens, broccoli, Brussels sprouts. (I recommend that most adults supplement their diets with 1,000 mg of vitamin C/day)
Vitamin B_3	19 mg	Beef, broccoli, brown rice, carrots, chicken, eggs, halibut, oats, rainbow trout, salmon, tuna, turkey breast
Vitamin B_6	2 mg	Bananas, beef, blueberries, cabbage, chicken, eggs, fish, green peas, spinach, sunflower seeds, walnuts
zinc	15 mg	Oysters, clams, crabmeat, liver, turkey leg or thigh, pumpkin seeds, sunflower seeds, black-eyed peas
selenium	70 mcg	Garlic, shrimp, oats, scallops, Brazil nuts
manganese	N/A	Brown rice, Brazil nuts, almonds, oatmeal, pineapple, green peas, blackberries

Food storage and preparation affect nutrient content. Vitamins E and C are destroyed by high heat. Vitamin E is destroyed during prolonged storage. Vitamin A in food becomes *more* available when vegetables are cooked, however. Boiling vegetables removes minerals, unless the water used for boiling is also consumed.

ficult to implement, but you may want the help of a nutritionist or a physician with training in nutritional medicine.

To choose a qualified nutritionist, look for three characteristics: education, experience, and attitude. The person you consult should have an advanced degree: an M.D., a Ph.D. in nutrition or biochemistry, a master's degree (M.S.) in nutrition, or a Doctor of Naturopathy (N.D.) from a nationally accredited college of naturopathy. The individual you choose should be someone who keeps abreast of recent developments in this rapidly changing field. Robert Crayhon, author of *Robert Crayhon's Nutrition Made Simple,* suggests that you ask your nutritionist what recent developments in nutrition research have been most exciting to him or her. As Crayhon insightfully says, "A good nutritionist will follow the latest research like a stockbroker follows the stock market. Someone who doesn't have an answer to this one should be avoided." He also recommends that you ask, "Have you ever dealt with someone who had this problem before? What is your success rate?" You will get the best results from a more experienced practitioner.[19]

For referral to a practitioner who has been trained in the tenets of Functional Medicine, you can call the HealthComm referral service at (800) 245-9076.

Level One: Nutritional Density

Nutritional density refers to the concentration of specific nutrients in foods as compared to the calories contained within the food.[20] Most Americans can substantially improve their health, vitality, and longevity by eating foods of high nutrient density. Foods that supply calories without also supplying vital nutrients are injurious to health. The main sources of these "empty calories" are the sugar, refined flour, and processed fats or oils added to manufactured foods, especially snack foods.

The healthiest foods to eat, from the perspective of nutritional density, are:

1. Most vegetables, with the distinct exception of iceberg lettuce and cucumbers. The usual tossed salad has little nutritional value and does not meet anyone's need for vegetables. The most nutritious vegetables are (in alphabetical order): arugula, asparagus, beans of all types, broc-

---

VEGETABLES AND FRUITS MOST HIGHLY CONTAMINATED WITH PESTICIDES

Vegetables
bell peppers
spinach
celery
green beans
cucumbers

Fruits
strawberries
cherries
peaches
Mexican cantaloupe
apples
apricots
Chilean grapes

---

coli, Brussels sprouts, carrots, cauliflower, kale, romaine lettuce, mushrooms, onions, peas, potatoes (sweet and white, baked), spinach, sprouted beans and seeds, and tomatoes. Squash and green beans are fairly low in vitamin content but are rich in the carotenoids lutein, zeanthin, and alpha-carotene, which convey protection against cancer.[21]

How you buy and prepare vegetables will affect their nutritional density. Buy local vegetables in season. They will be cheaper, fresher, and less likely to be laced with pesticides than imported vegetables. Choose produce that is deeper in color. Paleness is usually associated with loss of nutrients. Wash vegetables thoroughly with water and a scrub brush, and peel when practical, to remove pesticides. Eat within a few days of purchase but wait until just before eating or cooking to wash and cut. Do not overcook. Steam lightly until tender but still crisp. The nutrients in lightly cooked vegetables are more easily absorbed than the nutrients in raw vegetables, but overcooking destroys vitamins. The use of microwave ovens to heat vegetables may also prevent destruction or washing away of nutrients, but microwaves do a poor job of killing bacteria.

VEGETABLES AND FRUITS LEAST CONTAMINATED
WITH PESTICIDES

Vegetables
> green peas
> broccoli
> asparagus
> romaine lettuce
> carrots
> radishes
> Brussels sprouts
> potatoes

Fruits
> nectarines
> blueberries
> raspberries
> blackberries
> oranges
> grapefruit
> tangerines
> watermelon
> seasonal domestic cantaloupe or grapes

Foods grown without the use of pesticides are increasingly available in supermarkets, natural food stores, and farmers' markets. To be really free of pesticides, they should be certified organic in compliance with standards set by a state certifying organization.

---

2. Fruits. Among the more nutritious are apricots, bananas, blueberries, cantaloupe, cherries, grapefruit, honeydew melon, kiwifruit, mango, nectarine, orange, papaya, pear, pineapple, plum, raspberries, strawberries, tangerine, and watermelon. Apples and grapes are not high in vitamins, but apples are a good source of boron, a mineral needed for healthy bones, and purple grapes are an excellent source of bioflavonoids, natural substances that combat heart disease. Wash all fruit thoroughly with water and a scrub brush (if possible) and, after washing, peel all waxed fruit, to minimize the content of pesticide residues. Local or domestic fruit in season will be cheaper, more nutri-

tious, and less contaminated by pesticides than imported fruit. About 4 percent of imported fruits tested by the FDA contain pesticides so toxic they are prohibited by U.S. law.[22]

In November 1995, the Environmental Working Group, a research and advocacy organization in Washington, D.C., rated forty-two fruits and vegetables for pesticide contamination, based upon a study of fifteen thousand samples conducted by the FDA during 1992 and 1993. They used seven rating criteria, including the percentage of each crop with detectable pesticide residues and the known toxicity of each type of residue. The group calculated that 50 percent of food pesticide exposure occurs through consumption of twelve foods. The vegetables with the greatest contamination were bell peppers, spinach, celery, green beans, and cucumbers. They recommended substituting less contaminated vegetables for these. The safer vegetables included green peas, broccoli, asparagus, romaine lettuce, carrots, radishes, Brussels sprouts, and potatoes.[23]

According to this same report, the commercial fruits most highly contaminated with pesticides were strawberries, cherries, peaches, Mexican cantaloupe, apples, apricots, and Chilean grapes. Less contaminated fruits included nectarines, blueberries, raspberries, blackberries, oranges, grapefruit, tangerines, watermelon, and seasonal domestic cantaloupe or grapes.

3. Whole grains, especially oats, brown rice, and barley. In choosing bread, choose 100 percent whole wheat bread; other varieties contain mostly refined flour. Buckwheat is technically a vegetable, a relative of rhubarb, but from a culinary and nutritional perspective behaves like a grain. It is an excellent source of vitamins and minerals.

4. Nuts and seeds, fresh and raw, especially walnuts, almonds, sesame, sunflower, and pumpkin seeds. Peanuts are not really nuts; they are legumes, in the same family as beans. I do not advise my patients to consume peanuts or peanut butter, because of their potential for contamination by toxic molds (see page 169).

5. Fish are an excellent source of protein, B-vitamins, and minerals, and fatty cold-water fish are an excellent source of omega-three EFAs. Although most studies indicate that fish-eaters live longer than those who don't eat fish,[24] the contamination of fatty fish with pesticides and PCBs is cause for concern.

Recent alarms have been raised by worldwide pollution with chemicals known as *organochlorines*. They include: the pesticide DDT, banned in the United States in 1972 but still sold by U.S. corporations to other countries and still found in our own soil and water; the herbicide dioxin; and polychlorinated biphenyls (PCBs), which have been widely used in making electronic equipment, plastic, inks, adhesives, rubber, and carbonless duplicating paper. Food, milk, and water everywhere contain organochlorines.

Organochlorine contamination may have seriously affected the safety of seafood. Although fatty fish are an excellent source of essential fatty acids, most pollutants tend to accumulate in fatty tissue, so that fatty fish are no longer safe to eat on a regular basis, especially if they come from lakes or rivers. Larry Skinner, wildlife ecologist for the New York State Department of Environmental Conservation, told *Nutrition Action Newsletter:* "Your chance of getting cancer from eating a weekly eight-ounce meal of trout caught in Lake Ontario is about the same as your lifetime risk of being murdered in the United States today—about one in two hundred."[25] Jeffery Foran, an environmental health expert at George Washington University, told a *Time* magazine reporter, "If you're pregnant or nursing, you should probably avoid most kinds of fish."[26] Freshwater fish are still home to DDT and PCBs, even though DDT has been banned in the United States since 1972, and PCB manufacturing has been banned since 1979.

In the ultimate environmental horror story, organochlorine contaminants have been found to either mimic or block the effects of human sex hormones. Hormonal effects of organochlorines have been blamed for increased rates of spontaneous abortion, toxemia of pregnancy, endometriosis, breast cancer, and testicular cancer.[27] If male fertility really is declining, as some scientists assert, organochlorines may be to blame.[28] The high levels of organochlorines found in human milk raise frightening questions about the safety of breast-feeding. I urge my patients not to lose weight while breast-feeding, but to eat heartily. Weight loss releases organochlorines stored in body fat, which travel into the blood and from there into breast milk. Lose weight *after* weaning, *not* before. Because organochlorines appear to be most toxic to infants in the womb—but the effects of this toxicity are not apparent until adulthood—the extent of the organochlorine catastrophe will not be evident for at least another generation.[29]

The landscape of the industrialized world is clouded by a highly di-

CONTAMINANTS IN FISH

Contaminant	Found In	Examples
Organochlorines (includes DDT, PCBs, and dioxin)	Fatty freshwater fish	rainbow trout,* lake trout, eel, catfish,* carp
	Fatty shoreline feeders	bluefish, striped bass
Methylmercury	Freshwater fish caught in newly formed lakes and reservoirs	lake trout, pike, bass
	Large ocean fish	swordfish, tuna, shark
Ciguatera (a toxin produced by tropical plankton)	Tropical fish	grouper, red snapper, amberjack, barracuda
Histamine poisoning from breakdown of fish protein	Improperly refrigerated fish, especially scromboid fish	mahimahi, fresh tuna
Hepatitis virus, Norwalk virus (causes gastroenteritis), Vibrio bacteria (cause diarrhea)	raw shellfish	clams, oysters, mussels

*Contamination of farm-raised trout and catfish depends upon source.

lute vapor of mercury gas, produced by coal-burning electric power plants and municipal refuse incinerators, which washes out in rain and snow, entering rivers and lakes. The mercury content of the sediment extracted from remote lakes in northern Minnesota has tripled in the past century. (Mercury in disposable batteries contributes more than half the mercury emitted by incinerators. Recycle your batteries. Don't throw them in the trash.) Once mercury vapor is dissolved in water, algae convert it into organic methylmercury, which is far more toxic.

Because fish are relatively insensitive to mercury, they can accumulate toxic quantities in their flesh. Saltwater predators like swordfish and tuna are usually contaminated with mercury and daily consumption of tuna can quickly raise the mercury level in hair, suggesting an increase in total body burden of the metal.[30] The concentration of methylmercury in freshwater game fish can reach extremely high levels, especially if the fish are caught in newly formed artificial lakes and reservoirs. Decomposing foliage in the bottom of these lakes makes methylmercury concentrations soar to twenty times the level at which advisory warnings are issued to anglers.

The safest fish to eat are low-fat fish caught offshore, such as cod, haddock, pollock, flounder, and yellowfin tuna. According to Jon Rudd of the Freshwater Institute in Winnipeg, saltwater fish are safer to eat than freshwater, because their high selenium levels tend to counteract methylmercury toxicity.[31] Many fish farms are found in agricultural areas where drifting pesticide sprays and agricultural runoff can be a serious problem, so, if you eat fish from farms, you must know your source.

Problems of contamination do not end once the fish has been caught. Fish is one of the most perishable foods, readily spoiled by bacteria and by natural enzymes contained in the fish's flesh. An investigation by *Consumer Reports* in 1992[32] found that almost half the fish they tested were contaminated with fecal bacteria, a sign of improper food handling. When you buy fish, make sure they smell fresh. Cook them well, within a day of their purchase.

6. Dairy products, eggs, and red meat have come in for much vilification over the past thirty years, some of it undeserved. The high fat content of these foods increases the need for omega-three EFAs. Nonetheless, they are excellent sources of protein, vitamins, and minerals. Consumption of dairy fat has declined considerably over the past hundred years; dairy consumption cannot be held accountable for any of the chronic diseases that have flourished during the twentieth century, except among those individuals who are hypersensitive to components of milk protein. Decisions about consumption of meat and dairy must be highly individualized. Cuts of beef or poultry with the lowest fat content will usually contain the lowest levels of environmental pollutants.

By eating meals and snacks of high nutritional density and avoiding junk, you not only increase your consumption of vitamins, minerals, and bioflavonoids, but also decrease your exposure to the *antinutrients* with which junk food is loaded. As the term implies, antinutrients actually interfere with the body's healthful functioning. Aside from alcohol, the most important antinutrients in the U.S. diet are salt (specifically, sodium) and *trans*-fatty acids, which are produced by the partial hydrogenation of vegetable oils. The small amounts of sodium or of *trans*-fatty acids that occur naturally in food pose no health hazard. It is the addition of sodium chloride to food that raises the sodium concentration to levels that are unsafe for many people. High-sodium foods are those that taste salty or that contain sodium chloride as an ingredient, listed on the food's label. Most *trans*-fatty acids enter our diets from the addition of partially hydrogenated oils, which are usually listed on the label.

High sodium intake causes a loss of calcium and magnesium in urine and contributes to the development of high blood pressure in susceptible individuals. In this way, high sodium intake is antinutritional. Nonetheless, there are some individuals for whom high sodium intake may be beneficial. Researchers at Johns Hopkins University studied a group of patients with chronic fatigue syndrome and compared them with healthy individuals. They found that 95 percent of the patients had problems keeping their blood pressure high enough. As their blood pressure dropped, the patients experienced severe symptoms of nausea, fatigue, and trouble concentrating. Almost half the patients experienced a marked improvement of their chronic fatigue when their blood pressure was raised by a combination of high salt intake and drugs. The researchers noted that three-fifths of the patients with chronic fatigue were following low-salt diets which they believed to be healthy, even though they had low or normal blood pressures.[33] The Johns Hopkins research contains an important nutritional message: There are always a few people who are the exceptions to the rule. Since sodium is an essential mineral, one can anticipate that there will be some people who require high sodium intake to stay healthy.

Unlike sodium, *trans*-fatty acids are not essential nutrients and appear to play no beneficial role in human nutrition. Most of the *trans*-fatty acids consumed today are artificially produced by food manufacturers. The dangers of *trans*-fatty acids in the diet have recently received scientific attention that is long overdue. To understand the toxic potential of *trans*-fatty acids, you have to know how they affect the body's use of EFAs.

EFAs have a chemical structure that is polyunsaturated. Technically, this means that each molecule of an EFA has two or more double chemical bonds. The double bonding twists the molecule, giving it a serpentine shape. When incorporated into a cell's membranes, the snakelike EFA molecules add fluidity and flexibility to the membrane. EFAs, unfortunately, are rather unstable when exposed to air. The double bonds break down rapidly, producing a toxic form of fat that can be detected in food by its rancidity. Preservatives may be added to food to prevent this breakdown from occurring, thereby increasing the shelf life of the food. A natural preservative for fatty acids is vitamin E (alpha-tocopherol), but the most commonly used preservatives are the synthetic antioxidants BHT and BHA.

A more efficient way to prolong shelf life, however, is to hydrogenate the fatty acids, destroying the EFAs. In hydrogenation, the double bonds are broken by hydrogen gas and the unsaturated fatty acids become saturated with hydrogen. This means that all sites for chemical bonding are filled. Naturally saturated fatty acids are commonly consumed in meat and dairy products. They are also manufactured in your liver and stored in your body's fat cells. Saturated fatty acids are straight, not twisting, in shape, and impart stiffness and solidity to membranes. Human cell membranes usually have one saturated fatty acid lined up alongside one unsaturated fatty acid, producing just the right blend of stiffness and flexibility for responding properly to signals sent from other cells.

In present-day food processing, the hydrogenation of vegetable oils is usually not complete. It is partial. Partially hydrogenated oils are easier to work with and produce a softer foodstuff than fully hydrogenated oils. Chemically, partial hydrogenation converts EFAs into *trans*-fatty acids, which are unsaturated fatty acids that twist abnormally. *Trans*-fatty acids do not have the serpentine shape and fluidity of naturally unsaturated fatty acids (which are called *cis*-fatty acids). *Trans*-fatty acids are stiff and straight, like saturated fatty acids, but because they are unsaturated, they replace natural *cis*-fatty acids in the cell membranes. The result of *trans*-fatty acid consumption is stiff cell membranes, abnormal response to signals from other cells, and an increase in dietary requirements for EFAs. Partially hydrogenated vegetable oils, which are ubiquitous in manufactured foods, are loaded with these antinutrients.

In the first edition of *Superimmunity for Kids*, written ten years ago, I warned parents about the dangers of raising their children on margarine and other foods built from partially hydrogenated oils. My arguments derived from research on the chemical effects of *trans*-fatty acids and knowledge of how this chemistry could distort cell function. Clinical studies have vindicated the warning. High consumption of *trans*-fatty acids raises cholesterol levels and increases the risk of heart attack, especially among women.[34] Dr. Walter Willett, chairman of the department of nutrition at Harvard University's School of Public Health, estimates that consumption of *trans*-fatty acids in the United States accounts for thirty thousand premature deaths per year.[35]

Level Two: Balancing EFAs and Antioxidants

Eating foods of high nutrient density and avoiding antinutrients like *trans*-fatty acids does not guarantee physiological balance or an adequate intake of EFAs for each individual. Some indications that an EFA deficiency or imbalance is present are:

- dry skin
- the need to use moisturizing creams and lotions
- "chicken skin," the presence of tiny rough bumps, usually on the back of the arms
- dry or unruly hair
- dandruff
- soft, fraying, or brittle nails
- menstrual cramps
- premenstrual breast tenderness

If you have these symptoms, you will often find that they improve by supplementing an otherwise healthy diet with the appropriate oil. Discovering the appropriate oil requires a bit of personal experimentation. Most people in the United States and Europe are short on omega-three EFAs and will benefit from supplementing their meals with flax oil (one tablespoon a day). Because it spoils quickly, flax oil should be

GOOD SOURCES OF ESSENTIAL FATTY ACIDS

Food Source	Omega-three Percentage	Omega-six Percentage
Flaxseed (linseed) oil	55	25
Walnut oil	10	40
Soybean oil	8	45
Wheat germ oil	8	40
Salmon oil	35	15
Safflower oil	1	65
Sunflower oil	1	45
Corn oil	1	45
Sesame oil	1	40
Primrose oil	1	60
Black currant oil	1	55
Borage oil	1	65

Fish that tend to be rich in omega-threes include salmon, sardines, albacore tuna, anchovies, herring, mackerel, and rainbow trout.

Exact EFA concentrations vary with climate. Cold, northerly conditions favor more EFAs in general, and a greater quantity of omega-threes in particular. Warm, southerly conditions favor lesser quantities of EFAs, even within the same species.

Processing also affects the quality of the oil you consume. EFAs are damaged by heat, light, and oxygen, which help to turn oils rancid. The seed oils you buy should be expeller-pressed without the use of solvents. They should be unrefined, unbleached, undeodorized, stored in opaque containers, sealed with an inert gas like nitrogen. Because oils accumulate pesticides, the seeds from which they are pressed should be certified as organically grown. The seeds should not have been cooked or tempered prior to pressing. Store oils in the refrigerator or freezer and discard six weeks after opening the bottle.

bought in small quantities, stored in the dark, and kept refrigerated; it should not be used for cooking.

Because EFAs are polyunsaturated, containing two or more double chemical bonds, they are prone to rancidity, not merely in foods but also in the human body. Rancidity occurs when the double bond is broken by oxygen, producing an oxidized fatty acid. Oxidized fatty acids not only taste bad, they behave badly, disrupting the normal functioning of the cell membranes of which they are a part. Oxidized fatty acids are rapidly generated from the process called free radical–induced cell damage (see pages 204–205).

To protect EFAs from harmful oxidation, it is essential to consume adequate levels of dietary antioxidants, especially vitamin E. Consumption of a nutrient-dense diet will assure a higher-than-average intake of all antioxidants. Foods especially rich in antioxidants are listed in the tables "Nutrients Needed for EFA Utilization" (p. 134) and "Top Dietary Sources of Antioxidants" (p. 206). Depending upon the specific foods you choose, however, where those foods have been grown, your efficiency of digestion and absorption, your individual need for EFAs, and the presence of inflammation within your body, you may need to supplement your diet with additional antioxidants. If you take fish oil or flax oil supplements you should consider an antioxidant supplement in addition. For adults, I generally recommend one tablespoon (ten grams) of flax oil or three grams (usually three capsules) of fish oil, plus four hundred milligrams of vitamin E, two thousand milligrams of vitamin C, and one hundred micrograms of selenium, in addition to—not instead of—a nutrient-dense diet.[36]

Although most Americans consume more than enough omega-six EFAs, there is a small but significant proportion of the population (about 15 percent, if my patients are in any way representative) who are unable to properly metabolize omega-six EFAs and will benefit from supplementation with oils that are rich in omega-sixes. The three most useful omega-six-rich oils are evening primrose oil, borage oil, and black currant seed oil, all of which are sold in capsule form. These oils contain a special EFA called gamma-linolenic acid (GLA), which allows the body to overcome the most common impediment to proper utilization of omega-six EFAs. Although experimental data indicate

that consuming large doses of omega-six-rich oils such as corn oil or safflower oil can promote the growth of cancer, there is no evidence that
consuming GLA in the form of primrose oil contributes to cancer.
Quite the contrary, primrose oil behaves like the omega-three-rich oils
(flaxseed and fish) in actually preventing tumor growth in experimental animals.[37] The usual requirement for GLA among those who need
it is supplied by taking four to six capsules of evening primrose oil, two
to three capsules of borage oil, or three to four capsules of black currant
seed oil every day (assuming each capsule contains five hundred milligrams of oil). I generally reserve GLA supplements for people whose
dryness does not respond to omega-three supplementation. Because
the omega-three and omega-six EFAs compete with one another in the
body, feeding fish oil to a person who needs GLA may actually increase
that person's omega-six deficit, making the skin dryer or the breasts
more tender. An increase in these symptoms with omega-three supplements is almost surely a sign to switch to GLA. Lack of response is usually a reason to add GLA. Controlled studies have demonstrated
therapeutic benefits for people suffering from arthritis, eczema, and
premenstrual syndrome.[38] What is important in making therapeutic decisions, however, is not the disease but the patient. EFA therapy does
not treat disease, it improves cellular function.

Linda Samuels is a petite, cheerful young woman with a scary medical
history. At the age of twenty-five she developed pain in her eyes and
blurred vision. An ophthalmologist told her she had an inflammation
of the optic nerve, a condition called optic neuritis. She was given a
short course of prednisone (a form of cortisone), which suppressed the
inflammation and cleared away her symptoms. Two years later, her
blurred vision and eye pain returned, and again disappeared with prednisone. Optic neuritis is frightening not only because it can cause
blindness, but because it can be a forerunner of multiple sclerosis
(MS), an inflammatory disorder of the brain and spinal cord that tends
to strike people in the prime of life.
    The way in which MS is defined is almost the opposite of the way in
which schizophrenia is defined. Schizophrenia is a clinical syndrome
in which there are no consistent pathological abnormalities in the tissues of the body. MS is defined by its pathological lesions—multiple

patches of hardening (sclerosis) of nerve tissue, caused by a loss of the oily insulation (myelin) that coats and protects most nerve cells. Loss of myelin, in turn, is caused by inflammation of the nerves. The cause or causes of MS are unknown. The dominant theory today is that MS results from an autoimmune reaction that attacks the brain and spinal cord, provoked by an unknown infection, probably due to a virus. The consistent pathology of MS is responsible for its being considered a discrete disease entity, even though its clinical pattern is highly variable and unpredictable. Tingling in the hands and feet or complete numbness with loss of feeling indicate damage to nerves involved in registering sensation. Weakness of muscles, which can progress to total paralysis, is a sign of damage to nerves controlling movement. Double vision or slurred speech indicates impairment of the nerves to the head. These symptoms may wax and wane, disappear completely, or relentlessly progress.

Linda was working as a clerk in a community hospital in Massachusetts and had seen the devastation that MS could bring to a healthy adult. She was terrified. When both her feet began to feel as if they were on fire at all times and her left foot began to drag when she was running, Linda panicked. She consulted two neurologists and had two thorough examinations, including a spinal tap and an MRI. One told her she had MS; the other told her she didn't. The results of the MRI were in dispute. One radiologist believed he could see the patches of inflammation on the scan; another read the scan as "probably normal." Her condition appeared too mild and stable to warrant prolonged administration of cortisone, so no treatment was recommended. Linda, however, had to care for two young children and was *not* about to do nothing while she waited to see if her condition worsened. After researching MS, she began to follow a very-low-fat, nutrient-dense diet, which had first been recommended in 1950 by Dr. Roy Swank of the Oregon Health Sciences University. Swank had reasoned that MS, like coronary heart disease, appeared primarily in countries with a high consumption of animal fat and might be caused by the stiffness of cell membranes and sludging of blood that such diets encourage. He advocated a largely vegetarian diet, devoid of animal fat, supplemented with small quantities of vegetable oil. The complete absence of MS among the Inuit (Eskimos), who have a very high intake of fish oils, led Swank to advocate cod liver oil as part of the treatment. Linda had followed

Swank's directions carefully and added flax oil as an additional source of EFAs. Although Swank's data indicate that patients who followed his regimen fared better than those who did not,[39] neither low-fat diets nor EFA supplements have become standard therapy for MS. In fact, there has been no standard therapy for MS, because no drug has been shown to alter the long-term prognosis.[40]

During five years on the Swank diet, Linda fared pretty well. She had no further episodes of optic neuritis and no progression of muscle weakness. She even recovered enough strength in her foot to be able to walk or run without a limp. After running, however, her legs would feel weak and seemed to move slowly, and her feet continued to burn every day.

Linda came to see me because she wanted another opinion. She wanted me to tell her that she did not have MS after all. Unfortunately, Linda's reflexes were distinctly abnormal. When I tapped her knees, her lower leg jerked forward with such startling force that it made her laugh.

"How long have your reflexes been like that?" I asked.

"I don't know," she replied. "I know they weren't so strong when I was first examined five years ago."

A hyperactive reflex of this type does not necessarily mean the patient has MS, but it may indicate damage to the nerves that descend from the brain to the spinal cord (called *upper motor neurons*). When I pushed on the sole of her foot, flexing the foot upward, her foot responded by snapping downward and then shaking up and down several times, uncontrollably. This reflex action, which is called ankle clonus, is very unusual in individuals who do not have damage of the upper motor neurons. My heart sank. I hated to see these results.

"Linda," I explained, "I know you want me to say that you don't have MS. I can't say that. Your reflexes are abnormal, your feet burn and tingle, your legs are weak, and you've had optic neuritis. Clearly, something is damaging nerves. Fortunately, this damage is mild and has stayed mild. Maybe you've controlled it with the Swank diet. What I can do is to help identify factors that may stimulate healing. Even when MS appears to be certain, vitamin B_{12} injections can be helpful.[41] Let's look at *you*, without attempting to put a more definite label on your disease, and see if there's a way to help heal your nerves."

One of Linda's most striking characteristics was the dryness of her hands, which had the consistency of sandpaper. Her skin in general was dull and lacking in luster, her nails appeared frayed, and her hair was stiff.

"How long has your skin been like this?" I asked.

"I don't know." She shrugged. "A long time, I guess."

"Has it gotten worse over the past five years, since you've been on the low-fat diet? What was your skin like before?"

She looked at her husband, who stood attentively by the side of the examination table. "Maybe it's worse now," he said, "but you've been using hand cream as long as I've known you."

"The Swank diet seems to suit you well," I said to her, "but it may be short on essential fatty acids. You're avoiding saturated fat and *trans*-fats, which is good. The extra oils you're eating should give you a fair intake of omega-three EFAs; these are important for the nervous system. But this program is not doing anything for your skin. You may not be getting enough of the omega-six EFAs. Try taking primrose oil for a few weeks. Let's see what happens."

When I examined Linda again four weeks later, the burning sensations in her feet had virtually disappeared and the skin on her hands was barely peeling, although it was still somewhat dry. I was thrilled to find that her reflexes were normal now; there was no hyperactivity and no ankle clonus. Linda remained without symptoms for three years, as long as she maintained her use of primrose oil. When she stopped, her hands again began to peel and her feet to tingle and burn.

I do *not* consider primrose oil to be a treatment for MS. I have seen many patients with MS who showed no response to the Swank diet or any EFA supplementation. Primrose oil is a treatment for *Linda*; it meets her own, individual metabolic needs, and in so doing it provides her with a chemical balance that reverses both the symptoms and signs of neurologic damage.

The right nutritionist will help you determine if your diet includes the correct balance of EFAs and antioxidants.

Level Three: Balancing Calcium with Magnesium

Magnesium is the fourth most abundant mineral in the body. Calcium is the most abundant. At many levels of the cell, magnesium opposes calcium, blocking its effects.[42] Just as EFAs, as precursors of the prostanoids, are natural guardians of cell function, so is magnesium, as nature's calcium blocker. If excess free calcium produces a state of cellular responsiveness that is excessively *yang*, the effects of magnesium can be seen as favoring *yin*. It is not surprising that the modern diseases that run rampant through Western society, like heart disease, high blood pressure, asthma, and migraine headaches, are often accompanied by magnesium deficiency.[43]

Americans generally consume diets that are low in magnesium and that fail to meet the government's recommended daily allowance, 300 to 350 milligrams.[44] Magnesium intake is lower than average among people who develop heart disease or asthma, and the administration of magnesium by intravenous injection can ameliorate the symptoms of asthma or the complications of a heart attack.[45] But people become magnesium-deficient even when their diets are quite adequate and, for many of my patients, a diet of high nutrient density is unable to correct magnesium deficiency. The key to this mystery appears to be the intimate, reciprocal association between magnesium depletion and stress.[46]

The most exacting research on the stress/magnesium relationship has been done in Berlin and Paris, using human volunteers. Men and women who are exposed to chronic noise, either traffic noise or occupational noise in a factory, develop irritability, fatigue, and loss of concentration. Levels of adrenaline, a stress hormone, increase in their blood. Under conditions of mental or physical stress, magnesium is released from cells and goes into the blood, from which it is excreted into the urine. Chronic stress depletes the body of magnesium. The more stressed the individual, the greater the loss of magnesium. The lower the person's level of magnesium at the beginning of the observation period, the more reactive to stress the individual becomes and the more his or her magnesium level is lowered in stressful situations. Administering magnesium as a nutritional supplement raises blood levels of the mineral and buffers the response to stress. Magnesium supplements can build resistance to the effects of stress.

Personality has an effect on this cycle. Students who must take an exam while being distracted with noise may also lower their magnesium levels. This effect occurs only in students who show the "type A," competitive, heart-disease-prone behavior pattern; it does not occur in their less competitive colleagues. It appears that the body's magnesium economy is an integral part of the stress response system. When stressed for any reason, the body's hormonal response causes an outpouring of magnesium from cells into the blood. This outpouring is a bit like taking magnesium by injection, except the source is internal. The effect of the sudden increase in magnesium is both energizing and calming. Magnesium is needed to burn sugar for energy; it also calms the excitation of cells produced by the stress-induced release of calcium. If there is insufficient dietary magnesium, or if there is insufficient rest in between episodes of stress, the body's magnesium stores are slowly depleted. The hormonal response to stress disintegrates. The blood level of magnesium does not elevate in response to stress as it should, so that the energizing/calming effect of magnesium isn't available to counter the nerve-jangling effects of adrenaline and other stress hormones. Consequently, your stress is intensified and your ability to cope is impaired.

Laboratory tests for magnesium may not be useful in evaluating the need for magnesium, because blood magnesium levels fluctuate, depending upon where you are in the cycle of stress responses and magnesium depletion. Your symptoms are a better guide. Muscle tension, spasm, and twitching are the most characteristic symptoms of magnesium depletion, followed by palpitation and breathlessness. Irritability, fatigue, trouble falling asleep, and hypersensitivity to loud noises are also common. The presence of migraine or tension headache, unexplained chest pain, strange sensations of the skin (like insects crawling), and abdominal pain or constipation are further indications of magnesium deficiency. If these symptoms do not respond to a diet of high nutrient density, your nutritionist might want you to try magnesium, in addition to other treatments that may seem appropriate.

The best-absorbed dietary supplement is magnesium glycinate, which is available in tablets, but there are many forms of magnesium available in drugstores and health food stores, and they may all be helpful to some people. The dose needed varies from one hundred milligrams to about five hundred milligrams per day of elemental magnesium. Magnesium is never sold as magnesium alone; it comes combined with another type of molecule (chloride, carbonate, oxide, gluconate, etc.). Most of the weight of the compound is not due to magnesium but to the other substance. Magnesium chloride, for example, is only one-fourth magnesium and three-fourths chloride. So, four hundred milligrams of magnesium chloride contains one hundred milligrams of elemental magnesium. Too much magnesium can cause diarrhea, which is its main and virtually its only side effect. Magnesium taken by mouth in quantities no greater than five hundred milligrams daily is generally very safe, except in people who suffer from kidney disease or are severely dehydrated. These people may develop levels of magnesium in blood that are too high; that's why you should only take magnesium supplements under strict medical supervision. Just as magnesium taken at bedtime can induce sleep, so high blood levels of magnesium may cause drowsiness and lethargy.

There are occasional individuals with symptoms of magnesium depletion who do not respond well to magnesium supplements. Either the symptoms of deficiency are not corrected or they actually seem to intensify. These people often benefit from calcium supplementation. It seems paradoxical that taking calcium should have the same effect for some people that taking magnesium has for others. There are elements of balance that are hard to measure or even to understand. Calcium

---

TOP DIETARY SOURCES OF MAGNESIUM

Vegetables
> buckwheat (kasha), mature lima beans, navy beans, kidney beans, green beans, soybeans (tofu), black-eyed peas, spinach, Swiss chard

Grains
> oats, whole barley, millet

Fruits
> bananas, blackberries, dates, dried figs, mangoes, watermelons

Nuts, Seeds
> almonds, Brazil nuts, cashews, hazelnuts

Seafood
> shrimp, tuna

TOP DIETARY SOURCES OF CALCIUM

Dairy Products
  skim milk, low-fat yogurt, hard cheeses

Seafood
  sardines, canned salmon, shrimp, scallops, oysters

Fruit
  calcium-fortified orange juice

Nuts, Seeds
  almonds, Brazil nuts, hazelnuts

Grains
  tortillas

Legumes
  calcium-fortified soy products, lentils

Vegetables
  arugula, kale, broccoli spears, bok choy, collards,
    dandelion greens, turnip greens, mustard greens
    (spinach and Swiss chard are rich in calcium but
    also rich in oxalic acid, which prevents calcium
    absorption)

---

supplements have been shown to be capable of lowering blood pressure, even though the effect of raising the calcium concentration in blood is to raise blood pressure. The reason for this paradoxical effect appears to be that—for some people—taking extra calcium by mouth actually stimulates the body to inactivate calcium more efficiently. The response to calcium supplements is then an anticalcium response that may behave much like the effects of magnesium supplements. Each person must ultimately serve as his own experimental control under his doctor's supervision. If symptoms such as muscle spasm, palpitation, and anxiety do not respond to magnesium alone, then add calcium.

Although calcium is best absorbed when taken with meals, calcium blocks the absorption of other minerals in food, especially iron and zinc. Taking calcium supplements with meals every day may result in iron or zinc deficiency. It is safer to take calcium an hour before meals or at bedtime. However, if you don't take them with food, most calcium pills are not well absorbed. The best form to take is, therefore, calcium citrate or calcium apatite, because they do not require stomach acid to render them soluble. People who need calcium supplements generally have to take 750 to 1,200 milligrams of elemental calcium per day. If the label does not specify the amount of *elemental calcium* in each dose, it may be referring to the total amount of the calcium compound in each pill. Calcium citrate and calcium hydroxyapatite are each only about 15 to 20 percent calcium by weight, so each pill will contain only 150 to 250 milligrams of calcium. There are some calcium supplements I do not recommend. These include chewable tablets containing talc, like Tums, and "natural" supplements of bone meal, dolomite, and oyster shell. Talc promotes tumors in animals, and bone meal, dolomite, and oyster shell are sometimes contaminated with toxic metals like lead.

Much has been written about the need to balance the calcium/magnesium ratio when taking supplements. However rational or irrational that notion may be in the abstract, in real life there is no set ratio that applies to everyone. People who take magnesium supplements do not automatically require extra calcium. In France, where therapy with magnesium pills has been widespread for thirty years, calcium is rarely given in conjunction with magnesium. There is no evidence that magnesium pills interfere with calcium absorption. Calcium and magnesium are absorbed into the body by distinct and separate mechanisms. Similarly, people who benefit from calcium supplements do not necessarily have to take extra magnesium, although many women who are taking calcium for the purpose of preventing osteoporosis may well need magnesium in addition. There is a growing body of evidence that magnesium in the diet is as important for prevention of osteoporosis as is calcium.[47] The rule with regard to calcium and magnesium is the same as the rule for EFAs. First, follow a diet of high nutrient density. Next, base supplementation on your specific symptoms and adjust your dosage according to how those symptoms change after you begin taking supplements. Allow about a month for changes to occur.

To nourish the cells of your body for optimal function:

- Read labels. Avoid foods that contain added sugar (including dextrose and corn sweetener), salt, or fat (including partially hydrogenated vegetable oils).
- Eat at least three servings of vegetables and two servings of fruit a day (iceberg lettuce, potatoes, and cucumbers should not be counted as vegetables, or you shortchange yourself).
- Buy fresh local produce in season.
- Just before eating, wash and peel produce or scrub clean with a soft brush.
- Eat nuts and seeds either whole or ground into nut butters: almonds, walnuts, sesame, sunflower, and pumpkin seeds are the most nutritious.
- Eat whole grains like brown rice and oatmeal and low-fat ocean fish like cod or haddock.
- If you suffer from dry skin, dry hair, brittle nails, dandruff, painful menstrual cramps, or premenstrual breast pain, supplement your diet with organic flaxseed oil, one tablespoon a day, plus vitamin E 400 mg/day, vitamin C 1,000 mg/day, and selenium 100 mcg/day. If flax oil does not help, add evening primrose oil, six capsules/day.
- If you suffer from a combination of common symptoms that include muscle spasm or tension, palpitations, irritability, anxiety, insomnia, fatigue, or frequent headaches, add a supplement of magnesium supplying 200 to 400 mg of elemental magnesium/day. (Too much magnesium may cause diarrhea.) If the symptoms do not improve, add enough calcium to supply 750 to 1,200 mg of elemental calcium/day. (Too much calcium may be constipating.)

My advice is to stay attuned to your own body's signals. A one-size-fits-all diet plan cannot by design fit your individual needs. You will need to work closely with your doctor/nutritionist to create the diet that suits you best.

EXERCISE

Exercise is a second component of *díaita* that has received attention from scientists. Moderate-intensity exercise, such as brisk walking thirty minutes a day, improves immune function and mood, prevents migraines, lowers blood pressure, and decreases the disability that affects inactive people as they age.[48] Both the level of activity and the general level of fitness are important. In Norway, where I now know that snacking is rare, a study was done in which apparently healthy middle-aged men had their exercise capacity (aerobic fitness) assessed by pedaling a stationary bicycle. Sixteen years later, the medical records of all men were inspected. Those whose exercise capacity placed them in the lowest quarter at the beginning of the study were twice as likely to have died by the study's end than those in the highest fitness category.[49]

The intensity and duration of physical activity needed for promoting optimal health is not known. The Centers for Disease Control and Prevention recommend thirty minutes a day of moderate-intensity exercise for everyone. It is estimated that a quarter million deaths per year in the United States could be prevented by regular physical activity at this level of intensity. Walking at a rate of three to four miles per hour is moderate intensity for most adults. So is cycling at a speed of five to ten miles per hour, swimming at modest speed, calisthenics, racquet sports (including doubles tennis and Ping-Pong), golfing without a power cart, mowing the lawn with a power mower, general housecleaning (but not vacuuming, which is less demanding). The activity need not be performed continuously, but can be broken up into three to four bouts of eight to ten minutes each. Although this level of activity is quite modest and easily attainable, fewer than 25 percent of U.S. adults meet it.[50] Moderate activity for more than thirty minutes a day yields greater benefits than being active for less time, but it is not yet certain whether vigorous activity has greater health benefits than moderate activity. Vigorous activity includes running, cycling at speeds faster than ten miles per hour, fast swimming, singles tennis, racquetball, or the use of aerobic exercise machines like stair climbers. One study, which followed the death rates of Harvard alumni, found that those who engaged in vigorous sports for three hours a week were healthier than those who performed moderate-intensity exercise.[51] Exercise appears to influence health by acting on levels of chemical mediators. Aerobic fitness increases the activity of the endorphin system, a complex of chemical mediators with natural morphinelike actions, which modulate stress responses, mood, and immune function.[52] Increased endorphin levels with exercise are thought to account for the "runner's high."

Despite the pleasurable effects of physical activity, many people find it too hard to stick to an exercise routine. My view is that people are not machines, there are too many "should's" in life to begin with, and the best course for most of us is to find one or more activities that are enjoyable or necessary enough to be incorporated into our daily lives. Walking is an excellent place to start and you can share it with friends at different levels of physical fitness. One recent study found that brisk walking for thirty to forty-five minutes three times a week decreased the risk of heart attack among postmenopausal women by 50 percent![53] To markedly increase the intensity of exertion at any speed of walking, wear a small backpack and place five to ten pounds of anything in it. A study done with Israeli army recruits found that walking with a pack was highly effective at increasing fitness.[54]

The main problem with walking is that it does little for agility, coordination, flexibility, or general muscle strength. Some additional activity, such as dancing, low-impact aerobics, yoga, calisthenics, or t'ai chi, performed once or twice a week, can enhance and maintain fitness from youth into old age.

SLEEP AND RELAXATION

Sleep and relaxation, the third component of *díaita*, should concern more modern physicians. We tend to think of sleep in negative terms, as a time when we are not awake. Sleep is an active time, however, during which the body restores itself. Unfortunately, over 50 percent of Americans are sleep-deprived, failing to regularly obtain the amount of sleep they need. Signs of sleep deprivation can be easy to spot. If you doze off readily in a boring meeting or lecture or if you cannot awaken in the morning without an alarm clock, you are probably operating with insufficient sleep. Getting more sleep is a normal response to infection and appears to favor recovery. Sleep deprivation of experimental animals increases their susceptibility to viral and bacterial infection, and in humans, insomnia reduces natural killer cell activity.[55] Healthy young men awakened from sleep between 3:00 and 7:00 A.M. show a 30 percent dip in natural killer cell activity the next morning.[56] The natural sleep requirement of adults varies from as little as six to as much as ten hours per day, with most people needing seven to nine hours, preferably without interruption. Incredibly, hospitals—the places where patients need the most sleep—seem designed to induce sleep deprivation, because of their noise levels, their lighting, and the usual routines of patient care.

Daytime relaxation also has important health benefits. A period of quiet, focused relaxation each day may lower blood pressure, relieve anxiety, improve nighttime sleep, and decrease the discomfort of chronic headache and other painful conditions.[57] Relaxation includes meditation, prayer, or systematic relaxation of all voluntary muscles in the body. Dr. Herbert Benson, of Harvard University, developed the theory that focused relaxation stimulates an integrated response in the brain, which actively buffers stress responses. He called this the relaxation response.[58] One mechanism by which the relaxation response buffers the effects of stress may be through reducing the body's responses to the effects of stress hormones like adrenaline.[59] The evocation of a relaxation response is not dependent upon the use of any particular technique. Dr. Charles Stroebel of the Institute of Living in Hartford, Connecticut, who used the term "quieting response," found that people who learn to induce this response regularly can relax briefly but deeply at will, and may automatically relax themselves several times a day, even in the midst of a busy schedule.[60]

7

THE THIRD PILLAR:
YOUR ENVIRONMENT

MIASMATA

Sidney Shaw had just retired from his job with a Milwaukee insurance agency when he had his first heart attack. He was relaxing in front of the television set after spending three hours at his favorite pastime, refinishing old furniture down in his basement. A crushing pain, like an elephant stepping on his breastbone, sent him into a sweat. He called his personal physician, who met him at the emergency room of the local hospital. Sidney had been stripping paint from an antique oak chest. Thinking that the chemicals in the paint stripper might be irritating his lungs, he brought the bottle of paint remover with him to the hospital. His doctor read the label, which identified the main ingredient as methylene chloride and cautioned that it should only be used with adequate ventilation. The doctor informed Sidney that the problem was not the paint stripper; it was his heart. The electrocardiogram showed that he was having a minor heart attack, a small myocardial infarction, which is the death of a segment of heart muscle, usually caused by lack of oxygen resulting from a blocked artery. Sidney was admitted to the coronary care unit and started on treatment with oxygen.

Sidney recovered rapidly. A week later he was sent home and two weeks later he returned to his basement to finish stripping paint from the oak chest. After another three hours in his workshop, the crushing chest pain recurred. His wife called an ambulance and he was rushed to the emergency room, this time suffering from a major heart attack, complicated by cardiogenic shock. Once again he was lucky. He was among the 20 percent who survive cardiogenic shock. After three weeks in the hospital, he returned home, on medication intended to control his heart failure, and began a program of cardiac rehabilitation with slowly increasing exercise. Despite the extensive damage to his heart muscle, he progressed well, and within six months was ready to resume his previous level of physical activity.

Sidney's next trip to the basement was his last. Six months after his second heart attack, he decided to finish the job of stripping paint from the oak chest, working slowly with the help of his wife to minimize his physical exertion. He died before the ambulance arrived. Had his doctor bothered to investigate the toxicity of methylene chloride, he would have learned that it is rapidly converted in the body to carbon monoxide, a deadly poison that prevents the blood from carrying oxygen. Carbon monoxide kills people by internal suffocation. It can cause heart attacks in people whose blood vessels are narrow but not fully blocked, because it deprives the heart of oxygen.[1]

Sidney Shaw's untimely death illustrates two important, related shortcomings of contemporary medical practice. The first, and more obvious, is the general disregard of physicians for environmental triggers of disease. The second, and more profound, is the reason for this disregard: diseases are thought of as entities that exist independent of context. "Environmental diseases" exist as a category of disease entities that do not ordinarily include heart attacks. Once the doctor had made a diagnosis—myocardial infarction—he assumed that he knew all he needed to know about his patient.

Dismissal of environmental influences on illness has changed little in the twenty years since Sidney's death. Consider the strange case of Kim O'Shea.

Kim is a slim and athletic beautician who couldn't understand why she was gaining so much weight at the age of twenty-six. She cut back on her snacks and increased her exercise. It didn't help. In one month she gained over thirty pounds. Her ankles swelled, then her thighs. When her abdomen became so distended that she couldn't breathe, her boyfriend took her to an emergency room. The problem was obvious: fluid retention (edema) so drastic it produced a condition that at one time was called "dropsy." Edema starts in the toes and builds up—like water filling a well—until it reaches the thighs, fills the abdominal cavity, and begins invading the chest. The cause was also obvious: kidney disease. Kim was losing massive amounts of protein in her urine and retaining huge quantities of water and salt. This condition is called "nephrotic syndrome" or sometimes just "nephrosis." It has many causes.

Kim was admitted to a large community hospital near her home and treated with a strong diuretic drug called Lasix. She lost twenty pounds of fluid within three days and was able to breathe comfortably, but her blood pressure dropped so low she couldn't stand up. A kidney specialist (a nephrologist) was called in. Because nephrotic syndrome usually results from autoimmunity, he prescribed cortisone to suppress Kim's immune system. Initially this proved very helpful. Within a week there was no swelling in Kim's legs and no protein in her urine. Then her face started to swell, turning round as a pumpkin. She gained fifteen pounds of fat. These were side effects of cortisone. The nephrologist tried to lower the dose. Every time he lowered it, nephrotic syndrome would flare up, the first sign being a large amount of protein in her urine. The nephrologist prescribed another drug, Cytoxan, which is a stronger immune suppressant than cortisone. As its name implies, Cytoxan is a highly toxic drug, ordinarily used to treat leukemia. Kim refused to take it and allowed her uncle, a dentist, to bring her to New York to see me.

I hadn't treated a patient with nephrotic syndrome in many years, but for me the issue was not the disease but the patient. Was there something I could discover about Kim and the context in which her sickness had occurred that would suggest an alternative therapeutic strategy? What I learned was critically important.

About six months before developing nephrotic syndrome, Kim had developed asthma. She had been treated at the local hospital and referred to an allergist who found that she was allergic to dust and mold and most of the common airborne allergens. She was treated with drugs to help her breathing and with allergy shots. At the time she developed asthma, her main work as a beautician was applying artificial nails, using acrylic adhesives. Fearing that these may have caused her asthma, she stopped working with nails and started doing facials, but the asthma continued without abatement. When she started taking cortisone for nephrotic syndrome, her asthma disappeared, because cortisone blocks the inflammation of the bronchial tubes that occurs with asthma.

Asthma is often considered to be an allergic disease; nephrotic syndrome is not. The way that doctors think about nephrotic syndrome reveals a good deal about what is wrong with the practice of medicine. Nephrotic syndrome is thought to be caused by a cluster of different diseases, with each disease representing a "distinct clinico-pathologic entity."[2] What this means is that the pathology (visible patterns of abnormality in the tissue) seen in the kidney determines the nature of the disease. After a kidney biopsy, the pathologist studies the kidney cells under the microscope and classifies the pathology as separate diseases. They are given names like "minimal change nephritis," "membranous nephritis," and "segmental glomerulosclerosis," based upon the pattern of visual abnormalities. Specialists believe that to effectively treat nephrotic syndrome, one has to know its cause, and the "cause" is usually minimal change, membranous or segmental disease.

Over the years, I have developed a very different way of thinking about pathology. Pathology does not *cause* disease. It is merely another *manifestation* of the disease process, no more significant than the symptoms the patient describes or the external signs identified by the doctor. Pathology is an inadequate explanation for sickness and frequently is unrelated to the presence or severity of signs or symptoms.[3] In the case of nephrotic syndrome, those patients with the worst fluid retention and protein loss usually have the least visible pathology in the kidney.

I approached Kim's sickness by disregarding her pathology and examining her *story*. The key fact was that the development of nephrotic syndrome was probably preceded by occupational exposure to a toxic substance that had provoked an allergic disease.

Acrylic adhesives are capable of damaging the lining of the respiratory tract,[4] and the solvents that are used to remove them may be capable of damaging the cells of the kidneys.[5] With regard to Kim's lungs, the damage had resulted in her developing allergic asthma, which had continued even after exposure to the damaging chemicals had been stopped. Why shouldn't her kidney ailment involve a similar mechanism?

These thoughts rushed through my mind as I wrote down the details of her story. I remembered reading some letters in the highly regarded British medical journal *The Lancet*, written by physicians who had seen cases of nephrotic syndrome provoked by allergic reactions to food. What is fascinating about these reports is that food allergy provoked nephrotic syndrome with different types of kidney pathology. Some food allergic reactions caused "minimal change disease"; some caused "glomerulosclerosis." The pathology was irrelevant. Patients with any type of pathology improved if the offending food was eliminated from the diet. It was the patients' specific sensitivities, *not* the disease category, that mattered.[6]

"If you want to avoid Cytoxan," I told Kim in earnest, "you're going to have to try a drastic experiment. It's not harmful, but it will take a great deal of discipline. We'll know whether it works in less than a week." I explained my thoughts about the possible allergic basis of her illness and recommended two major environmental changes: First, she would temporarily leave her dust-laden, mold-ridden apartment and stay with her cousin's family. Second, she would give up her usual food and drink. Instead, she would follow a modified fast, consuming nothing but water and a specially prepared powder called UltraClear,[7] which is practically nonallergenic. She would slowly lower the dose of cortisone and would check her urine for protein every day using a commercially available kit.

I anxiously awaited our first follow-up appointment a week later. The experiment had worked! There was no protein in her urine, she had lost nine pounds of fluid, and she was soon able to discontinue cortisone. Encouraged by this outcome, Kim slowly reintroduced food, one item each day, and continued to check her urine for protein. Eggs appeared to be the main culprit. The morning after reintroducing eggs into her diet, she was leaking protein into her urine for the first time in three weeks. When she avoided eggs, protein again disappeared. By avoiding eggs, she has been perfectly well for three years, off all medication, with no recurrence of nephrosis or asthma. Kim needs to be very careful about what she eats, of course, because eggs are a hidden ingredient in numerous foods, especially pastries and sauces, and she exercises great caution with exposure to chemicals at work.

SICK BUILDINGS, SICK PEOPLE

In the industrialized nations of the world, people spend 90 percent of their time indoors, and the greatest airborne health risks may be posed by indoor air pollutants. Occupational exposures are common. A survey of outpatients seen in the primary care clinic of a Midwest hospital found that three-quarters of the men interviewed had been exposed to at least one potentially toxic agent at work and over 30 percent had been exposed to more than four potential toxins. Chemical fumes, solvents, pesticides, and asbestos were the most common exposures.[8] For many of my patients, the presence of an indoor toxic exposure has gone unnoticed until after illness develops: A school undergoes construction while classes continue, causing a high rate of sickness among students and teachers. At another school with a poorly vented furnace, children come home smelling of soot and their school performance deteriorates. In one concert hall in which the air intake vents leading to the orchestra pit are located above the loading dock where trucks idle, the musicians become sick. In a bedroom in which the condensation beneath a waterbed is slowly disintegrating the particleboard frame, releasing fumes of formaldehyde, the residents suffer insomnia, profound fatigue, and bouts of coughing.

Toxic exposures to specific chemicals encountered at work account for 70,000 deaths a year in the United States, with 350,000 new cases of occupationally related environmental illness appearing each year.[9] Beyond disease caused by individual toxins lies a broad spectrum of health problems caused by the buildings in which people work.

The World Health Organization has defined the "sick building syndrome" as a group disease, the occurrence of excessive work- or school-related illness among workers or students in buildings of recent construction.[10] The symptoms may include lethargy, dry or sore throat, stuffy nose, headache, irritation of the eyes, chest tightness, impaired memory and concentration, dizziness, nausea, itching, skin rash, and shortness of breath.[11] In about one-quarter of the cases, a specific source of indoor air pollution can be found: either an accumulation of motor vehicle exhaust or contamination of a humidification system with mold, producing allergic reactions among the building's occupants.[12] In most cases, however, no single source of contamination can be identified. Yet a survey of nine thousand office workers in three European countries found that 50 to 80 percent of those working in modern office buildings reported symptoms typical of the sick building syndrome. At any one time, ten to twenty-five million workers in a million U.S. office buildings suffer from building-related illness. The personal and economic impact of this modern miasma is considerable, because symptomatic workers feel lousy, have reduced productivity, and are absent more.[13]

The original name of sick building syndrome was "tight building syndrome." It was believed that tightly sealed buildings, which do not allow much outside air to seep in, acted like sumps to concentrate the level of indoor air pollutants. This theory has not been borne out. Increasing the supply of outdoor air does not prevent or relieve the symptoms of people working in sick buildings.[14] It appears that sick building syndrome is caused by the presence of chemical toxins or airborne microbes that cannot merely be diluted away.

Two broad categories of pollutants have been implicated as the culprits. The first category are *volatile organic compounds* (VOCs), invisible gases emitted from paints, adhesives, carpeting, wall coverings, new furniture, building materials, solvents, cleaning solutions, copy machines, and laser printers. Studies using experimental chambers have shown that VOCs can cause irritation of the respiratory system in humans and animals at levels one hundred times weaker than permissible exposure levels or the World Health Organization Indoor Air Guidelines. Controlled experiments with people who describe themselves as sensitive to VOCs confirm that VOC exposure causes headache, fatigue, and difficulty concentrating. People who deny such sensitivity also experience symptoms but do not experience mental impairment when exposed. Air samples of buildings with and without sick-building complaints have established an association between VOC exposure and human sickness.[15]

The second category of sick-building culprits are the *bioaerosols*, which consist of living bacteria or fungi (molds and yeasts) or their toxic by-products or fragments, circulating in the air supply. If live microbes circulate as aerosols, respiratory infection may occur. Legionnaires' disease is the best-known example. An epidemic of pneumonia (182 cases, with 29 deaths) disrupted an American Legion convention in a Philadelphia hotel during the summer of 1976. The epidemic was traced to a bacterial species, subsequently named *Legionella pneumophila*, which contaminated the hotel's air-conditioning system. At least 20,000 cases of Legionnaires' disease occur in the United States every year. There are twenty different species of *Legionella* bacteria. They all thrive in stagnant water and have caused epidemics of flulike illness in resorts and hotels throughout the world.

Some scientists believe that fungal or bacterial *toxins* may be responsible for the more common symptoms of sick building syndrome. European studies reveal that sick building syndrome is more likely to occur in air-conditioned buildings than in buildings with natural ventilation. This has generated the theory that accumulation of water in ventilation ducts supports the growth of microbes, which disperse fragments of their membranes or toxic secretions into the air ducts.[16] A recent study from the Georgia Environmental Technology Consortium found that samples of fungi (molds) growing in sick buildings actually produce their own VOCs identical to the VOCs originating in building materials.[17]

VOCs and fungi can cause disease in private homes as well as public buildings. In 1991, I served as consultant to the New York State Attorney General's Office in an investigation of dozens of cases of sickness that followed the installation of new carpeting in homes. The major symptoms were those of sick building syndrome. The attorney general's report listed over a hundred VOCs given off by new synthetic carpet, some of them known to cause brain dysfunction or cancer. The normal emissions from some commercial carpets are toxic enough to cause disease in laboratory animals.[18] The extent of human sickness resulting from household pollution with VOCs is unknown, because these substances have not been present at high concentrations in homes for more than a generation. It is worth noting, however, that benzene derivatives, which may be given off by a variety of household products, including nylon carpet, moth crystals, and "air fresheners," can initiate and promote the growth of cancer.[19]

THE DANGERS OF MOLD

In contrast to VOCs, mold is an ancient pollutant, and a source of many different human ills. Moses warned the Israelites that, as punishment for disobedience, "The Lord shall smite thee with consumption and with fever, and with swelling, and with the fiery head, and with the sword, and with *mildew* . . ." (Deuteronomy 28:22).

A study conducted in Scotland, where mildew and dampness are abundant, found that people who lived in housing that was judged to be damp or showed visible mildew had a higher rate of sickness than people whose housing was free of dampness or visible mold growth. These differences were not dependent upon smoking habits, occupation, or income; they seemed to be related to the dampness itself.[20] Damp homes breed both mold and dust mites. Indoor levels of mold spores can reach concentrations that are ten thousand times greater than those likely to be reached outdoors.

Mites are microscopic insects living in dust. Not only are they potent airborne allergens, but they secrete an enzyme that is directly damaging to the lining of the bronchial tubes. Heavy exposure to dust mites and mold in childhood increases the rate of allergic reactivity.[21] Allergy may account for some of the symptoms that make people sick when they live with dampness.[22] Allergic reactions to mold can cause sinusitis, asthma, pneumonia, eczema, hives, muscle and joint pain, fatigue, spaciness, and depression. I have also seen many patients in whom mold allergy aggravated autoimmune disorders such as rheumatoid arthritis.

It was mold that almost destroyed Philip Dustin's career. A freelance graphic designer, Philip had rented a house in Connecticut with a studio in the basement. Within weeks he and his wife, Sharon, began to experience severe fatigue and difficulty concentrating. They fell prey to every virus in the community. Once a month, both of them were bedridden with one infection or another. She would feel better when she left home for work, but he noticed burning of his skin and nose while in the basement. Within six months he was unable to work at all. At first, Philip and Sharon attributed their fatigue to the stress of a new marriage and a new home. I asked them to examine their house carefully and to obtain whatever records of floods and repairs the landlord would make available. We discovered that the house had experienced several leaks and floods over the past five years. There was thick mold growth on the gypsum board in the basement and abundant mold spores were readily cultured from the air in every room. Several months after breaking their lease and moving into a new apartment, the

Dustins began to regain their health. Unfortunately, Philip's graphic supplies, folios, and office equipment had become contaminated with mold during the six months he had used the basement as a studio. Everything had to be replaced.

The cascade of illness that plagued the Dustins involved more than allergy. Cultures from Philip's studio grew species of mold that produce toxins, called *trichothecenes*, that suppress the immune system. Trichothecene toxicosis has caused other cases of sick home syndrome.[23] Dampness and marked fluctuations in temperature produce ideal conditions for mold growth and toxin formation. Cancer-causing mold toxins have been found in homes where more than one inhabitant has developed leukemia.[24]

Trichothecenes, like most mold toxins (mycotoxins), were originally discovered as contaminants of food. A trichothecene called DON (deoxynivalenol), which may suppress the immune system and increase the rate of cancer, frequently turns up in U.S. breakfast cereals. Although Canada and Russia have established limits for DON contamination of grains, the U.S. government has failed to do so, relying instead on a letter advising food manufacturers to limit the DON levels in wheat products to one part per million. A sample of seven-grain cereal from a natural food store contained sixteen parts per million of DON.[25]

Aflatoxins are mycotoxins produced by *Aspergillus* species growing on peanuts and corn, rice, and other grains. They suppress immune function and are among the most potent cancer inducers in nature.[26] Exposure to aflatoxins in food appears to promote the development of liver cancer among people with preexisting hepatitis.[27] All peanuts and peanut butters are contaminated with aflatoxins. Levels are lowest in the major brands and highest in the fresh-ground peanut butters found in health food stores and supermarkets.[28] Although *Aspergillus* grows inside the peanut shell before harvest, prolonged storage increases the opportunity for mold growth and toxin production. In southern Georgia, heavy consumption of peanuts and grains likely to contain high levels of aflatoxins was associated with an increased rate of mental retardation among local children.[29] Aflatoxin production is inhibited by treating food with sorbic acid, a naturally occurring antifungal, first isolated from unripe berries of mountain ash trees in 1859. Peanut butter preserved with sorbic acid is safer than "fresh" peanut butter.

ALLERGY AND ASTHMA

Biologist Marc Lappé believes that allergy began as a defense against mycotoxins in food and air.[30] In reviewing the large number of natural allergens that provoke asthma, Lappé observes that they all thrive in environments that encourage mycotoxin production. Although we are accustomed to thinking of allergic disorders as inherited diseases, the widespread occurrence of allergy throughout the world indicates that allergy must have some protective value to human beings, and the increasing prevalence of allergy in most parts of the world implies that environment is more important than inheritance in evoking the allergic state. One theory holds that the part of the immune system responsible for allergy originated as a defense against infection with worms. This theory does not account for the increasing rate of allergic illness in industrialized countries[31] and the ineffectiveness of allergic immune responses in ridding the body of worms. It makes allergy into a vast immunologic mistake, which it is not.

Margie Profet, a biochemist at the University of California at Berkeley, finds in allergic reactions an "adaptive design" that limits the exposure of the affected individual to the provoking allergen.[32] Sneezing, coughing, spasm of the bronchial tubes, scratching, watering of the eyes, vomiting, and diarrhea—the major symptoms of allergic reactivity—all serve to shield the body from penetration by foreign substances or to shed them from the body's surfaces. The cost of this protection is high; allergic reactions can be incapacitating or even fatal. They are adaptive, believes Profet, because most naturally occurring allergens are *not* innocuous; they are either toxic themselves (like bee venom or metallic nickel or even pollen grains) or they are encountered in association with toxins. Peanuts—the food most likely to provoke fatal allergic reactions—are usually contaminated with aflatoxins.

Allergy is a last-ditch defense, a high-risk emergency reaction designed to be activated when the person encounters a toxin that has previously entered the body in sufficient quantity to evade the normal low-risk mechanisms for toxin avoidance and destruction. The appearance of allergy in childhood may represent a defect in nonallergic methods for protection against environmental toxins[33] or defective regulation of cell signaling.[34] Histamine, a chemical released during allergic reactions, not only causes sneezing and itching, which are protective responses, it stimulates the cellular enzyme systems involved in detoxification. The protective role of allergic reactivity against environmental toxins may explain the results of highly publicized Canadian studies that showed that prolonged administration of *anti*histamines to experimental animals promoted the development of cancer.[35]

When understood as an adaptive response to environmental toxicity that compensates for heavy exposure or defects in primary protective mechanisms, allergic "diseases" begin to make sense, and a rational plan for prevention and treatment can be constructed. The existing disease-based theory of allergy has been a disaster, especially with regard to asthma, a disorder that affects at least ten million people in the United States.[36] Over the past thirty years, the frequency and severity of asthma in the U.S. population, the rate of hospitalization, and the death rate have all increased to a frightening extent, especially among children.[37] During the past decade alone, the incidence of asthma has increased by 50 percent. About half the cost of medical care for asthma (six billion dollars a year) is due to emergency treatment of asthmatic crises.

The conventional view is that asthma is a disease produced by spasm and inflammation of the bronchial tubes. The disease is treated with drugs that block bronchial spasm (bronchodilators) and drugs that block bronchial inflammation (chiefly, cortisone).[38] There is considerable evidence that the conventional, disease-based treatment approach to asthma actually *contributes* to its increasing severity and mortality.

Prior to 1940, the death rate from asthma in industrialized nations was quite low. With the introduction of bronchodilator therapy in the 1940s, the death rate promptly increased.[39] Although bronchodilators are useful for the emergency relief of breathlessness, the regular use of bronchodilators causes deterioration in lung function[40] and increases the risk of death and near-death from asthma.[41] Respiratory therapists, who are exposed to airborne bronchodilator sprays as part of their work, develop asthma at a rate almost five times greater than expected, *after* entering their profession.[42] In other words, occupational exposure to bronchodilators actually creates asthma where it did not previously exist.

The increasing severity of asthma produced by bronchodilation makes sense if one understands that asthma is not a disease; it is a protective response to environmental toxicity. Abolishing that response without changing the environment aggravates the underlying processes that cause disease. In contrast, a cleaner environment ameliorates the underlying condition. Prolonged avoidance of dust mites, for example, not only relieves asthmatic symptoms, it also decreases the asthmatic reactions people experience when exposed to chemicals that ordinarily provoke asthma. The key to long-term control of asthma is not drugs,[43] but environmental control coupled with intensive support of the protective mechanisms that defend against toxicity.

No single environmental factor alone is responsible for the increasing prevalence of asthma. If you want to clean your environment, you must decrease the *total load* of allergens, irritants, and toxins resulting from outdoor and indoor air pollution.[44] Toxins like ozone (produced by photochemical smog), nitrogen dioxide (released outdoors by vehicle exhaust and indoors by gas stoves and dryers), and sidestream tobacco smoke act by increasing the sensitivity of the respiratory tract to inhaled allergens more than by direct irritation.[45] Allergens like dust mites and molds contain toxic proteins that directly damage the lining of the bronchial tubes.[46]

Nutrition may also influence the development of asthma by regulating the activity of protective mechanisms.[47] A high-sodium diet aggravates asthma.[48] Diets that are relatively low in vitamin C, zinc, magnesium, or selenium predispose to wheezing, bronchitis, and respiratory complaints.[49] The association between nutritional deficiency and asthma means that rational nutritional therapy can improve your condition.

Asthmatic patients studied in England, New Zealand, and Sweden have shown reduced selenium levels in blood or decreased activity of selenium-dependent antioxidant enzymes in their blood cells.[50] Dietary supplementation with selenium improves their antioxidant enzyme levels and asthmatic symptoms.[51]

The program presented below and in the next chapter is designed to lower your toxic load and support your resistance to environmental toxicity, prevent sickness, and support the healing process, whatever your state of health might be. The program is focused on toxins encountered indoors in air, food, and water, because that is the source of your greatest exposure and the domain over which you can exercise your greatest control. If you have already developed allergic sensitization, you'll probably need more extensive controls than those who have not. Your particular needs are discussed in Appendix A.

CREATING AN ENVIRONMENTALLY SAFE HOME

Most people spend half their lives at home, much of it in sleep, a condition of increased vulnerability. Making your home an environmental oasis is one of the most important steps you can take to protect your family's health and your own. Although outdoor air pollutants may be found inside homes, most of the air pollution in your house or apartment is created *inside* your home by *you* and is, therefore, under your control. General principles for safeguarding your home:

1. Stop Smoking

Don't smoke at home. Exposure to tobacco smoke, whether your own or someone else's, increases your risk of developing lung cancer, bronchitis, and heart attacks and your child's risk of developing frequent colds, allergies, asthma, and recurrent ear infections. Smoking inside your home or allowing visitors to smoke inside your home is an invitation to sickness. Invest in a stop-smoking program; it's the single most important step you can take to safeguard your health and that of your family. If you or your friends are addicted and unable to stop, smoke outdoors only.[52]

2. Kick Off Your Shoes

Remove your shoes upon entering your home. This Japanese custom is well worth importing. Turkish hosts, in fact, present their houseguests with a pair of slippers upon arrival. In homes where people do not routinely remove their shoes, the house dust is loaded with lead and pesticides tracked in from outdoors. Carpeting holds up to a hundred times the amount of dust as bare flooring; the deeper the pile, the harder it is to remove the dust. Dr. David E. Camann of the Southwest Research Institute in San Antonio, Texas, isolated dangerous pesticides and wood preservatives from carpet dust five years or more after these had been sprayed outside homes. The lead levels in carpet dust often exceed levels requiring cleanup at Superfund sites.[53] Toxins trapped in home carpets pose a particular hazard to crawling toddlers.

3. Control Moisture

Maintain a relative humidity of 30 to 45 percent in each room of your home. Relative humidity is the percent saturation of the air with water vapor. The ability of air to hold water increases with the temperature of the air. Furnaces heat the air without increasing its water content; therefore, they decrease the relative humidity, producing the dryness of homes in winter. When this warm air meets a cold windowpane and cools, relative humidity increases so dramatically that moisture condenses on the windowpane. Condensation often drips down into wall spaces, causing structural damage and mold growth. Common sense dictates that any sign of moisture buildup in your home should be analyzed and corrected, including seasonal condensation in basement, attic, or living space, and leaks from any source.

Relative humidity can be measured with an inexpensive meter, available in hardware stores. Relative humidity of 55 percent or greater encourages the breeding of dust mites. At 70 percent or more, mold and mildew have a field day. Excess humidity is, ideally, controlled by removing its source, but often the source is poor architectural or environmental design. Shade from overhanging trees, a poorly drained building site, or an inadequate moisture barrier between home and ground are causes of excess humidity that can be very expensive to change. Ventilation, temperature control, and dehumidification may be more practical solutions.

Ventilate the attic and the basement and use exhaust fans to remove the moisture that builds up when cooking or bathing. Don't seal your house tightly in winter; keep windows cracked open to prevent condensation inside. Unless your home is quite dry, don't set the nighttime thermostat down more than 8 degrees below the daytime temperature; as temperature drops at night, relative humidity increases. In warmer weather (temperatures above 65 degrees), dehumidifiers can effectively lower the relative humidity to 40 percent. Clean their condensation bins frequently to prevent buildup of bacteria, algae, and fungi. Air conditioners are more effective at dehumidifying if they are relatively less powerful and must run continuously to cool a space than if they are too powerful and can cool the space quickly and then shut off.

Don't use carpeting in areas prone to dampness, like bathrooms and basements. Any material that harbors fungal growth—rotten food, old wood, furnishings or building materials that have been damaged by water—should be removed from the house. Surfaces where mold regularly grows, especially shower stalls and curtains and the damp areas beneath sinks, should be cleaned weekly with an antiseptic solution such as hydrogen peroxide diluted with an equal part of water.

Refrigerators are a haven for mold, which loves to grow on bruised fruits and vegetables. If a hard food that is *uncooked* becomes moldy, cut and discard the moldy part and at least one inch of the food in each direction from the site of mold. ("Hard" foods include apples, broccoli, carrots, cauliflower, hard cheese in chunks, garlic cloves, onions, pears, potatoes, squash, and turnips.) If a soft food, juice, or cooked leftover becomes moldy, throw it all away; do not attempt to salvage any of it. Refrigerated leftovers not consumed within forty-eight hours should be discarded even if they are not visibly moldy.

There is surprisingly little evidence to implicate *lack of humidity* as a source of human ills. If the relative humidity is less than 30 percent, your skin may become dry and your nose and throat may become irritated. Before you rush out to buy a humidifier, however, try lowering the thermostat a few degrees. The hotter you keep your home, the more moisture you need in the air. Humidifiers are dangerous breeding grounds for mold and bacteria. Antifoulants added to the water in a humidifier are worthless in controlling bacterial growth and themselves pose a health hazard if inhaled.[54] The standard medical advice to humidify the air to improve respiratory problems has little evidence to support it. Only humidify your home air if you notice a definite improvement in preexisting respiratory complaints; otherwise the risks outweigh the benefits. If you must use a humidifier, use a cool mist or ultrasonic room unit that is not connected to your central heating system. It will be much easier to clean. Use only *distilled* water in the reservoir and drain the unit daily, cleaning it with hydrogen peroxide diluted one-to-one with distilled water.

4. Monitor Sources of Combustion

Stoves, heaters, and dryers that burn fuel of any kind may generate carbon monoxide, nitrogen dioxide, and formaldehyde, all highly toxic gases. An improperly maintained or vented appliance can cause carbon monoxide poisoning. Severe carbon monoxide exposure can cause heart attacks (as in the case of Sidney Shaw) or silent death, the fate that befell tennis star Vitas Gerulaitis when sleeping in a friend's guest cottage. Carbon monoxide is the commonest cause of death by poisoning in the United States. Acute carbon monoxide intoxication may produce headache, lethargy, hyperactivity, irritability, confusion, bizarre behavior, shortness of breath, chest pain, nausea, blackout spells, and seizures. Acute poisoning may be followed by evidence of brain damage two to four weeks later. The delayed symptoms include memory loss, unclear speech, visual disturbances, unsteady gait, and personality changes. Chronic low-grade exposure may cause subtle deterioration in mental function and hearing loss. Sometimes the first signs of carbon monoxide toxicity in the home are morning headache or dizziness and difficulty concentrating. If you remotely suspect carbon monoxide toxicity, have your heating and venting system professionally inspected. Seepage or backdraft of exhaust gas from flues is a common problem. I recommend you install a carbon monoxide detector. Although carbon monoxide itself is odorless and invisible, the water vapor that travels with it may condense and drip into the basement. The unexplained condensation of water near a furnace indicates that flue gases are not properly vented and should prompt an investigation. Information on low-cost carbon monoxide detectors is available from the Consumer Products Safety Commission (800-638-2772).

Nitrogen dioxide is a respiratory tract irritant that can cause sore throat or cough and increase the rate of allergic sensitization. Its main indoor sources are appliances that burn natural gas and kerosene space heaters. Nitrogen dioxide emissions in homes are greatly reduced by venting appliances to the outside and by the electrical ignition of gas stoves rather than the use of a pilot light.

5. Avoid Exposure to Formaldehyde

Because of the extensive use of building materials and furnishings that release it, formaldehyde exposure is almost inescapable in modern indoor environments. The greatest levels are given off by the glue that holds together fiberboard, particleboard, and plywood paneling. New houses with particleboard subflooring and mobile homes are loaded with formaldehyde. Although formaldehyde emission eases with time, high humidity or moisture disintegrates the glue and increases formaldehyde release. Formaldehyde is used to stiffen fabrics of all types, so that new clothing, carpeting, and upholstered furniture may emit considerable formaldehyde for days or weeks. Other sources of formaldehyde in household air are foam insulation, urea-formaldehyde finish coatings on furniture and flooring, fresh latex paint, space heaters, new paper or plastic products of any type, and cosmetics (including nail polish, skin creams, and hair sprays).

Acute exposure to low doses of formaldehyde may cause burning of the eyes, nose, and throat, tearing, nausea, dizziness, cough, chest pain, and shortness of breath. Chronic exposure has been causally associated with headache, drowsiness, memory loss, menstrual irregularities, and two types of human cancer.[55]

You can test the formaldehyde concentration in any room of your home with a home testing kit. Kits may be obtained from REEP, Inc., by calling (800) 733-7462, or from Environmental Construction Outfitters, (212) 334-9659. Testing should be done when all doors and windows are closed and heat and humidity are high, to eliminate false negative readings. When the source of formaldehyde cannot be removed (e.g., in mobile homes), surface treatments of pressed-wood sources with a hard lacquer may significantly reduce emissions.[56] Lacquers should be applied with care, because they give off their own emissions when drying. A safe choice is Safe Seal from AFM Enterprises, available through sources listed in Appendix B.

6. Use the Right Household Products

Consumer goods release hundreds of chemicals into the air, many of them irritating or unpleasant, some potentially dangerous. Cleaning solutions may contain ammonia or chlorine, each of which can be irritating to eyes, nose, and throat. Never mix ammonia products with chlorine-containing products. The resulting chloramine fumes are highly toxic. Dozens of VOCs have been identified in residential air. They are released by building materials, such as caulking and adhesives, latex paint, polyurethane varnish, vinyl floor and wall coverings, floor wax, furniture polish, mothballs, air fresheners, toilet bowl deodorizers, and plastics. Some of the VOCs found in indoor air are suspected of promoting cancer in humans. Concern over the safety of cleaning solutions and VOCs has created a demand for less-toxic alternatives. Information about these products can be obtained from sources listed in Appendix B. Good dust control can help lower VOC levels because dust particles absorb VOCs and increase their concentration in the air.[57]

7. Check Your Water

Chlorination of municipal water supplies was first introduced in Jersey City, New Jersey, in 1908. It dramatically reduced the death rate from typhoid fever, a bacterial infection spread through drinking water. But chlorination has drawbacks. Chlorine reacts with organic matter dissolved in water to form cancer-promoting substances such as the trihalomethanes (THMs), of which the best known is chloroform. Drinking chlorinated water increases the risk of developing cancer of the rectum or the bladder; the more water you drink, the greater your risk.[58] A preventive solution: filter your tapwater through activated charcoal, which removes the vast bulk of chlorinated compounds. Charcoal filters also remove other chlorinated contaminants of tapwater, like trichloroethylene (TCE), a degreaser that enters municipal water supplies after being dumped in the soil. TCE contamination of the municipal water supply in Woburn, Massachusetts, was blamed for an epidemic of childhood leukemia in the early 1970s. (This tragedy is retold in Jonathan Harr's *A Civil Action*, Random House, 1995.)

THMs and TCE are volatile; they evaporate from water during cooking or when showers are running and contaminate the air in homes,[59] so filter your water before you boil it. (For more on water purification, see pages 214–215.) Showerhead filters that remove chlorine will help to prevent the release of chloroform gas during hot showers (see Appendix B).

Fluoridation of water increases the likelihood that water will leach aluminum from cookware into food.[60] Increased serum levels of aluminum were described in a group of children with hyperactivity and learning disorders,[61] and elevated levels of aluminum in drinking water are associated with 50 percent greater risk of developing Alzheimer's disease.[62] Filtration of tapwater can remove aluminum from drinking water.

8. Get Out the Lead

Under pristine conditions, the earth's surface is almost lead-free. Mining extracts lead from the bowels of the earth, and patterns of human use disseminate it throughout the air and water. Today's humans harbor a body burden of lead that is absent from ancient skeletons. For four million U.S. children below the age of six, levels of lead in blood are high enough to threaten normal development.[63] Chronic low-level lead toxicity contributes to many different, allegedly unrelated disorders, which are commonly classified as separate diseases. These include hyperactivity and learning disabilities in childhood; kidney disorders, high blood pressure, and gout in adults; immune system dysfunction with frequent infections and cancer; stillbirths; anemia, chronic fatigue, depression, and muscle pain.[64] Among people with a high lead exposure, these separate "diseases" may all be manifestations of the same toxic process. Ask your pediatrician how often your children's blood should be tested for lead. Any level over 25 micrograms indicates a problem.

The commonest source of chronic low-level lead exposure for children is lead-contaminated house dust. A great deal of attention has been focused on old, lead-based paint, peeling and flaking from walls and ceilings, as a source of this contamination. It is less well known that roadside soil is still poisoned with lead deposited by gasoline fumes emitted before the ban on leaded petroleum additives, or that the soil around houses becomes contaminated with lead during new home construction or home renovations. This lead is tracked into the house, elevating lead levels in air. You can buy home kits for testing lead on surfaces. Taking your shoes off upon entering the home, wet-mopping all surfaces (including windowsills) to control dust, and regular handwashing markedly lowers the blood lead concentration of children living in homes with high lead exposure.[65]

Although lead has been banned from house paint, it may still be used in printer's ink, along with other toxic metals. Burning newspapers or magazines can liberate lead into the air. Lead can also contaminate drinking water, usually entering from pipes, fixtures, and solder.

Low-lead spigots are now available. Bulk-delivered water stored in tanks has poisoned children in the Southwest.[66] Charcoal filtration removes most of the lead from tapwater and, for reasons mentioned above, should be a routine in every household that uses tapwater for food preparation. If your water is not filtered, run the faucet for a minute or two before removing drinking water from it. Always take drinking water or water for cooking from the cold-water tap; the hot-water line contains more dissolved lead. You can have your water tested for lead by the local utility or EPA office.

Foods from cans with lead-soldered seams contain more lead than fresh food.[67] Lead can also enter food from ceramic ware, and is most likely to be leached out by acidic foods like tomato sauce and applesauce. The Environmental Defense Fund has tested the lead content of bowls and dishes and offers a consumer guide. They can be reached at (202) 387-3500.

9. Check Your Home Office

With more people working from home, the use of computers, copiers, fax machines, and printers in houses and apartments will continue to dramatically increase. All these office machines, including laser printers, emit VOCs during their operation. To decrease your exposure, I recommend that you keep all printers and copiers in one room (preferably not a bedroom), run them at a time of day when you or members of your family can leave the room, and run an exhaust fan after printing or copying more than just a few pages at one time.

To safeguard your home from environmental toxins:

- Don't allow tobacco smoking inside your home.
- Remove shoes upon entering your home from outside.
- Maintain a relative humidity of 30 to 45 percent in each room of your home.
- Do not carpet areas like kitchens and bathrooms that are prone to dampness.
- Dust frequently and clean all horizontal surfaces with a damp rag or wet mop twice a week.

- Remove moldy foods from the refrigerator promptly.
- Make certain that all stoves, heaters, and dryers are properly maintained and vented. Do not use gas appliances that run with a continuous pilot light.
- Test home air for carbon monoxide and formaldehyde. Call the Consumer Products Safety Commission at (800) 638-2772.
- Filter tapwater through activated charcoal to remove aluminum, lead, and cancer-promoting derivatives of chlorine.
- Use air filters and environmentally safe consumer products; consult the resources and suppliers listed in Appendix B.

8

THE FOURTH PILLAR:
DETOXIFICATION

POISONS FROM WITHIN

At first glance, the woman sitting across from me did not look sick. She looked robust and told me her story with clarity and self-assurance. She had lots of experience. Lauren Sands had been a TV newscaster in Los Angeles before her illness and had seen two dozen physicians in the past three years.

Her problems had started insidiously in the spring of 1990. At first, she had trouble waking up in the morning. A full night's sleep no longer left her feeling refreshed. Then muscles and joints all over her body began to ache. Her whole body felt stiff and exercise became a chore. She stopped playing tennis and jogging and swimming. Massage was painful and gave no relief. Despite extensive testing, no cause for her sickness could be found. Finally, a rheumatologist rendered a diagnosis of fibromyalgia, a mysterious ailment with no definite cause and no definite treatment.

The syndrome of fibromyalgia was first clearly described over 150 years ago and affects about 5 percent of the total population in the United States. Nonetheless, until the last decade, it received little serious attention from the medical community, for two reasons: first, fibromyalgia was not considered to be a disease; there are no consistent pathological changes in the blood or the tissues. Second, three-quarters of its victims are women. Because the symptoms of fibromyalgia—pain and tenderness of muscles all over the body, fatigue, and poor sleep—may be accompanied by depression, it was easy for doctors to dismiss fibromyalgia as a form of depression, hysteria, or personality disorder.

A distinctive finding in fibromyalgia are the *trigger points*, exquisitely tender spots in the muscles of the body. Dr. Janet Travell of Washington, D.C., was one of the pioneers who demonstrated that pain and fatigue could be greatly improved by injections of local anesthetics like novocaine, along with salt water, into these tender spots. She treated President Kennedy during his years in the White House, her trigger point injections allowing him to maintain an exhausting schedule.

Lauren's specialist began a series of trigger point injections, which eased the pain in her back and shoulders. He prescribed antidepressant drugs, which she stopped because of side effects, and physical therapy, which she pursued with great determination. The pain of working her muscles was agonizing, and the progress was terribly slow. She left her job and began an odyssey to spas and health centers throughout North America and Europe, received pain relievers, hydrotherapy, acupuncture, vitamins, minerals, chiropractic, homeopathy, and Shiatsu massage.

Slowly, Lauren's pain diminished and her sleep improved. She returned to work part-time. Despite this progress, when she first came to see me in 1993, her arms and legs burned and tingled continually, her neck and shoulders ached, her ability to exercise was one-quarter of what it had been before her illness, and she needed pain medication almost daily.

"I've been lucky," she confided. "I was able to leave my job and return to it. I had the money to afford a huge variety of treatments. I think each one helped a bit. But no one has gotten to the cause of this sickness and there has to be one." Her tone changed abruptly. "Well, you have a reputation for being a good medical detective. That's why I'm here."

"Fibromyalgia is not a single disease," I explained. "It's a name given to a set of symptoms for which there can be various causes. More than fifty different abnormalities have been described in association with fibromyalgia—chemical disturbances in the function of the brain or the muscles, abnormal activity of the immune system, chronic infection, allergy."

"I've always had allergies," she interrupted. "I saw an allergist in Beverly Hills. He said I was allergic to six or seven foods. I tried avoiding them. It didn't help my pain but it did clear up my constipation."

"How long have you had bowel problems?" I asked.

"They started a few years ago," she said. "I think it was after a trip to Mexico. We were shooting a story in Baja and I got pretty sick. I had diarrhea for a week. It stopped with Pepto-Bismol. I've been constipated ever since."

"Were you ever tested for parasites?" I asked.

"I think they tested me when I returned to Los Angeles, but the test was negative."

"What year was that?"

"We shot that story in '89 or '90."

"Before you developed fibromyalgia?"

She looked at me intensely and nodded.

I doubted that Lauren had a parasite living in her blood or muscle, but I thought it possible that she had an intestinal parasite, provoking muscle pain by remote control, activating an allergic reaction in a woman prone to allergy. I tested her for parasites, even though her previous test had been negative. The results confirmed my suspicion. Lauren was infected with *Entamoeba histolytica* (the same organism that caused John Gerard's colitis, described in Chapter Five).

I couldn't be sure that amoebic infection was the prime trigger for Lauren's symptoms. Her symptoms were not typical of amebiasis the way that John's were. Perhaps she was just a carrier. Millions of people throughout the world carry *E. histolytica* in their bowels; the organism can be found in stool samples but it does not seem to make them ill. The variability of pathogenic potential recalls Pasteur's challenge to the French Academy: do the causes of disease lie within the microbe or do they lie within the host?

I discussed antiparasitic therapy with Lauren, but I also recommended dietary changes that I thought would alter the internal environment in her favor: avoidance of alcohol, sugar, fatty foods, and all foods to which she had previously tested allergic. The usual drug used to treat amoebas is metronidazole (Flagyl), a potent antibiotic with many side effects. Lauren was afraid of drug side effects and requested an alternative. I prescribed a herb, *Artemisia annua*, which kills several types of parasites and also destroys the bacteria that feed them. For over two thousand years, Chinese physicians have prescribed *Artemisia* for the treatment of fever. Recent research has shown that *A. annua* has great activity against malaria. Its most active ingredient, artemisinin, is administered intravenously in Vietnamese hospitals to cure patients who are dying of malaria in the brain.

Three days after Lauren began her treatment, I received an emergency phone call. All her original symptoms had returned at their full intensity. She was bedridden once again. I knew that this was not a direct side effect of the herb.

"This is actually a good sign," I said, hopefully. "If you were allergic to dust, and you decided to dust your room, you would cough and sneeze. This treatment is comparable to dusting the parasites out of your body. As they are killed, the allergens or the toxins they contain that are making you sick are liberated and your exposure goes up. Give this treatment another week and call me if you're not better."

A month later she was back in my office, buoyantly happy. "It happened exactly the way you said it would!" She beamed. "I was terribly sick for almost a week, and then I suddenly started to feel better. Within two weeks I had almost no pain at all. A few days ago I played an hour of singles tennis in ninety-degree weather. I haven't done that in three years. Now I'd like to get off this diet."

The diet proved to be a problem. Although Lauren had found no benefit from restricting her diet before we treated the parasite, once the infection was gone she had to remain on a restricted diet to feel really well. Small indulgences produced considerable pain. It was a full year before she could sip her favorite wine or eat two slices of bread without hurting for days after. During that time, she did her best to comply with a positive nutritional prescription, designed to balance the responses of her cells to signals: choosing foods of high nutrient density, supplementing with flax oil, antioxidants, and magnesium. Today, she is healthier than before she became sick.

COLONIES WITHIN

The human intestine maintains within its inner cavity a complex, crowded environment of food remnants and microbial organisms (called *the intestinal flora*) from which the body derives nourishment and against which the body must be protected. The relationship between the human host and her army of microbes is described by the Greek word *symbiosis*, which means "living together." When symbiosis benefits both parties, it is called *mutualism*. When symbiosis becomes harmful, it is called *dysbiosis*.[1] The first line of protection against dysbiosis and intestinal toxicity is strict control of *intestinal permeability*, the ability of the gut to allow some substances to pass through its walls while denying access to others. The healthy gut selectively absorbs nutrients and seals out those components of the normal internal milieu that are most likely to cause harm, except for a small sampling which it uses to educate and strengthen its mechanisms of immunity and detoxification.

Bacteria form the largest segment of the intestinal flora. The number of bacteria in the large bowel (about a hundred trillion) exceeds the number of cells in the human body. Intestinal bacteria perform some useful functions, so that our relationship with them is normally one of mutual benefit. They synthesize half a dozen vitamins, supplementing those obtained from food. They convert dietary fiber—that part of food which humans cannot digest—into small fatty acids that nourish the cells of the large intestine. They degrade dietary toxins like methylmercury, making them less harmful to the body. They crowd out pathogenic bacteria like *Salmonella*, decreasing the risk of food poisoning. They stimulate the development of a vigorous immune response. Four-fifths of the body's immune system is located in the lining of the small intestine.

Bacteria can be dangerous tenants, however, so that dysbiosis is a common problem. As powerful chemical factories, bacteria not only make vitamins and destroy toxins, but also destroy vitamins and make toxins. Bacterial enzymes can inactivate human digestive enzymes and convert human bile or components of food into chemicals that promote the development of cancer. Some by-products of bacterial enzyme activity, like ammonia, hinder normal brain function. When absorbed into the body, they must be removed by the liver. People whose livers fail this task, because of conditions like cirrhosis, develop progressive neurologic dysfunction, resulting in coma and death. For them, antibiotics, which slow the production of nerve toxins by intestinal bacteria, can be life-saving.

The immune reactions provoked by normal intestinal bacteria may be harmful rather than helpful. Inflammatory diseases of the bowel, including ulcerative colitis and Crohn's disease (ileitis),[2] and several types of arthritis have been linked to aberrant immune responses provoked by intestinal bacteria. Two types of aberrancy have been described. First, intestinal bacteria contain proteins that look to the immune system very much like human proteins; they confuse the immune system and may fool the body into attacking itself. Second, fragments of dead bacteria may leak into the wall of the intestine or into the bloodstream because of a breakdown in the mechanisms that regulate intestinal permeability. Circulating through the body, bacterial debris is deposited in tissues such as joints, provoking an attack on those tissues by an immune system trying to remove the foreign material.[3]

Bacterial colonies in the human intestine coexist with colonies of yeasts, which are no less dangerous, just far fewer in number. Bacterial colonization prevents yeasts from expanding their niche. Frequent or prolonged use of antibiotics decimates bacterial colonies, removing the natural brake on yeast growth. The most obvious effects of yeast overgrowth are local infections, like vaginitis, produced when yeasts invade and disrupt cells that line the body's surface. Intestinal yeast infections can cause chronic diarrhea, although gastroenterologists often fail to recognize this.[4] Yeast can also provoke allergic reactions, precipitating asthma, hives, psoriasis, or abdominal pain.[5] If you experience allergic symptoms or the aggravation of a preexisting allergy following the use of antibiotics, you should always consider yeast overgrowth as a potential trigger. Neglect of this factor by allergists has left countless patients trapped in a spiral of increasing allergic reactivity, augmented each time antibiotics are prescribed.

In addition to bacteria and yeast, most of the world's five billion people are also colonized by intestinal parasites. Contrary to popular belief, parasitic infection is not unusual in the U.S. population. It is a common occurrence, even among those who have never left the country.

Unlike bacteria, parasites appear to serve no useful function. The part of the immune system they stimulate does not strengthen the organism to resist serious infection; instead it contributes to allergic reactions, so that parasitic infection increases allergic tendencies. There are two general groups of parasites. The first consists of worms — e.g., tapeworms and roundworms — that attach themselves to the lining of the small intestine, causing internal bleeding and loss of nutrients. People infested with worms may have no symptoms or may slowly become anemic. The second category is the *protozoa*, one-celled organisms like the amoeba that played a role in Lauren Sands's debilitating case of fibromyalgia. The first protozoa were discovered over three hundred years ago by van Leeuwenhoek. When the inquisitive Dutchman set about to examine everything in the world that would fit under the lens of a microscope, he found organisms in his own stool that closely match the description later given to *Giardia lamblia*.

Giardia is the major cause of day-care diarrhea. Twenty to 30 percent of workers in day-care centers harbor *Giardia*. Most have no symptoms; they are merely carriers. A study at Johns Hopkins medical school a few years ago demonstrated antibodies against *Giardia* in 20 percent of randomly chosen blood samples from patients in the hospital.[6] This means that at least 20 percent of these patients had been infected with *Giardia* at some time in their lives and had mounted an immune response against the parasite.

In 1990, I presented a paper before the American College of Gastroenterology that demonstrated *Giardia* infection in about half of a group of two hundred patients with chronic diarrhea, constipation, abdominal pain, and bloating. Most of these patients had been told they had irritable bowel syndrome, which is commonly referred to as "nervous stomach." I reached two conclusions from this study: (1) Parasitic infection is a common event among patients with chronic gastrointestinal symptoms. (2) Many people are given a diagnosis of irritable bowel syndrome without a thorough evaluation. My presentation was reported by numerous magazines and newspapers, including *The New York Times*. My office was flooded with hundreds of phone calls from people who were suffering with chronic gastrointestinal complaints. Most of them had been given a diagnosis of irritable bowel syndrome (IBS) by their physicians. The standard treatment for this syndrome had not helped them. All they had received was a label. Many had been told there was no cure. In evaluating these patients, I found that the majority had intestinal parasites, food intolerance, or a lack of healthy intestinal bacteria. These conditions were not mutually exclusive; many patients had more than one reason for chronic gastrointestinal problems. Treating these abnormalities as they occurred in various patients produced remarkably good therapeutic results. A year later, researchers in the department of family medicine at Baylor University in Houston reported findings similar to mine.[7]

Giardia contaminates streams and lakes throughout North America and has caused epidemics of diarrheal disease in several small cities by contaminating their drinking water. One epidemic, in Placerville, California, was followed by an epidemic of chronic fatigue syndrome, which swept through the town's residents at the time of the *Giardia* epidemic.[8] Possibly, this epidemic was due to failure of some people to eradicate the parasite. In 1991, my colleagues and I published a study of ninety-six patients with chronic fatigue and demonstrated active *Giardia* infection in 46 percent.[9]

Sometimes, the intestinal damage produced by giardiasis persists for months after the parasite has been successfully treated. The impairment of digestion and absorption that results from this damage may cause fatigue and other symptoms.

Bert Thomas is a forty-five-year-old geologist who was a world-class athlete and wilderness enthusiast. In the spring of 1994, he went backpacking in Wyoming with his three children. Although he attempted to boil or filter all drinking water, he developed diarrhea and fatigue soon after his return. He stopped the strenuous sports like rock climbing and mountain biking that had been a way of life for him, began to lose weight, and became dizzy and short of breath. In the fall of 1994, while the cause of his diarrhea was being investigated, he began having blackout spells and palpitations and was hospitalized. Monitoring of his heart rate indicated a serious abnormality of the heartbeat (an arrhythmia) called paroxysmal atrial fibrillation, which was thought to be responsible for his episodes of lightheadedness and his blackouts. He was started on medication to control the arrhythmia, but stopped it because of side effects. An extensive cardiac evaluation finally found that he suffered from an abnormality of the muscle fibers responsible for synchronizing the rhythm of the heart, a condition likely to worsen with time. After several months of sickness, he was treated for giardiasis with Flagyl and experienced dramatic relief of diarrhea and a lessening of fatigue. The palpitations continued, however, and seemed to be aggravated by his attempts to resume exercise.

He came to see me in February 1995, and asked three questions: "Is there any missed causation for this atrial fibrillation? Can anything be done? Do I have to give up sports forever?" When I reviewed his records, I was dismayed at the length of time that had elapsed between the onset of his illness and his treatment with Flagyl. His story said "*Giardia*" right from the start, but he had spent six months being treated for ulcers, having blood tests and abdominal scans and X rays, all because the initial stool specimen was falsely negative. My present concern was that no thought had been given to the possibility that the parasitic infection had anything to do with his susceptibility to arrhythmia, even though infection closely preceded the arrhythmia in time of onset.

I had Bert tested for parasites through a lab I trusted, to make sure that giardiasis had been successfully treated. It had been. Through the same lab I ran a test for intestinal permeability, to see whether the intestinal damage created by *Giardia* had healed. It had not. The intestinal permeability test indicated that poor absorption of nutrients was likely. This was confirmed when I found low levels of two minerals, magnesium and manganese, in Bert's blood. I prescribed supplements of these minerals, along with a multivitamin.

Within a month, Bert experienced a 90 percent reduction in the frequency of his attacks of palpitation and lightheadedness and he was able to resume his favorite sports. Two months later, I repeated the intestinal permeability test. It had improved considerably but was still highly abnormal. Only in July of 1995, nine months after he was cured of giardiasis, did his intestinal permeability return to normal. Until that time he had to take large doses of mineral supplements to prevent the nutritional deficiencies that contributed to his symptoms. Correcting his nutritional deficiencies did not cure Bert's heart condition. It gave him many months without symptoms and improved his ability to function normally.

THE TOLL OF INTESTINAL PERMEABILITY

When I first began presenting the results of my clinical research on parasitic infection in the mid-1980s, my reports were met with considerable skepticism. The present decade has witnessed an increased awareness of parasitic infection as a common public health problem in the United States, thanks largely to *Cryptosporidium*,[10] which recently achieved notoriety for contaminating Milwaukee's water supply, causing the largest epidemic of diarrhea in U.S. history, infecting four hundred thousand people and causing over one hundred deaths. Most municipal water supplies in the United States today are home to protozoa like *Giardia* and *Cryptosporidium*, and one in five Americans drinks water that violates federal health standards.[11] Every year, almost a million North Americans become sick from waterborne diseases; about 1 percent die. Further epidemics are inevitable.[12] A recent epidemic occurred in Clark County, Nevada, despite state-of-the-art municipal water treatment.[13]

How protozoa make people sick is not clear. Some directly invade the lining of the intestine; others provoke an allergic reaction that causes the damage. Bert Thomas suffered malabsorption of nutrients from intestinal damage. Lauren Sands had an illness that was probably caused by *excessive* intestinal permeability. It appears certain that humans coexist quite readily with their parasites as long as the barrier formed by the intestinal lining remains fully intact, so that the parasites cannot attach to the wall of the bowel. The attachment of the parasite initiates a series of injuries to the intestinal wall that increase its permeability, generating a cascade of reactions that can shatter a person's health in many different ways. Excessive permeability permits excess absorption of antigens and microbial fragments from the gut, overstimulating the immune response, fostering allergy and autoimmunity.[14]

Excess permeability also allows excessive absorption of toxins derived from the chemical activity of intestinal bacteria, stressing the liver. All materials absorbed from the intestine must pass through the liver before entering the body's general circulation. Here, in the cells of the liver, toxic chemicals are destroyed or else prepared for excretion out of the body. The cost of detoxification is high; free radicals are generated and the liver's stores of antioxidants are depleted.[15] (See below,

pages 204–205) The liver may be damaged by the products of its own attempts at detoxification.[16] This damage may extend to the pancreas
when free radicals are excreted into bile; this "toxic" bile flows into the
small intestine and can ascend into the ducts that carry pancreatic
juices, damaging the pancreas and aggravating malnutrition.[17]

The symptoms produced by excessive intestinal permeability may be
limited to the abdomen or may involve the entire body. They can include fatigue and malaise, joint and muscle pain, headache and skin
eruptions. The clinical disorders associated with increased intestinal
permeability include any inflammation of the large or small intestine
(colitis and enteritis),[18] chronic arthritis,[19] skin conditions like acne,
eczema, hives, or psoriasis,[20] migraine headaches, chronic fatigue, deficient pancreatic function,[21] and AIDS.[22] In most cases, it is incorrect
to think of excessive permeability as the *cause* of these disorders. Instead, excess permeability occurs as part of the chain of events that
causes disease and aggravates existing symptoms or produces new ones.

Just as excessive permeability may have many different effects, it may
also have many different causes, each of which may add to the effects
of the others. These causes include intestinal infection of any type
(viral, bacterial, or protozoan), alcohol, and NSAIDs (nonsteroidal
anti-inflammatory drugs), which increase permeability by decreasing
the body's synthesis of beneficial prostaglandins.[23] Allergic reactions to
foods also produce an increase in intestinal permeability.[24]

A Case in Point: Chronic Arthritis

The fate of people treated for chronic arthritis exemplifies the spiral of
problems caused by excessive intestinal permeability. Arthritis (inflammation of the joints) is the leading cause of physical disability in industrialized countries. Some forms of arthritis are *preceded* by increased
intestinal permeability. People with inflammation of the intestine are
prone to develop inflammatory arthritis, which may continue for many
years after the intestinal inflammation is healed. Fragments of intestinal bacteria have been identified in the joints in some cases.[25] In others, antibodies directed against intestinal bacteria may attack the
person's own joint tissue, causing an autoimmune reaction.[26]

For most people with chronic arthritis, however, excessive intestinal
permeability develops as a *result* of arthritis and its treatment and may

aggravate the arthritis, creating a vicious cycle. People with any type of severe arthritis usually take large doses of NSAIDs on a daily basis to control the pain, stiffness, and swelling in their joints; they rapidly develop increased intestinal permeability. Excessive permeability allows bacteria or bacterial by-products to penetrate the wall of the intestine, creating a smoldering inflammation in the intestinal wall (called enteritis), which in turn further increases intestinal permeability.[27] Enteritis develops in 70 percent of people taking NSAIDs daily for two weeks. The excessive permeability caused by drug-induced enteritis allows fragments of bacteria to enter the circulation, where they cause or aggravate more arthritis.[28]

Much of the research on intestinal permeability and NSAIDs has been conducted with people who suffer from rheumatoid arthritis, an inflammation that affects many joints at the same time and is especially noticeable in the hands. It typically strikes women in their twenties or thirties and lasts for life, crippling 30 percent of its victims with severe deformities of the affected joints and shortening their life expectancy by ten to fifteen years. Patients with rheumatoid arthritis taking NSAIDs develop antibodies against components of the normal intestinal bacteria.[29] Development of an abnormal or excessive immune response is called *sensitization*. Sensitization to intestinal bacteria may cause or aggravate arthritis.[30] When patients with rheumatoid arthritis take antibiotics that reduce the numbers of intestinal bacteria, not only does their enteritis clear up,[31] but their arthritis also improves.[32] NSAIDs, the standard treatment for arthritis, by increasing intestinal permeability, create a new problem that aggravates the old one.

Fasting and vegetarian diets have been shown to benefit patients with rheumatoid arthritis. Increased intestinal permeability explains this beneficial effect.[33] Fasting reduces the excessive intestinal permeability of patients with rheumatoid arthritis while at the same time dramatically improving symptoms.[34] Vegetarian diets alter the bacterial growth in the intestine, acting in a sense like natural, highly selective antibiotics. Those people who respond to vegetarianism with a change in the intestinal bacteria are the ones that benefit. Those people who do not change their intestinal bacteria as a result of changing their diets do not improve their arthritis by becoming vegetarians.[35]

There is a common belief that avoiding specific foods can benefit people with arthritis. One effect of the increased permeability produced by NSAIDs is to increase the absorption of antigens coming from food.[36] People with rheumatoid arthritis frequently become sensitized to food proteins.[37] Their arthritis often improves when they avoid specific foods and then flares up when they consume those foods.[38] I have treated enough patients with rheumatoid arthritis to know that food allergy is not *the cause* of rheumatoid arthritis. It is part of the cycle of immunologic sensitization, inflammation, and increased intestinal permeability that occurs in most patients with severe arthritis.

The treatments commonly used for chronic arthritis may temporarily relieve pain, but they help to maintain the vicious cycle. Perhaps this explains why the long-term outlook for patients with rheumatoid arthritis is so bleak and has not been improved by any of the drug therapies developed over the past thirty years.[39] Professor Ann Parke of the University of Connecticut has voiced an opinion not often heard from rheumatologists: ". . . maybe NSAIDs have had their day. We should, instead, be striving to *maintain* the integrity of the gastrointestinal tract in an attempt to prevent the disease at a potential source, rather than treating the complaints and risking perpetuating the disease."[40]

BUILDING RESISTANCE AND REDUCING RISK THROUGH DIET

If medicine is to regain its Hippocratic roots, preserving and restoring health, then physicians must learn the science of preserving and restoring normal intestinal permeability. By this, I do not mean attempting to "cleanse" the colon with laxatives or enemas or to correct constipation. In the early years of the twentieth century, it was medically fashionable to believe that people were poisoned by the waste products in their own large intestines. This condition, called *autointoxication*, was considered to be the cause of chronic fatigue, stomach ulcers, rheumatoid arthritis, high blood pressure, hardening of the arteries, breast cancer, and ovarian cysts.[41] The complex regulation of intestinal permeability was not understood, and autointoxication was attributed to "intestinal stasis," a fancy term for constipation. In keeping with the spirit of the times, it was treated invasively: enemas for mild cases, colectomy (surgical removal of the large intestine) in severe cases.

Even institutions as august as the Mayo Clinic sanctioned colectomies for autointoxication during the first two decades of the twentieth century.

The preservation and restoration of normal intestinal permeability rests on two principles: *building resistance* and *reducing risk*. A diet of high nutrient density, described in Chapter Six, is the cornerstone for maintenance of intestinal health. The intestinal lining has the fastest growth rate of any tissue in the body. Old cells slough off and a completely new lining is generated every three to six days. The metabolic demands of this normally rapid cell turnover must be met if excess permeability is to be prevented or if healing is to occur. Thorough chewing of food may be important. Saliva contains a substance called epidermal growth factor (EGF), which stimulates growth and repair of tissue. EGF has been used therapeutically to heal the intestine when injured or inflamed.[42]

Essential fatty acids also play an important role in maintenance of intestinal integrity. Fish oils limit the intestinal injury caused by toxic drugs,[43] and GLA (found in primrose, borage, and black currant oils) stimulates production of prostaglandins, which help to maintain normal permeability. See Chapter Six for the principles of EFA supplementation. Merely consuming large quantities of vegetable oils, however, is likely to be harmful to the intestinal lining. High intake of polyunsaturated oils increases the free radical content of bile, producing a toxic bile that may damage intestinal integrity.[44]

In addition to a nutrient-dense diet, I recommend several specific dietary *resistance factors* to preserve normal intestinal integrity. These should be part of any program for intestinal detoxification.

1. Fiber

Fiber is the indigestible remnants of plant cells. The usual sources are vegetables, whole-grain cereals and breads, nuts, seeds, and fruits. Eating a fiber-deficient diet increases intestinal permeability.[45] Although medical researchers have been recommending high-fiber diets for about twenty years, and sales of Metamucil and other bulk laxatives have gone up, there has been no significant increase in fiber consumption from food, and the fiber intake of Americans is far below recommended levels of twenty-five to thirty-five grams a day.[46] This is unfortunate, because the fiber found in food is far more complex than the purified powders sold in drugstores.

There are many different chemical types of fiber, but the most important distinction is between *soluble* and *insoluble* fiber. Soluble fiber dissolves in water, forming a thick gel. Fruit pectin, for example, is a highly soluble fiber. Psyllium seed, the commonest source of bulk laxatives, contains fiber that is moderately soluble. Wheat bran consists of relatively insoluble fiber that is most readily evident as "roughage." Although all fiber adds bulk to bowel movements, the chemical effects of the different types of fiber can be opposite.

Soluble fiber feeds the intestinal bacteria, which ferment it to produce chemicals called short chain fatty acids (SCFAs). SCFAs have a number of positive effects on the body: they nourish the cells of the large intestine, stimulating healing and reducing the development of cancer. When absorbed from the intestine, they travel to the liver and decrease the liver's production of cholesterol, lowering blood cholesterol levels.[47] Oat bran, for example, contains fibers of moderate solubility; eating oat bran can lower cholesterol levels.[48] Within the intestinal canal, SCFAs inhibit the growth of yeasts and disease-causing bacteria.[49] The effects of soluble fiber are not always beneficial, however. Eating high levels of soluble fiber supplements like guar gum encourages an overgrowth of the normal intestinal bacteria, which deprives the body of vitamin B_{12} and produces an increase in the concentration of bacterial toxins.[50] Although low-fiber diets increase gut permeability, excessive consumption of soluble fiber from supplements can also cause excessive permeability[51] and may create changes in the intestinal milieu that actually enhance the development of stomach or bowel cancer.[52]

Insoluble fiber does not feed bacteria well and is not readily fermented to SCFAs. Eating wheat bran, which is largely insoluble fiber, has no effect on blood cholesterol levels. Insoluble fiber inactivates many intestinal toxins,[53] however, and high intake of insoluble fiber is associated with a decreased risk of colon and breast cancer.[54] Supplements of insoluble fiber made from wheat bran or pure cellulose appear to decrease the risk of bowel cancer.[55] Insoluble fibers also inhibit the ability of disease-causing bacteria and parasites to attach themselves

TOP SOURCES OF DIETARY FIBER

Grains
    all whole grains, including whole wheat, oatmeal,
        brown rice

Vegetables
    acorn squash, beans (kidney, navy, pinto), broccoli,
        Brussels sprouts, cabbage, green peas, kale,
        radishes, spinach, winter squash, yams

Fruit
    apples, blackberries, blueberries, pears, raspberries

The fiber present in whole foods is a mixture of soluble and insoluble fiber. A predominance of insoluble fiber is found in wheat bran. A predominance of soluble fiber is found in psyllium seed, apple pectin, and guar gum.

    Beans supply about eight grams of fiber in a half cup (cooked). Most vegetables supply two to three grams of fiber in a half cup (cooked).

---

to the intestinal wall. Insoluble fiber plays an important role in preventing excess intestinal permeability.

    It should be obvious that humans need a mixture of soluble and insoluble fibers in the diet and that food, not supplements, is the best source. Eating high-fiber foods protects against the development of the major degenerative diseases of the modern world—heart disease and cancer—increases longevity,[56] and protects against the development of parasitic infection. The best sources of mixed fibers are unrefined cereal grains (oats, brown rice, whole wheat), peas, beans, and squash. Among fruits, one gets the most fiber per serving from apples and berries.

    Some high-fiber foods contain natural chemicals that help to maintain normal intestinal permeability by unique mechanisms. Carrots, carob, blueberries, and raspberries contain complex sugars (oligosaccharides) that interfere with the binding of pathogenic bacteria to the intestinal lining.[57] These have been used in Europe for centuries for the treatment or prevention of diarrhea. Synthetic oligosaccharides are presently being developed as drugs for treating infection. Brown rice is the source of gamma-oryzanol, a group of powerful antioxidants that have been tested extensively in Japan for their ability to heal intestinal and stomach ulcers and alleviate a variety of chronic gastrointestinal complaints. Gamma-oryzanol can be consumed in rice bran or rice bran oil or in pill form. The therapeutic dose is one hundred milligrams three times a day.[58]

If you become constipated when increasing dietary fiber, you may need more fluid. Drink eight glasses of liquid a day, between meals, not with meals.

2. Friendly Flora

A large body of research over the past ninety years has demonstrated the preventive value of eating foods fermented with *Lactobacilli* or their cousins, *Bifidobacteria*. Eating these friendly bacteria prevents intestinal infection due to viruses or pathogenic bacteria and preserves intestinal permeability in the face of infection or other types of injury, can prevent antibiotic-induced diarrhea and travelers' diarrhea, and can lower serum cholesterol levels. *Lactobacilli* and *Bifidobacteria* also show anticancer activity, by two mechanisms: they inhibit the growth or activity of cancer-promoting bacteria, and some strains actually produce chemicals that inhibit tumor growth.[59]

Declining levels of *Bifidobacteria* in the elderly allow accumulation of toxin-producing *Clostridium* species, which have been implicated in the development of cancer in the large bowel. Taking *Bifidobacteria* in a dose of three billion organisms per day lowers the level of *Clostridia* in the bowel and also reduces the concentration of chemicals that are thought to promote cancer.[60]

The growth of *Bifidobacteria* in the large bowel is strongly affected by diet. *Bifidobacteria* thrive on vegetable fiber and on the complex sugars that occur in certain vegetables. These complex sugars, known as fructooligosaccharides (FOS), are especially concentrated in garlic, onion, artichoke, asparagus, and chicory root. A synthetic form of FOS is available as a food supplement in the United States. Extensive re-

FRIENDLY FLORA

Name	Dietary Sources	Resides In
Lactobacillus acidophilus	acidophilus milk, some yogurts	small intestine
Lactobacillus bulgaricus	homemade yogurt	transient
Lactobacillus plantarum	sauerkraut	large intestine
Bifidobacteria	growth supported by soluble fiber and fructooligo-saccharides	large intestine
Saccharomyces boulardii	lichee nuts	transient

As a dietary supplement, the dose for each of these is 1–10 billion viable organisms/day.

---

search conducted in Japan, the United States, and Europe demonstrates that supplementing the diet with FOS encourages the growth of *Bifidobacteria* and discourages the growth of most undesirable bacterial species in the intestine.[61] One teaspoon a day of FOS lowers the concentration of toxic bacterial enzymes in the large intestine. These enzymes, called beta-glucuronidase and glycholate hydrolase, are able to convert normal constituents of the stool, derived either from food or from bile, into carcinogens (chemicals that cause cancer).[62] Regular consumption of foods rich in FOS may decrease the risk of colon cancer.

There are numerous species of *Lactobacilli* and many strains for each species. Some, like *Lactobacillus acidophilus*, are normal inhabitants of the human digestive tract. Others, like *L. bulgaricus*, which is a common starter for making yogurt, are not. *L. bulgaricus* disappears from the intestine within two weeks after yogurt consumption is stopped. Sauerkraut is sour because of *L. plantarum*, a beneficial organism that is normally found in the human intestine and that stays for a long time after being introduced. Commercially available fermented foods are, unfortunately, unreliable as sources of *Lactobacilli*, because the lactic acid and hydrogen peroxide that *Lactobacilli* naturally produce may kill the producers themselves if their concentration becomes excessive. A few years ago, the *Annals of Internal Medicine* published a study that proved what many women have known for years—that eating yogurt daily can help prevent vaginal yeast infections.[63] The researchers were lucky. The batch of yogurt they gave their patients was loaded with living *Lactobacillus acidophilus*. These organisms not only took up residence in the intestines of the women who ate it, but also colonized the vagina, preventing yeast infection. When the scientists attempted to perform the same experiment a year later, they found that the same brand of yogurt contained *no* living bacteria.

The most reliable way to supplement your diet with *Lactobacilli* is to make your own yogurt or sauerkraut, or to buy nutritional supplements that have been tested by an independent outside laboratory and that list the concentration of viable bacteria found on culture. *Lactobacilli* are killed by heat, moisture, and sunlight. The making of tablets generates heat, which lowers the number of viable organisms. *Lactobacilli* should be freeze-dried, in powder or capsules, in opaque moisture-proof containers, and stored in the refrigerator. They should be consumed with meals. The strains that have been most extensively tested for their viability in the human intestine are *L. acidophilus* strain NCFM-2 and *L. plantarum*.[64] *L. acidophilus* is well suited to growing in the small intestine, where it is normally one of the dominant bacterial species. *L. plantarum* has growth characteristics that lead it to grow especially well in the large intestine. The daily dose should be between one billion and ten billion viable bacteria. More may cause gastrointestinal irritation.

"Nutritional yeast" has been used as a dietary supplement for generations, as a source of vitamins and minerals and for treatment of digestive complaints. After treating hundreds of yeast-allergic patients, I was very reluctant to prescribe yeast for anyone, until I discovered a preparation the French call "Yeast Against Yeast." The yeasts that invade human tissues, causing yeast infection, are mostly members of the genus *Candida*. The yeasts used in baking bread or brewing beer belong to the genus *Saccharomyces*. Yeast Against Yeast is *Saccharomyces boulardii*, a microbe that inhabits the surface of many different plants and that was first isolated from lichee nuts in Southeast Asia by French scientists during the 1920s. *Saccharomyces boulardii* has been used in Europe for decades to treat acute diarrhea and controlled trials have

shown it effective in preventing or treating diarrhea brought on by antibiotics. *S. boulardii* appears to exert its beneficial effects by inactivating bacterial toxins and by stimulating intestinal immune responses.[65]
Products labeled *S. boulardii* have been available in natural food stores
in the United States since 1991. People who are allergic to baker's yeast
may also be allergic to *S. boulardii*, but for most people, including
women with chronic *Candida* infection, Yeast Against Yeast lives up to
its name. The dose required is about three billion live organisms twice
a day, taken on an empty stomach.

3. Spices

Before they were used as seasoning, culinary herbs and spices were
probably used for food preservation. Many varieties have natural antimicrobial activity and can retard spoilage. They are also used to mask
the flavor of spoiled food, so I suggest using them at home, where you
know the food they flavor is fresh.

The world's most extensively studied spice is garlic. Its medicinal use
predates recorded history. Garlic is mentioned in the earliest Vedic
medical documents, written in India over five thousand years ago. During an epidemic of plague in Marseilles in 1721, four condemned crim-
inals were enlisted to bury the dead. None of them contracted plague.
It seems that they sustained themselves by drinking a cocktail of
crushed garlic in cheap wine, which came to be called *vinaigre des qua-
tre voleurs* (vinegar of the four thieves). In 1858, Louis Pasteur demonstrated garlic's antibiotic activity. The bulb was used by Albert
Schweitzer for the treatment of amoebic dysentery at his clinic in
Africa. Antimicrobial activity of garlic has been repeatedly demonstrated against many species of bacteria, fungi, parasites, and viruses. In
addition, garlic lowers cholesterol and blood pressure and may protect
against cancer. The dose of garlic needed to obtain significant benefit
is at least ten grams (about three small cloves) per day.[66]

Onion, garlic's closest edible relative, has also been widely used for
medicinal purposes. Although it lacks the potency of garlic, it can be
consumed in much larger quantity, so that its antimicrobial benefits
may be equal to those of garlic if consumed regularly.[67]

Turmeric, a major ingredient in curry powder, is a natural antibiotic
that relieves intestinal gas by lowering the numbers of gas-forming bac-

MICROBE–FIGHTING SPICES

Name	Amount Needed in Food	Amount Needed as Supplement
garlic	3 small cloves/day	1,000 mg twice a day
onion	1 medium onion/day	N/A
turmeric	1/4 teaspoon/day	500 mg twice a day
ginger	1/2 teaspoon twice a day	N/A
cinnamon	1/2 teaspoon twice a day	N/A
sage	1/2 teaspoon/day	15 drops of tincture twice/day
rosemary	1 teaspoon twice a day	15 drops of tincture twice/day
oregano	1 teaspoon twice a day	500 mg after each meal
thyme	1/4 teaspoon twice a day	10 drops of tincture twice/day

The essential oils of oregano, rosemary, sage, and thyme are irritating and should not be consumed, except under medical supervision. The whole herbs are generally safe but may cause allergic reactions in susceptible individuals.

___

teria. It has antifungal activity and has been traditionally used for relieving inflammation. The effective dose is about one gram per day.[68]

Ginger, which contains over four hundred chemically active ingredients, has long been used for the treatment of digestive complaints. It protects the intestinal lining against ulceration and has a wide range of actions against intestinal parasites.[69] Cinnamon, which I recommend for sweetening the taste of ginger tea, has antifungal activity.[70]

Sage and rosemary contain the essential oil eucalyptol, which kills *Candida albicans*, bacteria, and worms. Oregano contains over thirty biologically active ingredients of which twelve have antibiotic, antiviral, antiparasitic, or antifungal effects.[71] Thyme has antiparasitic activity as well.

Meals seasoned with these pungent, aromatic herbs, consumed regularly, help protect against intestinal infection. However, heating at 200 degrees Fahrenheit for twenty minutes destroys the antibacterial activity of most of these spices. They should be added to food at the end of cooking, just before being eaten.[72]

NOTE: If high-fiber diets, friendly flora, or spicy food give you diarrhea, gas, or abdominal bloating, instead of improving digestive function, you may be changing your diet too rapidly, or you may have an allergy to one specific component of the regimen described here. Slow down and try again. Be methodical, making one change at a time. First, cut down on sugar and fat, then switch to whole grains, then add more vegetables. Give yourself a chance to know how each new food you try affects your body. It may take a few days. Then add nutritional supplements, one at a time, allowing yourself three or four days between each change. Experiment with different brands. For some people, one preparation of *Lactobacillus* will cause diarrhea, but another will not. If you still find that you cannot increase your consumption of fiber or flora without feeling worse, rather than better, you may have an overgrowth of bacteria or yeast in the small intestine that have adapted to using the fiber you are taking to expand their niche, rather than to limit their growth. Bacterial overgrowth of the small intestine is far more common than doctors suspect and most commonly results from a lack of stomach acid or from prior surgery. Yeast overgrowth usually results from taking antibiotics. Resources for dealing with these problems are listed in Appendix C.

DETOXIFICATION, PHASE ONE

Liver detoxification is generally divided into two phases: Phase One and Phase Two. Phase One requires oxygen. Toxins are burned, or oxidized, to render them more soluble in water. The enzymes active in Phase One detoxification are called the "cytochrome P450" system. They are located in special components of the cells called *mitochondria*, tiny biological furnaces designed to use oxygen efficiently. It is in the mitochondria that most foreign substances are destroyed and most of the body's energy is generated. Because many drugs are detoxified in mitochondria, they can interact with one another by inhibiting or stimulating the activity of mitochondrial enzymes. The most dramatic drug interactions occur when one drug inhibits the chemical transformation of another. Two popular antihistamines, for example, Seldane (terfenadine) and Hismanal (astemizole), are chemically changed by an enzyme called cytochrome P450-3A (CYP-3A). This enzyme also breaks down at least twenty-four other commonly used drugs, including many antidepressants, tranquilizers, and antihypertensives (drugs for lowering blood pressure). The activity of CYP-3A is blocked in people taking the antifungal drugs Nizoral (ketoconazole) or Sporanox (itraconazole) or the antibiotic erythromycin. It is mildly blocked if the drugs are taken along with grapefruit juice.[73]

The interaction between Nizoral and Seldane can kill people. If a person taking Seldane also takes Nizoral, the blockade of CYP-3A produced by Nizoral will greatly elevate the level of Seldane in the body. High Seldane levels can cause irregularities of the heartbeat, which can be fatal. The Nizoral-Seldane interaction received considerable notoriety a few years ago because of these dramatic effects. But dangerous drug interactions caused by cytochrome P450 inhibition are very common in people taking other drugs as well. To avoid these, doctors and patients need to know the effects on detoxifying enzymes of every drug that is taken, whether by prescription or over-the-counter. Future drug development must emphasize the production of drugs that have minimal effects on the major forms of cytochrome P450.[74]

Although inhibition of cytochrome P450 can cause adverse drug interactions, excessive activity of cytochrome P450 is also risky. No biochemical function shows more clearly the need for establishing balance. First, the process occurring here routinely generates *free radicals*, which have received considerable attention as a possible factor in aging and the development of degenerative diseases.[75] Second, some of the chemicals produced by the cytochrome P450 system are actually more toxic than the chemicals from which they are formed. The conscious support of healthy detoxification requires an understanding of the ways in which the body protects itself against the dangers of its own Phase One system. Foremost is defense against free radicals.

Simply stated, free radicals are by-products of *oxidation*, the process by which the body uses oxygen to burn food as fuel, producing energy, and to destroy harmful chemicals. The fires of oxidation often produce chemical sparks that fly off and start fires where they are not wanted.

These sparks are free radicals. Free radicals may damage the mitochondria themselves, compromising energy production. Mitochondrial damage occurs in many neurological and muscular disorders and appears to be an important factor for some people with chronic fatigue syndrome.[76] Free radicals generated in the liver also diffuse out of mitochondria into the cell substance, injuring liver cells, and spill over into the blood and the bile. Free radicals in the bile can damage the intestines and the pancreas. When free radicals reach the nucleus of a cell, where the DNA is stored, genetic damage may occur. One outcome of free radical–induced genetic damage is cancer.

To protect its cells from harmful oxidation and limit free radical–induced damage, the body employs a defense system composed of protective enzymes and circulating chemicals called antioxidants. Some of these antioxidants are manufactured in the body; many come only from food. Dietary antioxidants include vitamin E, vitamin C, vitamin A, carotene and related carotenoids, bioflavonoids, and the minerals selenium, manganese, copper, zinc, and sulfur (which is usually consumed as part of protein). Some antioxidants inhibit free radical–induced damage directly by quenching the sparks, in essence sacrificing themselves. Other antioxidants inhibit free radicals indirectly, by activating enzymes that convert free radicals to less destructive compounds.

Paradoxically, *any* antioxidant can actually spread the fire and increase free radical–induced damage, once it becomes damaged itself. In nature, antioxidants never work alone; they always operate as components of a complex and interactive system. Taking supplements of single antioxidants, which has been attempted in several recent human experiments, makes little sense. The entire antioxidant defense system must be supported to protect the mitochondria.

Many of the environmental pollutants that initiate cancer are believed to do so by activating the cytochrome P450 system, flooding the body with free radicals. Protection against the effects of environmental pollution, free radical–induced cell damage, and cancer is provided by dietary antioxidants.[77] Foods that are richest in these antioxidants are red, yellow, and green vegetables, uncooked nuts and seeds (like almonds and sunflower seeds), and fish.

The appetizing colors of fresh fruits and vegetables derive from the presence of special groups of antioxidants. *Carotenoids* are fat-soluble

---

TOP DIETARY SOURCES OF ANTIOXIDANTS

Foods generally rich in antioxidants
> red, yellow, and green vegetables, uncooked nuts and seeds (e.g., almonds, Brazil nuts, hazelnuts, sunflower seeds), legumes, whole grains (e.g., oatmeal and brown rice), garlic, shrimp, scallops

Foods rich in carotenoids
> apricots, broccoli, cantaloupe, carrots, collards, dandelion greens, kale, mustard greens, papaya, pumpkin, red peppers, sea vegetables (dulse, hijiki, kelp, nori, wakame), spinach, sweet potatoes, Swiss chard, tomatoes, winter squash

Foods rich in bioflavonoids
> beets, black cherries, blackberries, blueberries, cranberries, green asparagus tips, green tea, purple corn, purple onions, radishes, raspberries, red cabbage, red grapes, rhubarb, sweet potatoes, spices (ginger, parsley, rosemary, sage, thyme, turmeric)

---

compounds that range in hue from light yellow to deep orange. The flagship carotenoid is *beta-carotene*, the orange pigment evident in carrots and cantaloupe. In the body, beta-carotene is converted to vitamin A, but the importance of carotenoids for human health extends far beyond beta-carotene's role as a precursor of vitamin A. Dietary supplements of beta-carotene are ineffective in preventing cancer or heart disease, whereas *food* that is high in beta-carotene and other carotenoids does confer protection. Scientists have previously paid insufficient attention to these other carotenoids, like alpha-carotene, lutein, lycopene, and the xanthins. They do not serve as precursors of vitamin A, yet their consumption, along with beta-carotene in food, may explain why carotene-rich foods decrease the risk of cancer. The "other" carotenoids exert significant antioxidant effects of their own.[78] I do not recommend nutritional supplements containing beta-carotene to my patients. Instead, I recommend a diet high in mixed carotenoids, which includes many different varieties of fruits and vegetables: carrots, broccoli, spinach, tomatoes, winter squash, and papaya. Sea vegetables like kelp, wakame, dulse, hijiki, and nori are especially rich in mixed carotenoids. They can be quite tasty cooked or raw, along with rice or beans or in salad.

The darker colors of fruits and vegetables are supplied by a group of compounds called *bioflavonoids*, which typically range from bright yellow to deep purple in hue. There are over four hundred bioflavonoids in the human diet. They are widely distributed in fruits, vegetables, beverages, and spices. A typical North American consumes about one gram of bioflavonoids per day; Asians may consume over five grams per day, much of it coming from herbs and spices. Bioflavonoids are potent antioxidants that contribute not only to the health benefits of fruits and vegetables but also to the therapeutic effects of many traditional Chinese and Indian herbal remedies.[79] The bioflavonoids that give grapes their purple color are believed to be responsible for the protection against heart disease that is offered by red wine. Epigallo-catechin gallate (EGCG), the bioflavonoid that is the main constituent of green tea, is credited with the protection against cancer that results from drinking green tea.[80]

An antioxidant with specific activity in protecting mitochondria is coenzyme Q10 (ubiquinone), which is chemically related to vitamin E. Although coenzyme Q10 is present in many foods that also contain vitamin E, and is additionally synthesized in the human body, deficiency of coenzyme Q10 has been identified in groups of patients with a diversity of clinical problems, ranging from periodontal disease to high blood pressure and diabetes. Psychiatric drugs and anticancer drugs may also lower levels of ubiquinone in the body's tissues. Dietary supplementation with coenzyme Q10 in the range of thirty to two hundred milligrams per day has been of benefit to patients with high blood pressure, heart failure, angina, gingivitis, and chronic fatigue. In experimental animals, ubiquinone protects the liver from the effects of injected bacterial toxins. Its role in human detoxification can at present only be surmised from its known antioxidant effects in mitochondria.[81]

The hazards of detoxification require more protection than can be

offered by antioxidants alone, however. Cytochrome P450 may increase rather than decrease the toxicity of some of the chemicals it
transforms. Certain chemical carcinogens are more damaging to the
body *after* they are oxidized. The mineral zinc, at normal levels in
human tissue, inhibits components of the Phase One system that activate carcinogens, whereas zinc deficiency increases tumor-promoting
Phase One activity.[82] Good dietary sources of zinc are limited. They include liver, the dark meat of turkey, lean beef, shellfish, pumpkin seeds,
sunflower seeds, and almonds.

DETOXIFICATION, PHASE TWO

To rid itself of poisons produced by Phase One detoxification, the liver
employs a Phase Two system, in which the oxidized chemicals are com-
plexed with sulfur, specific amino acids, or specific organic acids, and
then excreted in bile or urine.[83] Amino acids are the building blocks of
protein; consequently a deficiency of protein will impair detoxification.
The most important amino acids for Phase Two detoxification pathways are cysteine and methionine, because they are also the main dietary sources of sulfur. Cysteine and methionine are widely distributed
in meat, fish, poultry, eggs, and dairy products. Vegetarians can obtain
adequate supplies from nuts, seeds, and beans. The adult RDA for cys-
teine/methionine is 700 to 1,000 milligrams per day. The amount a person needs is never fixed, however; it fluctuates with the liver's burden
of toxic compounds. The greater the toxic stress, the greater the demand, because the body's stores of these amino acids are depleted in
the detoxification process.

Perhaps the most important role for cysteine and methionine in
detoxification lies in their conversion to *glutathione*, which is a complex of three amino acids (a tripeptide). Glutathione is both an essential detoxifier and an important antioxidant. Fasting depletes the body
of glutathione, but a brief period of fasting followed by feasting actually elevates glutathione to a level higher than before the fast. Glutathione may also be directly absorbed into the body from foods,
especially fresh meats and nuts and vegetables like asparagus and avocado. Most forms of food processing, except for freezing, destroy glutathione.[84] Supplementing the diet with five hundred milligrams of

vitamin C per day elevates the level of glutathione in the blood of healthy adults, indicating that vitamin C protects glutathione from destruction.[85] In contrast, alcohol, acetaminophen (Tylenol), and a number of other drugs and poisons deplete the body of glutathione. Although the occasional use of Tylenol is generally safe, there are people who develop liver disease from taking as little as four grams (eight 500-mg pills) during a twenty-four-hour period. These people are usually depleted of glutathione because they have not been eating well or because they have been drinking alcohol.[86] Taking a nutritional supplement called N-acetyl cysteine (NAC), which is widely available in health food stores, restores glutathione levels in the body and protects against liver damage caused by a range of toxins, from Tylenol overdose to carbon tetrachloride poisoning.[87] N-acetyl cysteine should be taken only under a doctor's supervision. The effective dose may range from 500 to 8,000 milligrams per day.

A number of foods stimulate the body to produce more Phase Two enzymes. These foods have been shown to improve liver detoxification and to decrease the risk of developing cancer. They include members of the cabbage family (*Cruciferae*), which includes not only cabbage but broccoli, cauliflower, bok choy, and Brussels sprouts, and also green onions and kale. These vegetables contain compounds called aryl isothiocyanates, which directly stimulate the activity of an enzyme, glutathione S-transferase, an important component of the Phase Two system. Activation of Phase Two detoxification probably explains the highly publicized effects of broccoli, Brussels sprouts, and cabbage in preventing cancer in humans and experimental animals.[88]

Bioflavonoids may also stimulate glutathione S-transferase. In fact, bioflavonoids appear to be capable of stimulating or inhibiting every enzyme known. Some induce and some suppress the activity of various components of the cytochrome P450 enzyme system. As complicated as their actions are, the overall effect of bioflavonoids on the liver's metabolism of organochlorines and related pollutants appears to be beneficial.[89] Bioflavonoids found in soybeans have weak estrogenlike activity. If a woman is deficient in estrogen (if she's gone through early menopause, for example), consuming soy products can replace the missing estrogen and relieve hot flashes. If a person is exposed to an excess of estrogen, the flavonoids in soy act as estrogen blockers and lower the effects of estrogen. The low frequency of breast cancer in East Asia,

COMBATTING INTESTINAL TOXICITY

Body's Defenses	Function
Stomach/Intestines	
Stomach acid	kill pathogenic microbes
Intestinal immunity	kill pathogenic microbes, prevent attachment of microbes to intestinal lining, inactivate allergens
Motility (peristalsis)	prevent overgrowth of microbes
Friendly bacteria	kill pathogenic microbes, inhibit growth of pathogens, nourish the intestinal lining, stimulate immune responses
Impermeability	prevent absorption of toxins, allergens
Liver	
Phase One enzymes	oxidize drugs and toxins to make them less active, more soluble in water
Phase Two enzymes	alter drugs, toxins, and Phase One products to make them less toxic and easier to excrete in bile or urine

where soy is a major source of protein, has been attributed to the mild estrogen-blocking effect of soy flavonoids. Preliminary research indicates that soy flavonoids can block the estrogenic effects of dioxin.

Milk thistle, *Silybum marianum,* is an herbal folk remedy for treating liver diseases. Its active ingredients are a group of bioflavonoids col-

COMBATTING INTESTINAL TOXICITY

Strengthened By	Weakened By
protein, spicy food nutrient-dense diet, *Saccharomyces boulardii*	acid-lowering drugs cortisone, stress, malnutrition
fiber, spicy food	stress, lack of fiber, drugs (narcotics, cocaine, Donnatal)
soluble fiber, FOS, *Lactobacillus acidophilus*, *L. plantarum*, *Bifidobacteria*	antibiotics, lack of fiber
nutrient-dense diet, bioflavonoids, EFAs, antioxidants, fiber, thorough chewing (releases EGF)	parasites, drugs (aspirin, Advil), food allergens, malnutrition
antioxidants, zinc, coenzyme Q10	zinc deficiency, drugs (Tagamet, Nizoral, others)
cysteine, vitamin C, glutathione, cruciferous vegetables, bioflavonoids, milk thistle	alcohol, Tylenol

lectively called silymarin. Milk thistle is reportedly potent enough to protect against poisoning by the mushroom *Amanita phalloides* (death cap), which contains the most potent liver toxins known.[90] Milk thistle also protects against acetaminophen poisoning in rats[91] and many types of liver disease in humans.[92] The standard dose is 70 to 210 milligrams of silymarin three times a day. Even prolonged use has not been associated with toxicity.

Unraveling the complex chemistry of detoxification, understanding the effects of nutrition, environment, and intestinal toxicity on this chemistry,[93] and devising new treatment approaches to support it, are among the greatest challenges confronting clinical science at the present time.

RISK REDUCTION

Cut Down on Aspirin and NSAIDs

The most common, preventable causes of increased intestinal permeability are drugs and infections. If possible, don't take aspirin and other NSAIDs on a daily basis. Most people using NSAIDs daily are trying to relieve chronic headache or joint and muscle pain. I suggest you try instead alternative strategies for pain relief. The likelihood of benefit depends upon the location of the pain and the presence or absence of inflammation. Pain control strategies and resources are listed in Appendix D.

Reduce Your Alcohol Consumption

After NSAIDs, alcohol is the drug most likely to destroy normal intestinal permeability. More than one glass of wine or beer is likely to be detrimental.[94]

Don't Rely on Medication to Reduce Stomach Acid

The body's first line of defense against intestinal infection is the acid produced by a healthy stomach.[95] Stomach acid kills most of the bacteria and parasites that are swallowed along with meals. Strong suppression of stomach acid increases the risk of intestinal infection.[96] The widespread use of antacids is, therefore, a reason for concern, and the FDA's recent decision to make the acid-lowering drugs Tagamet, Zantac, Axid, and Pepcid available without a doctor's prescription is a terrible disservice to the American people. Most people who take treatments to buffer or reduce stomach acid do not need acid reduction and should avoid it. Tagamet and Pepcid are called H-2 blockers because they block certain effects of histamine in the body. (Conventional "antihistamines" used for treating symptoms of allergy are called H-1 blockers.) They were originally developed for the treatment of ulcers and they made huge profits for the companies that owned them. Doctors soon began using H-2 blockers for relieving stomach pain not caused by ulcers (this pain is called "nonulcer dyspepsia"), even though their efficacy for nonulcer pain was disputed.[97] The most common cause of nonulcer dyspepsia, by the way, is taking NSAIDs. If NSAID use is markedly reduced, the frequency of stomach pain and the need for H-2 blockers will also be reduced. Recently, it has become quite clear that most ulcers are triggered by a bacterial infection of the stomach and that antibiotics are superior to H-2 blockers for treating ulcers. As the need for H-2 blockers in the treatment of ulcers just about vanished, the FDA suddenly approved their nonprescription use for the treatment of heartburn. The truth is that H-2 blockers are rarely needed to treat heartburn, because heartburn is not caused by excess stomach acid. It is caused by reflux of normal amounts of stomach acid into the esophagus, which occurs when the valve responsible for preventing acid reflux is not working properly. Diet is the usual cause of this valve failure. Coffee, alcohol, chocolate, and high-fat meals prevent the valve from closing properly. Calcium, in contrast, makes it close more tightly.

Almost all people with frequent heartburn can get relief by eating small, low-fat meals, chewing a calcium tablet after each, and not eating for four hours before bedtime. It's a good idea to cut out coffee, alcohol, and spicy or irritating foods until the heartburn stops. Were these measures followed, the use of H-2 blockers and antacids could be cut by 90 percent.

Be Cautious About Taking Antibiotics

A second line of defense against intestinal infection is the normal intestinal bacteria, especially *Lactobacilli* residing in the small intestine. Antibiotics decimate *Lactobacilli*. In so doing, they may increase the risk of subsequent intestinal infection. Although antibiotics, when appropriately used, are the most important therapeutic discovery of modern Western medicine, they are often used inappropriately and the effects can be devastating. Whenever I prescribe an antibiotic, I always consider its possible effect on the beneficial intestinal flora. An antibiotic that is rapidly and completely absorbed in the stomach, reaching high levels in the tissues of the body and low levels in the small or large intestine, is least likely to harm intestinal ecology. I also administer *Lactobacilli* along with the antibiotics. *L. plantarum* is the only *Lactobacillus* not harmed by antibiotics and can be taken simultaneously with them.

A key component of risk reduction is maintaining a safe supply of food and drink. Epidemics of giardiasis and cryptosporidiosis from contaminated water and of food poisoning due to *Salmonella* in chicken or to toxic strains of *E. coli* in hamburger serve notice that the U.S. food and water supply is not safe. I give my patients certain guidelines to help them avoid infection when traveling to Asia and Africa. These same guidelines should be applied in the United States, at home or when dining out, because the food in the United States may be no safer than in many nonindustrialized nations. Although some of these guidelines may seem burdensome, they significantly reduce your risk of acquiring a food- or waterborne infection:

1. Always wash your hands carefully with soap and water when returning home from outside and before handling food. Hand-washing is a very effective way to remove pathogens. In day-care centers, where *Giardia* infection can be rampant, the parasite can be found on many surfaces, such as tables and chairs. Hand-washing by the staff drastically reduces the frequency of diarrhea. Regular hand-washing also protects against catching colds or flu from other people.

2. Don't drink tapwater that hasn't been properly filtered or kept at a rolling boil for at least five minutes. Chlorination does not kill the cyst forms of *Giardia* or *Cryptosporidium*, which are extremely hardy. The most effective way to remove *Cryptosporidium* from tapwater is to use a reverse osmosis system, which can be mounted under the sink or on a countertop. Reverse osmosis also removes many chemical contami-

nants from water but is slow and wasteful. A carbon-block filter with pores that are no larger than one micrometer is an effective way to remove chemicals and parasites. Water filters that effectively remove *Cryptosporidium* are certified by the National Sanitation Foundation (NSF), an independent nonprofit organization, under their Standard 53 for "cyst removal." No water filter practical for home use will remove bacteria. Have the bacterial concentration in your drinking water tested by an independent laboratory. Call the Water Quality Association at (708) 505-0160 or the American Council of Independent Laboratories at (202) 887-5872 for the name of a certified laboratory near your home.

The quality of bottled water is completely unregulated. Some bottled water comes from municipal water supplies. To discover the source of any bottled water, call the bottler and request documentation about the nature and purity of the source. Bottled water that comes from municipal water supplies or lakes should be treated by reverse osmosis before being bottled, if it is to be considered safe.

Avoid using ice unless you feel secure about the purity of the water from which it was made. Remember that automatic ice-makers use unfiltered tapwater. Freezing kills most parasites but does not kill bacteria.

Use pure water for brushing your teeth and rinsing your toothbrush.

3. Peel all fruits and vegetables, unless they are to be thoroughly cooked. Wash your hands afterward. If you cannot peel them, soak them for fifteen minutes in a solution made by adding one teaspoon of 3 percent hydrogen peroxide to two quarts of water and then rinse thoroughly with filtered water.

4. When eating out, only eat food that has been cooked just before it is served to you. In many restaurants and delicatessens, soups, sauces, and stews are frequently stored in large containers, often left uncovered on the floor and reheated in a microwave oven. Microwave cooking does not kill *Salmonella* and other strains of pathogenic bacteria. It is safest to eat food that is fairly plain and to avoid soup, unless you know how food is handled in the restaurant where you are eating.

5. Avoid salad bars. At first glance, salad bars seem like a good place to get healthy food in a hurry. Look again. Some years ago *The Wall Street Journal* sent a reporter to investigate the cleanliness of salad bars in different parts of the country. Problems were rampant, and they lay

not only with the restaurants but also with the clientele. People are un-sanitary in their use of salad bars. They sometimes sample food and put it back. The handles of the serving utensils frequently fall into the food trays, providing an opportunity for contamination.[98]

6. Do not eat food that has been prepared by a street vendor.

7. Avoid restaurants where there are flies. Flies can spread parasitic cysts and pathogenic bacteria.

8. Remember that uncooked meat, fish, and poultry are often con-taminated with pathogenic bacteria. When preparing your own meals, always keep raw flesh foods away from other food that will be eaten raw, like salad. Cook meat, fish, and poultry well and wash your hands after handling them. Also wash the utensils you use to cut them. People have become ill by handling chicken contaminated with *Salmonella* (as most American chicken is), and then using a contaminated knife or contaminated fingers to prepare other food that was not to be cooked. To kill *Salmonella* on utensils, soak them in a bleach solution for fif-teen minutes, then make sure you rinse the bleach thoroughly away. Do not use dishrags to wipe off kitchen counters, stoves, sinks, and ta-bles. Dishrags actually spread germs around. Use recycled paper towels to mop up the bacteria-laden juices from meat, poultry, and fish and use either paper towels or sponges to wipe surfaces. Run the sponges through the dishwasher every day to thoroughly remove bacteria.

Tofu is increasingly popular as a substitute for meat. Tofu that is bought floating in water often has high levels of bacterial contamina-tion. Wrapped and sealed tofu is safer. To kill bacteria, tofu should be cooked to an internal temperature of 160 degrees.

9. Have your pets de-wormed regularly. Wash your hands after han-dling your pets. Do not let your children crawl on ground where pets are free to roam.

For people traveling to places where a safe food supply cannot be as-sured, despite the implementation of all the precautions listed above, I recommend the use of antimicrobial herbs after each meal. My prefer-ence is a combination of berberine (the active ingredient in the herb goldenseal), 200 mg, and artemisinin (the most active ingredient in *Artemisia annua*), 100 mg, after each meal. This combination can help to prevent or treat bacterial and parasitic infection.[99] Do not take these herbs if you are pregnant, however; they can induce miscarriage.

There is a novel approach to control of intestinal pathogens, which derives from their need for iron. Virtually all bacteria, except for *Lactobacilli* and *Bifidobacteria,* require iron for growth. Animals protect themselves from infection by making chemicals that bind iron so that the microbes cannot use it. Iron-binding proteins called *lactoferrins* are concentrated in human milk and are found inside human white blood cells. The high lactoferrin in human milk protects breast-fed infants against intestinal infection. Pure lactoferrin is now available in capsules and has proved to be very useful for the prevention and treatment of intestinal infection, without side effects. It inhibits the growth of pathogenic bacteria and protozoa by starving them for iron, while improving iron absorption by the human host. I recommend that travelers and other people who cannot control the cleanliness of their food supply take one thousand milligrams of lactoferrin at bedtime and the artemisinin-berberine herbal mixture after meals.

To protect your body from intestinal toxins:

• Consume high-fiber foods daily: brown rice, oats, whole wheat, beans, peas, squash, nuts, and seeds.

• Eat freshly fermented foods like yogurt and sauerkraut or supplement your diet with friendly flora like *Lactobacillus acidophilus* and *Lactobacillus plantarum.*

• Spice your food liberally with garlic, onion, turmeric, ginger, sage, and rosemary. Add herbs and spices to food at the end of cooking, just before eating.

• Keep your use of drugs like alcohol, aspirin, and ibuprofen to a minimum.

• Avoid the use of antacids and acid-lowering drugs.

• Wash your hands carefully with soap and water when you return home from outside and before eating or handling food.

• Do not drink tapwater that has not been filtered by a carbon block or reverse osmosis or been kept at a rolling boil for five minutes.

• Peel all fruits and vegetables that are not going to be thoroughly cooked, or soak them for fifteen minutes in dilute hydrogen peroxide.

• Avoid salad bars, street vendors, and restaurants where there are flies.

• Wash your hands after handling raw food and soak utensils that you use on uncooked meat, poultry, or seafood for fifteen minutes in a solution of bleach.

• Do not wipe kitchen surfaces with dishrags; use disposable towels.

9

PLAGUES REVISITED

As I walked past a newsstand at Kennedy Airport, the cover of *Newsweek* demanded my attention. KILLER VIRUS, it warned. BEYOND THE EBOLA SCARE. WHAT ELSE IS OUT THERE?[1]

I thought about the words: *out there*. They say a great deal about the way we view infections. Infectious agents are *out there*, attacking us from a hostile environment which is beyond our control. At one time, we thought we had them beat.

INFECTIOUS DISEASES: IN HERE OR OUT THERE?

In 1969, the U.S. surgeon general, Dr. William H. Stewart, optimistically told Congress that it was time to "close the book on infectious diseases."[2] A decade later, AIDS would erupt in the United States and other sexually transmitted diseases would sharply increase. Lyme disease and Legionnaires' disease would be discovered, along with the bacterial cause of peptic ulcers. After another decade, measles would menace underimmunized college students and tuberculosis would surge again, threatening millions in crowded cities. Toxic shock syndrome, flesh-eating strep, and hantavirus would horrify the American

public, presaging the Ebola scare. Most terrifying of all, we would discover that our arsenal of antibiotics could not last forever, that bacteria
were developing resistance with frightening speed.

Although the war against infection is the arena in which modern
medicine has shown its greatest power, the war is so ill conceived that
it can never be won. Its premise is that microbes attack from *out there,*
that *they* are the causes of infectious disease. It disregards ecology and
evolution and ignores the precept that infection and disease are not the
same. Infection is unavoidable. We share the world—we share our own
bodies—with microorganisms that are hardier and more adaptable
than we are. Health results from stable coexistence, a condition called
symbiosis, not from a germ-free environment.[3] Infectious disease is the
failure of symbiosis. The symptoms and the pathology that accompany
infection are not produced by the microbe itself. They are the products
of our own immune responses, as we attempt to reestablish the symbiosis that has been disrupted. The assumption, supported by Koch's
discovery of the tubercle bacillus, that infectious disease is *caused* by
microbes, and that the response of the human host is of secondary importance, has lulled medical thinking to sleep.

The common symptoms of acute infection are protective, even if
they make us feel sick. Fever stimulates the activity of white blood cells.
Suppressing fever with aspirin slows recovery from colds and chicken
pox and may increase the likelihood that a person with severe bacterial
infection will go into shock.[4] Coughing and diarrhea expel microbes
from the body. Suppressing diarrhea with antidiarrheal drugs increases
the severity of bacterial dysentery. Pain and fatigue help to immobilize
the sick person, conserving energy and decreasing the likelihood that
infection will be spread through contact with others. Although the immune response to infection is generally beneficial, it may cause tissue
damage in the body. Extreme reactivity of the immune system almost
killed Miguel Benitez in the first few hours of his admission to Bellevue Hospital.

Miguel was infected with *Streptococcus pneumoniae* (colloquially
called *pneumococcus*), a species of bacteria that often grows in the nose
and throat of healthy people. The majority of children in the United
States experience at least one pneumococcal ear infection before the
age of five and recover without any complication, whether or not they
are given antibiotics. The mere presence of pneumococci in the body

is not enough to cause disease. First, the bacteria must attach to the cells lining the respiratory tract and induce these cells to separate from one another. When cells begin to peel apart, the respiratory lining is damaged, losing its integrity in the same way that the intestinal lining is damaged by the attachment of parasites. Live bacteria are not needed for damage to occur. Pneumococcal fragments will suffice, because these fragments transmit a chemical signal that activates the separation of cells. In a sense, the injury is self-induced.

White blood cells called *phagocytes* (literally, "cells that eat") are the best defense against further damage. They engulf pneumococci and their fragments and prevent them from provoking further peeling. If the work of phagocytes is hindered by alcohol, malnutrition, extreme cold, or a recent viral infection, the pneumococci are not restrained and are able to penetrate deeper. The tissues respond to this threat by forming tiny blood clots, flooding themselves with fluid, and emitting chemical signals that beckon more phagocytes to enter the area of penetration. This response is called *inflammation*. Its symptoms include fever and cough. Sometimes the lungs swell with so much fluid and such extensive clotting that they lose their lacelike honeycomb texture and turn into boggy lumps incapable of holding air. This is the classic pathology of pneumococcal pneumonia, and it still carries a death rate of 10 percent, despite the best available treatment.[5] In the case of Miguel Benitez, the white blood cell response was so ineffective that his pneumococci bypassed the lung, entering the bloodstream and provoking the clotting of blood throughout his body. Weakness in one component of the immune response allowed the activity of another component to carry him to the brink of death. In this way, infectious disease is not solely caused by infection. It is a self-induced process, in which the body's attempt to limit the spread of microbes causes much of the damage to tissue.

Specific Immunity

During every epidemic, however devastating, some people have seemed immune to sickness. Those who had survived a previous, similar epidemic were usually the least likely to succumb to the present one. From this observation came the technique of inoculation for smallpox, introduced in India among the aristocrats of the Brahman caste as early as the sixth century, spreading east to China by the eleventh century and west into Africa. A drop of pus from the sore of a smallpox victim was scratched into the skin on the arm of a child, producing a fresh sore and a—hopefully—mild form of the disease. The outcome was variable. One child out of fifty would die with smallpox, but the rest were never again troubled by the disease, which ordinarily killed off 10 to 15 percent of each new generation. The technique was introduced into the Americas by Cotton Mather, who learned of it from his African slave, Oneismus, and was brought to England at the instigation of Lady Mary Wortley Montagu, who was so convinced of its value that she arranged to have her six-year-old son, Edward, inoculated by an old Turkish woman, who used a rather blunt and rusty needle. Voltaire's recounting of the events made Lady Montagu internationally famous.[6]

In 1798, an English country doctor named Edward Jenner was told by a milkmaid that she had escaped smallpox by contracting cowpox from one of her animals. Cowpox is a mild disease of ruminants, which we now know is caused by a virus related to but far less dangerous than the virus of smallpox. Intrigued by the milkmaid's theory, Jenner began inoculating his patients with drops of pus from animals with cowpox. The technique was called *vaccination*, from the Latin word *vacca*, meaning "cow." Jenner published his technique, despite warnings from the Royal Society that it made no sense and would destroy his credibility. A public scandal ensued. Inoculating children with human pus was barely tolerable, but the use of cow pus was repulsive. Satirical cartoons depicted Jenner's patients growing horns, tails, and udders. But Jenner persisted, and the clear benefits of vaccination won him the support of Parliament. Vaccination rapidly spread around the world, enforced by Napoleon upon his troops and by the czar of Russia upon his people. Benjamin Waterhouse, an eminent Boston physician, performed the first New World vaccination on his five-year-old son in 1800. His support for the vaccination campaign cost him his professorship at Harvard and lost him many of his patients.

Vaccination eventually rid the world of smallpox. The last known case occurred in Somalia in October 1977. Eradication was made possible by three unusual characteristics of the smallpox virus: it has no animal reservoir, it is very stable and resistant to mutation, and one exposure confers lifelong immunity. As immunity spread around the world, the virus had no place to live. The last remaining specimens of smallpox virus are now frozen in liquid nitrogen and stored in maximum-security vaults in Atlanta and Moscow, awaiting their final destruction.[7]

Vaccination for smallpox exploits *specific* immunity, which is the ability of the body's lymphocytes to make antibodies that target a particular microorganism, either killing it or preventing its growth, before inflammation develops. The variability in specific immunity to various microbes among different populations has had profound historical effects. Smallpox was unknown in the New World prior to the Spanish explorations of the sixteenth century. It proved to be the main weapon of the *conquistadores*, decimating the Aztecs and the Incas, destroying their social organization and filling them with fear that the handful of strangers in their midst, immune to the devastation, were favored by the gods.

The epidemic of polio that brought panic to American parents in the mid-twentieth century reflects a changing pattern of specific immunity, paradoxically caused by improvements in sanitation. Paralytic polio was uncommon a hundred years ago. Outbreaks were recorded with increasing severity during the first two decades of the century, and the incidence of the disease steadily increased until just before the introduction of the Salk polio vaccine in the middle of the 1950s. The prevalence of infection with poliovirus did not change during that time. What changed was the frequency of polio, the crippling disease. In crowded urban slums, most children acquired the poliovirus before the age of three, either from other children or through contaminated water. Ninety-nine out of a hundred children would have no symptoms at all, and 1 percent would experience a mild flulike illness. Paralysis, which results from penetration of the virus into the spinal cord, was rare. With improved sanitation and the growth of suburbs, the onset of infection was postponed to late childhood, adolescence, or even adulthood. For reasons that are not understood, many viral infections, polio included, are least damaging in early childhood. Increasing maturity brings increasing severity of disease.[8] The virus doesn't change. It is the nature of the host that determines the outcome.

NONSPECIFIC IMMUNITY: THE TRIUMPH OF NUTRITION

Nonspecific immunity, the ability of an individual to resist the damage wrought by confrontation with a microbe, was the main factor responsible for the decline in mortality from infectious disease in the first half of the twentieth century. Its main determinant is nutrition. Along with housing and sanitation, nutrition, not medical care or the fruits of medical science, deserves credit for the increased life expectancy that followed the industrial revolution.[9]

Measles was the leading killer of children in nineteenth-century England, erupting with ferocious epidemics in the early and late decades of the century. During the twentieth century, long before a measles vaccine had become available, the severity of measles in the West began to decline. By mid-century, virtually all children in the United States and Britain still contracted measles but very few died. For African children, in contrast, measles remains a major killer. Despite the availability of measles vaccine, one million children die from measles each year. Most of them are poor and undernourished.[10] In fact, children in developing nations receiving measles vaccine experience an *increase* in mortality six to twelve months after vaccination, which is believed to be caused by immune suppression induced by the vaccine and amplified by malnutrition and chronic parasitic infection.[11]

For the past sixty years, we have known that vitamin A deficiency increases mortality of children with measles. Numerous studies have shown that administration of vitamin A to children in developing countries reduces measles fatalities by about 50 percent, and total mortality by about 35 percent. The declining severity of measles in developed nations over the past century has been due not to vaccination, but to our increased standard of living, which has made fruits and vegetables more widely available. In the United States today, the majority of children who develop measles have low levels of vitamin A. The relationship between measles and vitamin A is reciprocal. Vitamin A protects against the damage resulting from measles. Viral infection itself depletes the body's stores of vitamin A, because they are expended on recovering from the effects of infection. The more deficient the child, the sicker he gets and the more depleted. In this manner, a disease that is relatively benign among well-nourished children becomes fatal among those lacking a single nutrient. Dr. John Sommer of the Johns Hopkins University School of Hygiene and Public Health estimates that improving the vitamin A status of all deficient children worldwide would prevent as many as three million childhood deaths a year.[12]

The spread of tuberculosis in the industrialized world reached its peak in the late eighteenth century. At the start of the nineteenth century, half the world's population harbored the tubercle bacillus, fifty million people had active tuberculosis, and seven million people died of TB each year.[13] The spread of tuberculosis in Europe during the eighteenth and nineteenth centuries is often blamed on crowded housing, poor ventilation, and lack of sunlight, environmental conditions that foster the airborne spread of bacteria. Although crowded living conditions may increase exposure to the tubercle bacillus, they do not produce the disease. The death rate from TB began declining at the start of the nineteenth century, before improvements in housing occurred. In Britain, the death rate from TB dropped steadily and consistently from 1800 to 1950. The downward slope was interrupted twice, by World War I and World War II, which produced sharp but short-lived increases in TB mortality throughout Europe.[14]

The declining ferocity of the "captain of the men of death" is best explained by protein.[15] As early as the end of the eighteenth century, improvements in animal husbandry expanded the availability of meat and dairy products in Britain, and protein consumption slowly increased, even among the working poor. The growth of commercial fishing brought protein from seafood to the working classes, especially to men. By the middle of the nineteenth century, fish was a staple food of London dockworkers. The protein revolution came more slowly to women, whose portions of meat and cheese were only dispensed when their men were sated. Today, it is well known that women in the industrialized world have a greater life expectancy than men. In the last century, the opposite was true, and the shortened life expectancy of European women was almost wholly caused by their increased death rate from tuberculosis, the result of their lagging nutritional intake.[16]

With a phenomenal disregard for historical fact, medical science has taken credit for the decline of tuberculosis. In a recent book, Dr. Frank Ryan emphatically stated, "There can be little doubt that the discovery

of the cure for tuberculosis changed human history."[17] When streptomycin, the first antibiotic active against tubercle bacilli, was discovered
at Rutgers University in 1944, mortality from TB had already declined
from its peak level by 90 percent. Antibiotics merely accentuated the
trend. They steepened the slope of the decline in mortality and reduced the incidence of new cases of tuberculosis in North America and
Europe—for about thirty years.[18] The 1980s witnessed a resurgence in
the global spread of tuberculosis. By 1990, TB had again become the
world's leading cause of death due to infectious disease, claiming close
to three million lives per year.[19] The United States did not escape this
plague. Between 1985 and 1990, the prevalence of TB in the United
States increased by 20 percent. In New York City, the incidence of tuberculosis tripled from 1978 to 1992. Harlem today has a TB infection
rate that is higher than that of many underdeveloped countries.[20] The
resurgence of tuberculosis has been driven by factors that suppress immunity: increasing urban poverty and its companions—drug addiction,
alcohol abuse, and malnutrition—and the epidemic of AIDS.

THE SCOURGE OF AIDS

The naming of a new disease, like AIDS, does not mean that the microbes that provoke it are new. The origin of the virus associated with
AIDS is still unknown, and it may have been present for centuries before its rapid spread, which started in the late 1970s.[21] The first sign that
something terrible was about to happen was a report from the Centers
for Disease Control (CDC) in June 1981. An unusual form of pneumonia had killed five young homosexual men in Los Angeles. Their lungs
were filled with a parasite, *Pneumocystis carinii*, which was supposed to
cause disease only in people with severe immune deficiency, yet none
of these men had any known reason for immune deficiency. More reports followed quickly. *Pneumocystis carinii* pneumonia (PCP) was
found in association with thrush (a severe yeast infection of the mouth)
and an unusual form of skin cancer called Kaposi's sarcoma. The condition was initially called GRID (gay-related immune deficiency), and
its immune defect could be readily measured in the laboratory. A specialized group of lymphocytes called T-helper cells was decimated in
men with GRID. Loss of T-helper cells left victims of GRID subject to

infections with organisms like *Pneumocystis* that do not usually trouble healthy people. These are called "opportunistic infections." The term "opportunistic" implies that the causative agents are not ordinarily harmful, but take advantage of an impaired host to become aggressive. Opportunism is a relative concept. All microbes are opportunists and expand their niches as far as possible, depending upon the available resources for growth and the resistance offered by their environments.

GRID became AIDS (acquired immune deficiency syndrome) when its spectrum expanded. Opportunistic infections and depletion of T-helper cells soon appeared among heroin addicts, Haitian immigrants, people with hemophilia, the recipients of blood transfusions, and African prostitutes. Scientists searched for a new virus, one transmitted through the blood or by sexual intercourse. On April 23, 1984, the U.S. secretary of health and human services, Margaret Heckler, organized a press conference to announce the discovery of this virus, subsequently named the human immunodeficiency virus (HIV).

"Today," announced the secretary, "we add another miracle to the long honor roll of American medicine and science. Today's discovery represents the triumph of science over a dreadful disease."[22] She failed to mention that the virus had been isolated in Paris at the Institut Pasteur about a month before its isolation by scientists at the National Cancer Institute in Bethesda, Maryland. Robert Gallo, the NCI scientist whose team took credit for discovering HIV, promised that a vaccine would be available within two years. Twelve years later, four and a half million people have developed AIDS, more than nineteen million people are infected with HIV, eighty-five hundred new infections occur *every day*, and the number is still tragically increasing. In the United States, AIDS has become the leading cause of death among young adults.[23]

The discovery of HIV and the availability of blood tests for HIV antibodies slowly changed the concept of AIDS. It was possible to identify people infected with HIV who did not have opportunistic infections or Kaposi's sarcoma, or who were not even sick. A new concept emerged, called "HIV disease." The diagnosis of this disease was based solely on a laboratory test, the presence of antibodies to HIV. In 1990, the World Health Organization proposed a four-tiered staging system for HIV disease, which ranged from asymptomatic to advanced, with the criteria for advanced being the presence of opportunistic infections, Kaposi's sarcoma, or extreme debilitation. Intermediate staging was assigned to people with chronic fatigue, weight loss, skin rashes, swollen lymph nodes, or repeated bouts of sinusitis, thrush, or diarrhea.[24]

Except for the presence of HIV antibodies or HIV particles, none of the clinical or laboratory manifestations associated with HIV disease are specific for HIV infection. They have all been described in people without evidence of HIV infection. This is even true for the criteria originally used to define AIDS in America: Kaposi's sarcoma, PCP, and depletion of T-helper cells.[25] Each symptom or sign is given a new meaning, and a more ominous prognosis, when associated with the presence of HIV antibodies. For the person who is "HIV positive," every cold or flu is an omen, every pain a cause for alarm.

The problems posed by HIV disease profoundly challenge the way we wage the War on Infection. Most research has been driven by the quest for magic bullets: a vaccine against HIV and drugs that kill the virus or stop its replication.[26] HIV has confounded both approaches because of its high rate of mutation. Strains of HIV that are drug resistant emerge rapidly. Recent studies have demonstrated that multiple antiviral drugs, administered simultaneously early in the course of infection, may overcome this problem. The cautious optimism supported by these studies has given fresh hope to the community of people, scientists included, whose lives are enveloped by the tragedy of AIDS. Yet the limitations of the magic bullet approach to AIDS remain abundantly clear. Ninety percent of HIV infections occur in developing nations that lack the resources to pay for the enormous cost of treatment. In the United States and Europe, an international panel of AIDS researchers warns that "these agents do not guarantee that HIV transmission will be lowered and they raise the spectre that multi-drug resistant strains of HIV may be transmitted from infected to uninfected individuals."[27] Dr. Jay Levy of the University of California, San Francisco, cautions that "treatment directed at the virus alone is not sufficient,"[28] and Dr. Anthony Fauci of the National Institute of Allergy and Infectious Diseases advises, "Host factors have been shown to play a major role in the pathogenesis of HIV disease."[29]

There is a growing understanding among scientists that the development of HIV is multifactorial and that its pathology is not solely the result of immune deficiency induced by HIV infection. The immune system of people with all stages of HIV disease is chronically *overstim-*

ulated, releasing cytokines and prostanoids that damage the body's own
cells, cause weight loss and malnutrition, and prevent healing.[30] Even
those physicians who view HIV as the sole cause of AIDS recognize the
critical importance of infectious *cofactors* that are intrinsic to the development of HIV disease. It is the *other* infections affecting people
with HIV disease that make them sick: PCP, bacterial pneumonia, intestinal parasites, tuberculosis, and a number of fungal and viral infections. These *other* agents provoke most of the clinical disorders
considered a hallmark of advancing HIV disease.[31] They also increase
the rate of deterioration and the severity of HIV infection itself. Coin-
fection accelerates HIV disease by stimulating an imbalanced immune
system to produce cytokines that aggravate immune damage.

Infectious cofactors also play a critical role in promoting the initial
acquisition of HIV infection. Two-thirds of the world's HIV-infected
population live in sub-Saharan Africa, where parasitic infection and
malnutrition are endemic and sexually transmitted bacterial infections
are common. Antibiotic treatment of infections like gonorrhea and
syphilis markedly reduces the rate at which HIV is spread in rural
Africa.[32] Vitamin A deficiency, a common problem in Africa that contributes to the high mortality from childhood measles, also increases
the risk that a pregnant woman will transmit her HIV infection to her
newborn child.[33] Infection with amoebic parasites causes immune defects and can stimulate the growth of HIV in T-helper cells.[34] The epidemic of AIDS that swept through the gay communities of North
America was preceded by an epidemic of parasitic infection. Gay men
without HIV infection who were studied early in the AIDS epidemic already had a type of immune impairment that would increase their susceptibility to the virus.[35]

Those scientists who support the solitary role of HIV infection in
HIV disease usually cite as evidence the appearance of AIDS in people
who have received blood transfusions or injections of human clotting
factor concentrates for treatment of hemophilia. Presumably these
people are no more malnourished or likely to be drug abusers than the
population as a whole. But administration of human clotting factors or
of blood in itself alters immune responses, and people who have received blood transfusions have injuries or diseases that themselves impair immunity.[36]

The strongest case for a multifaceted understanding of AIDS is often overlooked: most people who are exposed to HIV do not develop HIV infection or HIV disease. The wives of men with hemophilia rarely become infected.[37] Of a thousand health workers stuck by contaminated needles, only three will show evidence of HIV infection. The majority of the others mount an initial immune response to the virus that prevents active infection.[38] The same is true of African women who resist infection after HIV exposure.[39]

HIV is itself an opportunist, spreading among people with preexisting immune dysfunction caused by drugs, medical treatment, parasites, or malnutrition. Nonetheless, when chronic HIV infection occurs, AIDS is not the inevitable outcome. A growing number of people in the United States have asymptomatic HIV infection that has lasted for ten to fifteen years without producing illness. These people maintain an active, organized immune response against the virus.[40] Most people with chronic, nonprogressive HIV infection have long abandoned their high-risk activities and use of drugs, and are consuming diets of high nutrient density supplemented with large doses of vitamin C, beta-carotene, and other antioxidants. Nutrition may not be the reason they have remained well, but higher nutritional intake early in the course of infection is associated with a better prognosis, and antioxidant supplementation has been advocated as a safe and rational strategy for immune support by scientists studying the effects of AIDS on the body.[41] Most people with nonprogressive HIV infection are passionately committed to their nutritional therapies.[42] This commitment may in itself have a beneficial effect on prognosis, because depression and denial are associated with an increased rate of disease progression.[43]

INFECTION AND SELF-CARE

Self-care for AIDS prevention has a social benefit beyond the improvement in individual survival. Virulence—the potency of microbes in causing disease—may be more strongly influenced by the characteristics of the host than by the microbe itself. Microbes like HIV, which undergo frequent mutation and are spread directly from person to person, tend to increase their virulence when their hosts make it easy for them to multiply and to spread. The mutation rate of HIV is so great that new strains with slightly altered characteristics emerge continuously. If host resistance is strong and interpersonal transmission is slow, those strains will survive that are least damaging to the host, giving each person the greatest opportunity to spread the organism to others. If, on the other hand, host resistance is weak and accelerated transmission is favored by extreme sexual promiscuity, the sharing of needles, or other behaviors, the opportunity is created for fast-growing, highly virulent strains to dominate. In this way, changes in the host create changes in the microbe, and new patterns of disease emerge. Improving the host's immunity and decreasing the high-risk behaviors that facilitate viral transmission not only decreases the spread of the virus but actually favors the evolution of reduced virulence, which can benefit everyone.[44]

Even the dreaded Ebola virus owes its lethal potency to human behavior. In the four known African Ebola epidemics, the fatality rate was close to 90 percent, making Ebola appear more formidable than any other infectious agent ever encountered. The disease would strike suddenly, with fever and malaise, like a bad case of the flu. Pain in the chest and abdomen, skin rash, diarrhea, and severe prostration would soon follow. Those few destined to survive would begin a slow recovery after one week of agonizing pain. The majority would lapse into coma and hemorrhage throughout their bodies, convulsive seizures bringing death. The global terror evoked by the 1995 epidemic was phenomenal.

The truth is that Ebola virus is not the unstoppable monster it appears to be. It is not readily spread from person to person and is rapidly killed by sunlight. People throughout Africa have antibodies to Ebola, signifying past exposure to the virus, possibly from infected bats. Epidemics occurred when people received medical treatment at ill-equipped, impoverished hospitals. The origin of the first epidemic, in 1976, was traced to five unsterilized syringes, each used to give one hundred injections per day to patients at a missionary hospital in Yambuku, Zaire. The initial case was a man from a nearby village who spent two days at the hospital, suffering from diarrhea and a nosebleed, and then walked home, leaving the virus behind. The epidemic started slowly within a week of his departure. Every victim was a patient or employee at the hospital, or a close relative who had washed the body of someone who had died. Unprotected exposure to contaminated needles and body fluids was apparently the sole mode of transmission. Each epidemic was stopped in its tracks by the implementation of standard hygienic techniques. The Ebola epidemics were not caused by a virus.

They were caused by poverty, ignorance, and lack of training among health personnel. The high fatality rate suggests that Ebola's virulence was dramatically amplified by the ease with which it disseminated in hospitals.[45]

The next plague is not going to attack the world from *out there*. It will be created by us. Like Ebola, it may well be a product of medical care.

ANTIBIOTICS AMOK

The most common way in which medical care disrupts symbiosis and alters the microbes that surround us is through the use of antibiotics. When antibiotics destroy the particular organisms that are sensitive to them, some organisms that are not sensitive survive. Because microbes tend to inhibit one another's growth, the survivors have the opportunity to flourish. The mutual inhibition among microbes proceeds by two mechanisms. First, they compete among themselves for food. Second, they secrete growth-inhibiting chemicals. Some of these chemicals are the waste products of microbial metabolism, like alcohol and lactic acid. The name *Lactobacillus acidophilus* means "the rod-shaped bacterium that loves lactic acid." Through their copious production of lactic acid, *Lactobacilli* curb the growth of other bacteria. The suppressive effect of lactic acid is not restricted to any particular species of bacteria. In fact, enough lactic acid will kill the *Lactobacilli* themselves, just as the alcohol in wine and beer kills the yeasts that originally produced it. Lactic acid accumulation is one reason that most of the yogurt bought in supermarkets has very few living *Lactobacilli* remaining and cannot be used as an efficient starter for a new crop of yogurt.

Microbes also inhibit the growth of other microbes by producing specific inhibitory substances. As early as 1870, several scientists had called attention to the implications of "antibiosis," the competitive struggle for existence among different microorganisms. In 1928, a Scottish bacteriologist, Alexander Fleming, discovered a mold called *Penicillium notatum* growing on a culture plate that had been left on his laboratory bench while he was on vacation. To his surprise, the bacteria with which the plate had originally been seeded failed to grow in the vicinity of the mold. Fleming juiced the mold and found that its antibacterial property lay in the juice. He published his results the next year, but made little effort to harvest mold extract for therapeutic use.[46]

With the outbreak of World War II, Howard Florey and Ernst Chain of Oxford University began searching for chemicals to treat or prevent wound infections. They extracted penicillin from Fleming's mold juice and quickly demonstrated its remarkable efficacy against the major bacterial species that infect the skin and the respiratory tract. Penicillin was soon worth its weight in gold, at least on the black market that developed before its industrial production in the United States made it easy to obtain. The commercial availability of penicillin produced a revolution in the treatment of pneumonia, tonsillitis, sinusitis, ear infections, and life-threatening infections of the skin, which formerly would spread through the blood and lymphatic system, poisoning the entire body, a condition referred to as *sepsis*.

Since World War II, over thirty different groups of fungal metabolites have been turned into important antibiotic drugs. Fungi secrete these antibiotics to limit bacterial damage to themselves and their food supply. Our appropriation of fungal by-products for medicinal use is both wise and "natural," but it has severe ecological consequences. Bacteria have lived with antibiotics for over a billion years. Not only have many bacterial strains developed methods for inactivating antibiotics (antibiotic resistance), they have developed methods for rapidly transferring this resistance from one bacterial species to another. Exposure to antibiotics activates the transfer of resistance genes, so that the application of a single antibiotic drug prompts the growth of bacterial populations resistant to many drugs at the same time. Since the 1940s, we have polluted our environment with industrially produced antibiotics at an alarming rate, stimulating the worldwide growth of bacteria that are resistant to multiple drugs (MDR-bacteria). The main sources of pollution have been the addition of antibiotics to animal feed and the profligate use of medicinal antibiotics by humans.

Antibiotics Enter the Food Supply

Antibiotics were first added to animal feed in the early 1950s, when it was discovered that they stimulated the growth of farm animals. Sound animal husbandry, however, obviates the need for antibiotic feeding. Animals reared under sanitary conditions and fed a nutritious diet do not grow better on antibiotics. The effect is seen only in runts and in animals who are malnourished.[47] Animals who are fed antibiotics become breeding grounds for resistant organisms that travel from them to farm personnel, food handlers, and eventually to consumers. Today, drug-resistant bacteria can be found growing on commercial fruits and vegetables. Healthy people who don't take antibiotics but who consume raw fruits and vegetables bought in supermarkets are heavily colonized with MDR-bacteria. When they cook all food before eating it, the levels of MDR-bacteria drop precipitously, indicating that the food transmitted the resistant organisms to healthy individuals.[48]

Antibiotic Resistance Flourishes

Within two years of penicillin's debut as a commercial drug, physicians witnessed the emergence of severe, resistant infections with unusual organisms, which struck their patients while they were still receiving penicillin.[49] Bacterial species that had rarely bothered humans in the past became major causes of infection acquired in hospitals. They spread to people from ventilation systems, pieces of medical equipment, and the unwashed hands of doctors and nurses, who, even today, refuse to practice the basic hygiene taught by Semmelweiss a hundred and fifty years ago, hand-washing in between the examination of patients.[50] It has been known for decades that the longer a person stays in the hospital, the more likely it is that he will become infected with resistant bacteria; and the more courses of antibiotics he receives, the more likely it is that he will die from an infection that no antibiotic can touch.

Infection with *Staphylococcus* (staph) is a major threat in hospitals, because staph grows readily on the skin and has a penchant for entering surgical wounds. In 1944, all *Staphylococci* were sensitive to penicillin. Resistance developed rapidly and pharmaceutical companies had to work assiduously, developing new forms of penicillin that could stay ahead of staph. Resistance has developed to each one. At the time of this writing (late 1996), there is only one antibiotic, vancomycin, that is universally effective against all strains of staph. But vancomycin has not only been used for treating staph infections; it is also used to kill other bacteria. By 1988, a few strains of *Enterococcus*, which is a distant relative of *Staphylococcus*, had learned how to defeat vancomycin. Over the next five years, the frequency with which vancomycin-resistant *Enterococci* were found in hospitals increased by 2,600 percent. Vancomycin use is now under stricter control, but it is not rolling back the numbers of resistant organisms.[51] If vancomycin resistance is transferred from *Enterococcus* to *Staphylococcus*, which is the nemesis of surgeons, the safety record of hospital-based surgery will plummet.

Infections that originate outside hospitals, in homes and communities, are also increasingly resistant to antibiotics. When I treated Miguel Benitez at Bellevue Hospital in 1968, I could be almost certain that his pneumococcal infection would respond to penicillin. In 1985, the prevalence of penicillin-resistant pneumococcus was still quite low. In the United States, only one person in five thousand with pneumococcal infection harbored a penicillin-resistant strain. By 1991, the prevalence had increased to five per hundred, and by 1994, it had reached twenty-five per hundred. At present, for white schoolchildren with respiratory infections caused by pneumococcus, the rate of penicillin resistance is over 50 percent, and one-quarter to one half are also resistant to the other antibiotics commonly used to treat childhood respiratory infections, such as erythromycin and co-trimoxazole (Bactrim/Septra). The rate is lower among black and Hispanic children, because their antibiotic exposure is less.[52]

Sadly, the response of doctors to this alarming trend is not to prescribe fewer antibiotics, but to prescribe more. Between 1980 and 1992, prescriptions for antibiotics in the United States increased by almost 30 percent, with the bulk of the increase going to the newest, most expensive antibiotics, the ones that are needed for treating resistant infections.

When Do We Really Need Antibiotics?

The scandal is that most of these antibiotics never needed to be prescribed.

The most frequent conditions for which doctors prescribe antibiotics are ear infections, upper respiratory infections (colds), acute bronchitis, sore throats, and sinusitis, with colds and bronchitis accounting for almost a third of out-of-hospital antibiotic prescriptions.[53] Rarely do antibiotics help patients recover from colds or acute bronchitis, because the infecting organisms are viral, not bacterial, and antibiotics have never been effective for viral infection.[54]

Sinusitis

The lack of benefit resulting from antibiotic treatment of sinusitis and ear infections is not as clear-cut, but there is a good deal of evidence that antibiotics are usually not needed to treat either of these infections. Sinusitis, for example, is most often a complication of the common cold. The majority of people with colds show evidence of sinusitis on sinus CAT scans and cure the sinusitis themselves, without antibiotics, within one to two weeks.[55] Even when bacteria infect the sinus cavities, the sensitivity of the bacteria to specific antibiotics and the response of the person to those same antibiotics do not match up, indicating that the bacteria may be growing there but are not the cause of the inflammation.[56] Most children with sinusitis fare no better if they receive antibiotics than if they don't.[57]

Middle Ear Infections

At the present time, the commonest diagnosis for which out-of-hospital antibiotics are prescribed in the United States is childhood ear infection (*otitis media*, which means inflammation of the middle ear). A virtual epidemic of otitis media is ravaging North American children. The incidence doubled between 1980 and 1990. Treatment costs for otitis during the 1980s averaged $3.5 billion per year. Antibiotics are always prescribed for this condition, even though children recover fully and almost as quickly without them.[58]

One reason that antibiotics are routinely used for acute otitis is the belief that antibiotics will prevent a complication of otitis called *mastoiditis* (infection of the mastoid bone, the part of the skull to which the ear attaches). In the decade before penicillin, mastoiditis often followed otitis. Today, mastoiditis is rare among middle-class children in the United States but still quite common in the inner cities. Contrary to medical mythology, antibiotics do not deserve credit for the dramatic reduction in mastoiditis. In Holland, children older than one year of age are no longer treated with antibiotics for acute otitis media. Antibiotic treatment was abandoned during the 1980s, yet the incidence of mastoiditis there has remained extremely low. It is likely that improved nutrition in early childhood, rather than antibiotics, accounts for the reduction in mastoiditis rates.[59]

One problem with antibiotic treatment of otitis media is its inappropriate use in children with *chronic* otitis, which is persistent fluid in the ears lasting for weeks, months, or years. Although bacteria are usually present in the middle ear fluid of children with chronic otitis, there is no evidence that antibiotics can cure this condition.[60] Over three-quarters of children with chronic otitis media have food allergies; the appropriate diet resolves the "infection" for 90 percent of them.[61] The treatment fiasco for otitis media is a glaring example of the error that occurs when doctors seek the cause of illness in a microbe rather than in the characteristics of the person who is sick.

The Alliance for the Prudent Use of Antibiotics cautions people to recognize that antibiotics are a precious resource, which must not be squandered. They advise:

DO'S

• DO maintain good sanitary conditions. A clean environment makes for healthier people and reduces infections and the need for antibiotics.
• DO maintain a healthy diet and adequate sleep. These measures are important in protecting your body from infection.
• DO take antibiotics for the complete duration of your doctor's prescription. Full-term use of the antibiotic is essential for a complete cure.
• DO tell your doctor of any allergies you have to drugs.
• DO tell your doctor of any reactions you have while taking an antibiotic.

DON'TS

• DON'T demand antibiotics from your physician.
• DON'T stockpile antibiotics for later use.
• DON'T take an antibiotic without knowing what the possible side effects could be.
• DON'T take antibiotics for simple diarrhea, common colds, or other nonbacterial or viral diseases. *They do not work!*

- DON'T take antibiotics to prevent a disease to which you think you might be exposed—you are only increasing your chances of picking up a resistant infection, and you will also change your body's physiology.

- DON'T play doctor. Do not give out unused antibiotics to family and friends.

(Source: Alliance for the Prudent Use of Antibiotics, P.O. Box 1372, Boston, MA 02117-1372.)

EATING RIGHT TO FIGHT INFECTION

The germ theory of disease, as formulated by Robert Koch, was brilliant science but poor medicine. Its narrow focus blinds physicians to the nature of the person who becomes sick and the characteristics of the environment in which sickness occurs.

The first goals of prevention and treatment of infection must be to enhance each person's general, nonspecific resistance and to create an environment that encourages the maintenance of symbiosis.

The leading cause of immune deficiency, worldwide and within the United States, is poor nutrition.[62] Its effects have been most readily measured in the elderly, who often consume poor diets, even when healthy and living independently.[63] When apparently healthy persons were followed for ten years, those people who had impairment on laboratory tests of immune function at baseline had twice the mortality rate of those with normal immunity.[64] Study after study has found that vitamin and mineral supplements improve the immune function of elderly Americans.[65] The specific nutrients with the most profound effects on immune function are EFAs, protein, zinc, vitamin A, vitamin B_6, folic acid, and iron. Among the healthy elderly, immune-boosting benefits have been demonstrated for antioxidants like zinc, selenium, vitamin E, and beta-carotene.[66]

As I stated in Chapter Eight, I don't recommend beta-carotene supplements to my patients because beta-carotene is readily available from fruits and vegetables, mixed with other beneficial antioxidants like the carotenoids and bioflavonoids. Beta-carotene supplements have been shown not to be useful in preventing cancer, whereas eating food high in beta-carotene does appear to be beneficial. The difference is that food rich in beta-carotene is also rich in other antioxidants and can support the whole antioxidant defense system in a way that pills of a single nutrient cannot.

I recommend you follow the dietary guidelines in Chapter Six as the first step toward achieving optimum resistance to infection. Not only will you reach adequate levels of all the essential nutrients for immune function, you'll minimize your exposure to pesticides, which impair immunity.[67]

Consume More Saponins

A high intake of vegetables increases the consumption of a group of natural chemicals called *saponins*, which have immune-stimulating and antibiotic effects. Saponins are the latest in a long list of plant chemicals that are not considered nutrients, the way that vitamins are, because no deficiency state has been identified, but which promote health. In plants, saponins seem to function as natural antibiotics, protecting the plant against microbial parasites. In humans, they may thwart cancer and ward off infection.[68] Saponins are most highly concentrated in soybeans, chickpeas, bean sprouts, asparagus, tomatoes, potatoes, and oats. They have a creamy texture and a sweet taste that separates them from other plant components. Some biotechnology companies are presently attempting to harvest saponins and use them as drugs.

Supplement Your Diet with Essential Fatty Acids

The nutrient-dense diet will also keep you from consuming too much fat and iron, which may impair immunity. Restricting dietary fat is especially important for building nonspecific resistance. The activity of a group of lymphocytes known as "natural killer cells" is enhanced by a low-fat diet and diminished by a high-fat diet.[69] Supplementing a low-fat diet with omega-three essential fatty acids (EFAs) supports normal immune function by two additional mechanisms: (1) omega-three EFAs increase the activity of phagocytes (the white blood cells that consume and destroy bacteria); (2) EFAs inhibit excessive reactivity of the immune system in response to infection.[70] This is crucial, because much of the damage associated with infection is caused by the immune system itself. A diet supplemented with fish oil, antioxidants, trace minerals, and the amino acid arginine has been shown to improve immune responsiveness in critically ill patients with severe burns, decreasing the rate of infection and permitting earlier hospital discharge.[71] For adults who are not critically ill, I recommend one tablespoon (about ten grams) of flax oil or three capsules (three to four grams) of fish oil concentrate per day. A controlled treatment study recently found that children experience fewer respiratory infections, less severe respiratory infections, and fewer days absent from school when supplementing their diets with two grams of flax oil a day.[72]

When supplementing your diet with EFAs, you'll usually need to take additional vitamin E. By increasing the generation of free radicals, EFA supplements taken without vitamin E may impair some important components of the immune response.[73] Vitamin E at a dose of only two hundred milligrams per day reverses EFA-induced immune suppression, even in people taking high doses of fish oil.[74] Combined treatment with vitamin E and fish oil is especially beneficial for the function of phagocytes. The optimum dose of vitamin E for improving immune function is probably in the range of two hundred to four hundred milligrams per day.[75] Higher doses are considered safe,[76] but I don't recommend their routine use because higher doses may actually impair the activity of phagocytes. The vitamin E levels of U.S. children are markedly lower than those of Japanese, German, Austrian, or Canadian children, suggesting that children in the United States may as a group suffer from a mild deficiency.[77] Healthy children with lower vitamin E levels have impaired immunity on laboratory testing.[78] The immune defects associated with a relative vitamin E deficiency in "healthy" children are the same deficits associated with increased mortality in the elderly.

The Role of Iron

After the wrong kind of fat, the nutrient most likely to cause rather than prevent infectious disease is iron. Iron is unique among essential minerals, because there is no mechanism for its excretion once it is absorbed into the body. Whatever iron is absorbed must be either used or stored, and excessive storage of iron in the body promotes the generation of free radicals. Excess dietary iron has been implicated by some scientists as a cause of cancer and heart disease. It also increases the risk of bacterial infection.

Except for the lactic acid bacteria like *Lactobacilli*, all microbes require iron for growth. Many of them produce special binding proteins to secure iron from their environments. Humans also produce iron-binding proteins that capture free iron so that microbes can't use it. An excess of iron overcomes this protective mechanism and increases susceptibility to bacterial infection. The amount of iron needed for optimal health reflects a delicate balance between deficiency and excess.[79]

The best-known effect of iron deficiency is *anemia*, which is the name given to a state in which the number of red blood cells is lower than normal. Anemia is not the same as iron deficiency, however. There are many different causes of anemia, which include folic acid deficiency, vitamin B_{12} deficiency, disorders of the bone marrow, and conditions that increase the rate at which red blood cells are broken down in the spleen. Iron deficiency, when mild, may not produce anemia but may still cause fatigue, immune defects, or fungal infections of skin.[80] There are probably twenty million people in the United States who are iron-deficient, and half of them are not anemic. Women with chronic fatigue and mild iron deficiency who are not anemic improve their energy after taking low doses of iron.[81] Twenty milligrams per day is all that's needed, no more. Low-dose iron supplements can cure people with recurrent boils on the skin, but only if those people have mild iron deficiency.[82] Presumably, correcting iron deficiency improves metabolism and immunity.

It is unfortunate that most commercial iron pills contain sixty to three hundred milligrams of iron, far more than are needed or than can even be absorbed from a single pill. High-dose iron supplements, taken orally or by injection, increase susceptibility to bacterial infection. Studies in Southeast Asia and in Africa demonstrate that even low-dose iron can be harmful. When Indonesian schoolchildren who are not iron-deficient take iron pills, they fail to grow normally.[83] When iron supplements are given to Somali nomads or Masai people, their rate of infection increases, even though their iron deficiency is corrected.[84] The high frequency of negative responses to iron supplements in Africa and Asia may reflect the interaction between iron and zinc.

Iron in food or pills interferes with zinc absorption and supplemental iron can aggravate zinc deficiency, which profoundly depresses immune function. The recommended daily allowance (RDA) for zinc, 12 to 15 mg/day, is based on the assumption that 40 percent of the zinc that is swallowed is absorbed into the body. Actually, only 17 to 35 percent of the zinc you eat gets absorbed, depending on what you eat with it. Starch and fiber interfere with zinc absorption, as do calcium and iron.[85] Lack of stomach acid, which may be caused by infection or acid-lowering drugs, also interferes with zinc absorption.[86] Zinc deficiency is common in parts of Africa and Asia where people consume large quantities of milk, which is high in calcium and low in zinc, and of starches and fibers, which interfere with zinc absorption. Administering iron to a zinc-deficient person is extremely risky. Not only does iron stimulate bacterial growth, but, by aggravating zinc deficiency, it weakens the immune system of the person being supplemented.

Never take iron supplements unless you have diagnosed iron deficiency. Pregnancy is the possible exception to this rule; check with your obstetrician. The best test for iron deficiency is a blood test called the *serum ferritin level*. Ferritin is a protein that carries iron, and low ferritin levels are a common sign of iron deficiency. Like all laboratory tests, the meaning of a ferritin level is subject to interpretation. Because the body has a limited capacity for iron absorption, it does not make any sense to take more than twenty milligrams of elemental iron at a time if you have a documented deficiency. Only take iron supplements for as long as your doctor recommends to correct a deficiency. This should take no longer than six months. Don't take iron as part of a multivitamin or multimineral preparation. Iron interferes with the absorption of the essential minerals zinc, manganese, and molybdenum; it destroys vitamin E; its own absorption is blocked by calcium and magnesium. Iron is best absorbed after a meal, with a small quantity of vitamin C (between one hundred and five hundred milligrams).

The second step in securing maximum immunity against infectious disease is assuring normal intestinal permeability, using the methods I described in Chapter Eight. Healthy intestinal bacterial flora stimulate immune responses in the gut, whereas depletion of intestinal bacteria with antibiotics suppresses immune responsiveness.[87]

Among the spices that protect normal intestinal permeability, garlic has the greatest immune-enhancing effect, stimulating activity of natural killer cells in healthy people and in people with AIDS. In one study, AIDS patients taking five to ten grams of aged garlic (equivalent to two to three small cloves) per day developed normal natural killer cell activity after twelve weeks, which was associated with clinical improvement.[88] The measures outlined in Chapter Eight for promoting intestinal hygiene not only improve immune function, but also guard against most food-borne infectious agents. The measures presented in Chapter Seven for protection against environmental toxicity not only offer protection against environmental hazards to the immune system, like mycotoxins, but also decrease the likelihood of being exposed to many of the airborne infectious agents.

OTHER MEASURES TO BUILD RESISTANCE

Adults, adolescents, and children may sometimes develop repeated infections despite a hygienic environment, a regular schedule of rest and exercise, and a diet of high nutrient density, appropriately tailored to their constitutional needs, supplemented with EFAs and antioxidants. There are many additional measures you can take to stimulate resistance to infections. I recommend these frequently to patients in my medical practice and have been impressed with their safety and efficacy:

1. Vitamin C, two thousand milligrams per day, taken in divided doses, increases the activity of phagocytes.[89]
2. Exposure to full-spectrum artificial light, ten thousand lux for thirty minutes per day, during the winter, can improve mood and the function of natural killer cells in people prone to winter depression.[90] You can buy an apparatus for delivering full-spectrum light of this intensity from Bio-Brite, Inc., Bethesda, Maryland, (800) 621-5483, or Hughes Lighting Technologies, Lake Hopatcong, New Jersey, (201) 663-1214.
3. Granular lecithin, two tablespoons a day, has been shown to improve the activity of phagocytes.[91] Lecithin is a common food additive and food supplement, derived from soybeans, readily available in natural food stores. I do not recommend lecithin for pregnant or nursing

women, because its safe use in pregnancy and nursing has not been demonstrated.

4. Dimethylglycine (DMG), an amino acid normally found in the body, has been shown to boost antibody responses to immunization in healthy human volunteers. The dose used was 120 milligrams per day.[92] I frequently recommend dimethylglycine for patients with recurrent bacterial infection. It is readily available in natural food stores. The safety of DMG during pregnancy or nursing has not been established.

5. Immune-stimulating herbs are becoming available in increasing numbers of locations. The following are safe and well studied, but should be avoided during pregnancy or nursing:

Echinacea species, popularly known as coneflower or Black Sampson, grow wild across the American Midwest from Wisconsin to Texas. All parts of the *Echinacea* plant have been used for centuries by Native Americans to treat wounds and snakebite. Recent studies on its effects reveal marked stimulation of many immune functions, including increased activity of phagocytes. *Echinacea* appears to be very safe.

The two main species, *Echinacea angustifolia* and *Echinacea purpurea*, are primarily recommended for acute treatment (ten to fourteen days) of colds or the flu. The dose needed is at least nine hundred milligrams per day, and I prefer *Echinacea purpurea* root to other preparations. The dosing of *Echinacea* tea is unreliable; use capsules or extracts. Some people with chronic or recurrent infections benefit from taking *Echinacea* for prolonged periods, especially during the winter. I recommend you take it continuously for eight weeks at a time, then stop for a week or two between each eight-week period to avoid tolerance.[93] *Echinacea* preparations are readily available at many natural food stores and some pharmacies.

In the treatment of acute respiratory infection, the activity of *Echinacea* is often enhanced by Chinese herbal mixtures traditionally used for treating fever. My favorite is called Isatis Formula. It is commercially available as an alcohol extraction of the leaves and roots of six plants. The adult dose is three droppersful three times a day. During heavy flu seasons, over three-quarters of my patients taking the *Echinacea* and Isatis combinations have made statements like "Everyone around me was sick for weeks, taking antibiotics. I usually get sick for three weeks with the flu, but I was better within a few days after starting these herbs."

Another cold remedy with promise is zinc lozenges. A recent study from the Cleveland Clinic confirmed the effectiveness of zinc lozenges in shortening the duration of cold symptoms like sore throat, cough, headache, and nasal congestion by about 50 percent. Lozenges contained 13 milligrams of zinc and were taken every two hours. Nausea was a possible side effect.[94]

Astragalus root is a component of many traditional Chinese herbal formulas, generally considered to be a strong tonic and resistance-builder. Contemporary studies reveal that *Astragalus* can increase natural killer cell activity.[95] I often recommend *Astragalus* for maintenance therapy of people with chronic or recurrent infectious diseases of any type, because of its high margin of safety. The effective dose is 250 to 500 milligrams three times a day. Astragalus may cause an increase in sweating or urination but side effects are otherwise rare.

6. Mushrooms. Fungi are powerful chemical factories that produce potent toxins and most of the world's antibiotics. Fungal extracts are widely employed in traditional Chinese medicine. Two fungi in particular, the mushrooms known by their Japanese names as shiitake (*Lentinus edodes*) and reishi (*Ganoderma lucidum*), contain complex sugars (polysaccharides) that increase natural killer cell activity and inhibit tumor growth in animals and in humans. Like *Astragalus*, shiitake and reishi are used in contemporary Chinese medicine as *fu zheng* remedies, which means they "support the normal," stimulating health rather than treating sickness. Shiitake mushrooms, which are quite tasty, are readily available in gourmet food stores. Both shiitake and reishi may be obtained in capsules. A dose that stimulates immune responses is nine hundred milligrams per day of each. For people with severe allergies, it is advisable to use reishi alone, as reishi may inhibit allergic reactivity and shiitake may increase it.[96]

7. If you're a woman with recurrent urinary tract infections (UTI), preventive regimens may help you avoid antibiotics. First, empty your bladder regularly, about every two hours. Loading up with fluids without regular bladder emptying will do more harm than good. Holding in urine and distending the bladder damages the lining and increases the risk of infection.[97] Cranberry juice inhibits the attachment of bacteria to the lining of the bladder. A single eight-ounce glass of sweetened cranberry juice every day decreases bacterial contamination of the urine. For those who dislike the taste of cranberries, freeze-dried cran-

berry juice extract is available in capsule form. Three to six capsules per day are quite effective at preventing urinary infection.[98] If cranberry juice is not effective, try bearberry leaf (*Arctostaphylos uva-ursi*) extract, which contains the urinary antiseptic arbutin. The dose needed is five hundred milligrams three times a day.[99] Do not mix *Arctostaphylos uva-ursi* with cranberry, because bearberry only works in an alkaline urine and cranberry renders the urine acidic. To achieve an alkaline urine when taking bearberry, avoid consuming meat, fish, poultry, or eggs. Vegetables, fruits, and dairy products create a relatively alkaline urine, because of the way in which they are metabolized in the body. Even orange or grapefruit juice, which are acid when swallowed, tend to create alkalinity in the urinary tract.

Our old friends the *Lactobacilli* not only colonize the intestinal tract but grow well in the vagina and the urethra, where they prevent growth of pathogenic bacteria.[100] The application of vaginal spermicides like nonoxynol-9, found in many contraceptive creams, may kill *Lactobacilli* and give pathogens more ready access to the urinary tract.[101] Taking *Lactobacilli* by mouth or inserting *Lactobacillus* capsules into the vagina may restore genital tract symbiosis and prevent infection.

If you do need to take antibiotics for bladder infection, remember that a three-day course of treatment usually works as well as a ten-day course.[102] (This is *not* the same as completing only three days of a ten-day course, which can promote the growth of resistant bacteria.) Avoid overtreatment.

Control Your Stress

Stressful life events and emotional distress impair immune function, increasing susceptibility to colds, strep throat, and reactivation of cold sores due to herpesvirus infection.[103] On the other hand, a program of relaxation and stress management has been shown to reduce the frequency of herpes infection.[104] An experimental study demonstrated that the activity of phagocytes could actually be improved by a form of self-hypnosis. Intriguing research has been done that demonstrates the ability of individuals to regulate their immune responses using visual imagery techniques. The unanswered questions provoked by this research are: can these effects be sustained, and will they prevent sickness?[105] The answers are not known. But it does appear clear that the *díaita* of modern Americans should include a daily period of quiet reflection, meditation, or prayer, as well as a daily period of exercise, for optimum immunity.

To support optimum resistance to infection:

• Follow a diet of high nutrient density (see Chapter Six), exercise for thirty minutes a day, and get enough sleep at night so that you can awaken in the morning without an alarm clock.
• Eat saponin-rich vegetables like soybeans, chickpeas, bean sprouts, tomatoes, potatoes, and oats, and fruits and vegetables rich in vitamins A and C like broccoli, carrots, tomatoes, and cantaloupe.
• Avoid foods with added fat.
• Do not use iron supplements unless you are pregnant or deficient in iron.
• Supplement your diet with flax oil 1 tablespoon a day, vitamin E 400 mg a day, vitamin C 2,000 mg a day, granular lecithin 2 tablespoons a day, dimethylglycine 120 mg a day, and the immune-stimulating mushrooms shiitake and reishi.
• Avoid the use of antibiotics for acute respiratory infections like colds, bronchitis, and sinusitis. They are demonstrated not to be effective for these conditions and their use only increases the rate of bacterial resistance to antibiotics. Instead use the herbs *Echinacea* and *Astragalus*, which have a high safety profile and work by improving immune responsiveness.

EPILOGUE: EACH PATIENT
IS A WORK OF ART

*Disease theory has no logical relation to person—in disease theory it
does not matter what person has the disease—therefore, the common
complaint that patients are overlooked in the treatment of their diseases
is another way of stating that in the intellectual basis of modern medicine patients and their diseases are not logically related.*[1]
                                                    —Eric Cassell, M.D.

The treatment of "diseases" without regard to the persons they afflict
has brought clinical medicine to a crisis of confidence as great as the
one it faced a hundred years ago, before the release of the Flexner Report. Throughout these pages, I have expressed dismay at the inadequacy of current clinical practice. Others have attacked its excesses.
The inappropriate use of drugs, for example, accounts for well over half
the episodes of cardiac arrest that occur in the hospitals of our university medical centers.[2] A Harvard research team studying iatrogenic
(doctor-caused) injuries concluded that 180,000 Americans are killed
in hospitals by their doctors *every year*, because of therapeutic mistakes.[3] In most cases, clinical errors occur because the doctor has overlooked the individual characteristics of the patient being treated.
Specialization, which was so dear to Flexner, is now decried as too
costly. The federal government has cut educational funding for specialists and mandated more training of general physicians. Yet there is
little understanding of the real skills required of generalists. Current administrative rules pressure them to act as double agents. Ostensibly responsive to the needs of their patients, primary physicians are
ultimately controlled by the demands of managed care corporations

and are penalized if they fail to control their patients' use of services.

The present crisis provides an excellent opportunity for reconstruct-ing health care. Disease theory has outlived its usefulness. Any regu-lated health care system that relies on rigid protocols for the treatment of disease will trample the individual needs of sick people. The only way out of the crisis is for the individual—not the disease entity—to be-come the focus of care. Physicians must be trained to understand the kaleidoscope model of health. We have learned enough about the me-diators, triggers, and antecedents of sickness that patient-centered diag-nosis can be fully integrated into the process of clinical evaluation. Generalist physicians must become experts at reinforcing the Pillars of Healing. They must be trained in creating a healing relationship with their patients and in analyzing each person's *díaita*, counseling indi-vidual changes. They must be able to instruct patients in establishing a healthful environment and understand the intricate chemistry of detox-ification, so that their treatments support the body's processes of repair, rather than hinder them. This must become the standard of care, for individual practitioners, for managed care organizations, and for regu-latory agencies. These endeavors will not fully replace crisis manage-ment, surgery, or the use of drugs. They *will* decrease the need for expensive and invasive treatments, decrease the frequency and severity of complications when such treatments are employed, and improve the overall effectiveness of care.

The crises afflicting mainstream medicine have stimulated interest in alternative medical therapies. About a third of the U.S. population consult alternative health practitioners. Americans spend more money out-of-pocket on unconventional health care than on conventional care.[4] People seek out alternative therapies because conventional, disease-oriented medicine does not meet their needs. Conventional medicine is too often impersonal, ineffective, or dangerous. Recogniz-ing that alternative therapies increase patient satisfaction and decrease cost, managed care organizations are starting to incorporate them among the services they offer. Several medical schools have added courses in alternative medicine to the curriculum and divisions of in-tegrative medicine are coming to life in major medical centers. Re-search projects have been initiated that utilize scientific methods to evaluate alternative healing techniques. These efforts alone will not have much impact on the practice of medicine. The strength of alternative medicine lies not in its varied techniques, which often fail to withstand scientific scrutiny, but in its fundamental approach to the patient. As a whole, alternative medical therapies rest on the traditional concept that illness results from imbalance or disharmony. Supporting the body's capacity for healing by restoring "balance" is their ultimate therapeutic goal. This traditional perspective must be restored to the practice of medicine and must guide the application of medical science to the care of patients. Fulfilling that mission is the purpose of this book.

The power to initiate change lies within you. It begins with your taking an active role in maintaining and promoting your own health. Whatever your age or your state of health, there are five steps you can take immediately, to begin the process of health enhancement. These steps have been woven into the stories and explanations that compose each chapter you have read. They are:

1. Eat consciously. Say "no" to snack foods, which for most North Americans supply one-third of daily calories. Ignore the latest dietary fads. *Nutrient density* is the key to healthy eating. Read food labels and avoid those foods that list sugar or oil as ingredients. Eat vegetables and fruits at every meal, especially those rich in disease-fighting antioxidants, flavonoids, carotenoids, saponins, and fiber (see pages 205–207). Spice your meals liberally with garlic, onion, ginger, turmeric, oregano, sage, thyme, and rosemary. Buy fresh local produce in season, wash and peel or scrub clean with a soft brush just before cooking or eating. Wash your hands thoroughly *before and after* handling food. Cook all meat, fish, or poultry well and thoroughly clean all utensils that contact uncooked food. Filter and/or boil drinking water as described on pages 214–215.

Most people will benefit from supplementing their healthy diets with flaxseed oil, vitamins C and E, magnesium, trace minerals, and friendly bacteria, like *Lactobacillus acidophilus* and *Lactobacillus plantarum*, following the guidelines presented in Chapters Six and Eight. Unless you are iron-deficient, avoid supplements that contain iron.

2. Get enough physical exercise. Commit yourself to thirty minutes a day of moderate- or high-intensity activity. Make exercise a family affair, or do it with a friend. Suggestions can be found on pages 157–158.

3. Explore meditation. A period of quiet contemplation, prayer, or deep relaxation once a day improves immune function and has remarkable recuperative power.

4. Create a safe home. The most helpful measures are described in Chapter Seven and Appendix B. Once your home is clear, turn your attention to the safety of your work environment and your children's school.

5. Avoid drugs that disrupt your body's ability to heal itself. Street drugs and tobacco have no redeeming qualities. Drugs that lower stomach acid increase your risk of intestinal infection. Alcohol and aspirin appear to have a two-tier effect on health. Very low doses may be beneficial; higher doses are potentially harmful, damaging the lining of stomach and intestine, increasing the entry of intestinal toxins into the liver. Antibiotics are the most important drugs ever developed, but their overuse has tragic consequences; it destroys the body's friendly flora and contributes to the emergence of antibiotic-resistant pathogens. Strategies for avoiding antacids, excessive use of pain relievers like aspirin, and unneeded antibiotics are presented on pages 212–214.

Implementing these five steps will do more than improve your health and well-being. It will equip you to change the nature of the medical care you receive. Health care can only change for the better if you, the patient, are an active participant in setting priorities for your own care. Taking charge of your own behavior empowers you to assume a collaborative relationship with your doctor. Inform your doctor of the steps you are taking to improve your health. Present your goals and expectations. Request the information that you need. If you are sick, explain the ways in which your illness has changed your life; express your feelings about the illness, and expect that your doctor will listen, acknowledge you, and treat you with respect. If your requests are not met with respect, change doctors and register your dissatisfaction with the managed care organization that employs or contracts with the doctor.

The foremost demand of patients is for health care that addresses their personal needs. That demand often remains unfulfilled, for the precise reason described by Dr. Cassell. The concepts that underlie modern medicine are concepts of disease, not of person. Patient-centered diagnosis allows the *person* who is sick to be at the center of health care. It sees through the obsolete notion that disease entities can exist in and of themselves. It unites science and humanism, allowing the power of science to consistently support the artistry of personal health care. It allows us to see, with the tools of science, that each patient is a work of art.

CONTROLLING ALLERGENS IN YOUR HOME

Common allergens in the home include dust, dust mites, animal dander, and mold. Mold and dust control is important for everyone and is detailed in Chapter Seven. People with allergy may also need to be careful about environmental exposure to dust mites and animal dander.

Dust mites are microscopic insects related to spiders. They thrive on dust and humidity and their feces contain important allergens. Carpeting and bedding are havens for dust mites. Remove carpeting, if possible. If you cannot remove it, use the following mite control measure: Once a month, apply a 3 percent tannic acid solution (available in drugstores) to the carpet, then vacuum. Tannic acid should not be applied to light-colored or white carpet, because it may stain it brown. Wear a cotton or paper mask while vacuuming. Use a dry vacuum cleaner with double vacuum bags and a HEPA filter over the vacuum's outlet.

Dander consists of minute scales that fall from the hair, feathers, and skin of all warm-blooded animals. There are no breeds of cats or dogs that are nonallergenic. Even "hairless" animals shed dander. Washing a pet once a month will decrease the shedding of dander. Do not use a vacuum with a water-filtration system. Animal dander attaches to water droplets from the filter and water vacuum cleaners actually increase the dander content in the air. Tannic acid solution will denature the animal dander attached to carpet and fabric, making it less likely to produce symptoms. If an animal is removed from the house, wash down the walls with water to remove adherent animal dander that might recirculate.

BEDROOM TIPS

Remove dust collectors like books, magazines, stuffed animals, paper, and miscellaneous clutter. Inch for inch, stuffed animals are among the richest sources of dust-mite antigen you can find. Do not use a computer printer in the bedroom; laser printers, in particular, emit irritating and allergenic VOCs when they print. Keep pets out. Encase pillows and mattresses in an impermeable fabric. These may be ordered by mail from Allergy and Asthma Shopper, P.O. Box 239, Fate, TX 75132, (800) 447-1100; or Allergy Control Products, 96 Danbury Road, Ridgefield, CT 06877, (800) 422-DUST. If you use plastic bedcovers, allow the plastic to air out and off-gas for a few days before sleeping on it. Avoid the use of feather pillows, wool blankets, or down comforters. Cotton, foam, or Dacron pillows are best. Wash new bedsheets before sleeping in them. New fabric is treated with formaldehyde, which will evaporate while you sleep. Wash all bedding, including sheets, pillowcases, blankets, comforters, and mattress pads, in water that is at least 130 degrees Fahrenheit (55 degrees Celsius) once every ten days.

Use an air purifier with a HEPA filter to remove particles and a carbon filter to remove fumes. A negative ion generator is also effective at particle removal but will tend to generate dirt because the negatively charged dust particles cling to walls and ceilings or to the air purifier itself. Never place a HEPA air purifier on carpet. Always place it on a bare floor. Dust regularly, using a damp cloth to avoid stirring up dust. Cover windows with washable blinds, not curtains. Use furniture that is not upholstered (leather, wood). If you have upholstered furniture, do not sleep or lie down on it.

ABOUT KITCHENS, BATHROOMS, AND OTHER DAMP PLACES

Never carpet a kitchen or bath or a concrete slab. Clean kitchen and bathroom tiles and grout frequently, using a solution of chlorine bleach. Control the cockroach population by placing "roach hotels" in corners and under sinks. The saliva, skin, and feces of cockroaches contain potent allergens. Clean regularly under sinks, inside cabinets, and behind toilets. Vacuum away cockroach detritus. Use unscented cosmetics and personal care products. Avoid the use of room deodorizers.

ENVIRONMENTALLY SAFE PRODUCTS FOR YOUR HOME

PUBLICATIONS

Books

Clean & Green, The Complete Guide to Nontoxic and Environmentally Safe Housekeeping, by Annie Berthold-Bond. Woodstock, N.Y.: Ceres Press, 1989.

Dan's Practical Guide to Least Toxic Home Pest Control, by Dan Stein. 1991. Hulogosi Communications, Inc., P.O. Box 1188, Eugene, OR 97440.

Green Groceries—A Mail Order Guide to Organic Foods, by Jeanne Heifetz. New York: HarperPerennial, 1992.

The Green Kitchen Handbook, by Annie Berthold-Bond. New York: Harper-Collins, 1997.

The Healthy Home: An Attic to Basement Guide to Toxin-Free Living, by Linda Mason Hunter. Emmaus, Pa.: Rodale Press, 1989.

Healthy Homes, Healthy Kids: Protecting Your Child from Everyday Environmental Hazards, by Joyce M. Shoemaker, Ph.D., and Charity Y. Vitale, Ph.D. Washington, D.C.: Island Press, 1991.

The Healthy House, by John Bower. New York: Lyle Stuart, 1989.

The Safe Shopper's Bible: A Consumer's Guide to Non-toxic Household Products, Cosmetics, and Food, by David Steinman and Samuel S. Epstein, M.D. New York: Macmillan, 1995.

Sustaining the Earth: Choosing Consumer Products That Are Safe for You, Your Family and the Earth, by Debra Dadd-Redalia. New York: Hearst Books, 1994.

Periodicals

ACTS Facts. Arts, Crafts and Theater Safety, 181 Thompson Street, #23, New York, NY 10012-2586. (212) 777-0062.

The Green Guide for Everyday Life (newsletter). Mothers & Others for a Livable Planet, 40 West 20th Street, New York, NY 10011.

Organic Gardening. Rodale Press, P.O. Box 7320, Red Oak, IA 51591-0320.

Safe Home Digest. Norwalk, CT 06840. (203) 227-1276.

INFORMATION AND ASSISTANCE

American Academy of Environmental Medicine, P.O. Box CN 1001-8001, New Hope, PA 18938. (215) 862-4544.

American College of Occupational and Environmental Medicine, 55 West Seegers Road, Arlington Heights, IL 60005-3919. (708) 228-6850.

American Council of Independent Laboratories, for a laboratory near your home that will test for impurities other than lead. (202) 887-5872.

American Lung Association, 1740 Broadway, New York, NY 10019. (212) 315-8700.

Environmental Protection Agency Drinking Water Hot Line, for referral to a testing lab. (800) 426-4791.

Environmental Protection Agency Indoor Air Quality Information Clearing House. (800) 438-4318.

National Lead Information Center. (800) LEAD-FYI.

National Pesticides Telecommunications. (800) 858-PEST.

U.S. Consumer Products Safety Commission. (800) 638-CPSC.

Washington Toxics Coalition, 4516 University Way NE, Seattle, WA 98105. An excellent resource for product analysis and recommendations.

WATER FILTERS

Turbo-Shower Filter to remove chlorine from water used in the shower. New Market Naturals, 1039 Overcrest, Fayetteville, AR 72703. (800) 873-4321. Fax: (501) 442-3867.

Water Factory Systems Drinking Water Appliances, reverse osmosis filter. Available through Allergy Resources, Inc., P.O. Box 444, Guffey, CO 80820. (800) USE-FLAX. (719) 689-2969 for information.

Water Pure carbon block filter removes organochlorines, chlorine, lead, and parasites. 15 Great Neck Road, Great Neck, NY 11021. (800) 313-7873.

CONSUMER PRODUCTS BY MAIL

Cleaning Products, Air Purifiers, General Merchandise

Allergy Resources, Inc., P.O. Box 444, Guffey, CO 80820. (800) USE-FLAX.

Environmental Construction Outfitters, 44 Crosby Street, New York, NY 10012. Air purifiers, building materials, paints. (212) 334-9659.

Environmentally Safe Products, 8345 Walnut Hill Lane, Suite 225, Dallas, TX 75231. (800) 428-2343.

N.E.E.D.S., 527 Charles Avenue #12-A, Syracuse, NY 13209. (800) 634-1380.

Non-Toxic Environments, Inc., P.O. Box 384, Newmarket, NH 03857. (800) 789-4348.

Seventh Generation, 1 Mill Street, Box A26, Burlington, VT 05401-1530. (800) 456-1177.

Personal Care Products

Coastline Products, P.O. Box 6397, Santa Ana, CA 92706. Orders: (800) 554-4111. Customer service: (800) 554-4112.

Logonia. (800) 648-6654.

Organic Food

Diamond Organics. (800) 922-2396.

Gold Mine Natural Foods. (800) 475-FOOD.

Jaffe Brothers. (619) 749-1133.

Walnut Acres. (800) 433-3998.

For local organic food co-ops, contact National Cooperative Business Association (NCBA) at (202) 638-6222, or the Co-op Directory Services at (612) 332-0417.

Natural Fiber Beds and Bedding

Crown City Mattress, 250 S. San Gabriel Blvd., San Gabriel, CA 91776. (818) 796-9101.

Heart of Vermont, 131 S. Main Street, Barre, VT 05641. (800) 476-3098.

The Natural Bedroom. (800) 365-6563.

Natural Carpet

The Environmental Home Center, 1724 Fourth Ave S., Seattle, WA 98134. (206) 682-7332.

Naturlich Floor Interiors, P.O. Box 1677, Sebastopol, CA 95473. (707) 824-0974.

Sinan Company, P.O. Box 857, Davis, CA 95617. (918) 753-3104.

I wish to thank Annie Berthold-Bond for help in assembling this list of resources.

APPENDIX C

THE GUT
FERMENTATION SYNDROMES

People who suffer from abdominal bloating and gas, which may be associated with pain, constipation, diarrhea, or clear-cut food intolerance, often experience their symptoms because of an overgrowth of bacteria or yeasts that ferment dietary starch and sugar. Gut fermentation syndromes are usually induced by insufficient stomach acid, injudicious use of antacids or antibiotics, or surgery. They can also occur as complications of numerous medical disorders, like diabetes, or of parasitic infection. Characteristics of this syndrome have been described in two recent studies:

K. K. Eaton, Gut fermentation: a reappraisal of an old clinical condition, diagnostic tests and management. A discussion paper. *Journal of the Royal Society of Medicine*, Vol. 11 (1991), pp. 669–71.

A. Hunnisett, J. Howard, and S. Davies, Gut fermentation (or the "autobrewery" syndrome): a new clinical test with initial observations and discussions of clinical and biochemical conditions, *Journal of Nutritional Medicine*, Vol. 1 (1990), pp. 33–39.

Bacterial overgrowth in the small intestine is most readily determined by measuring the amount of hydrogen and methane gas in a person's breath. This test is performed in many hospitals. It can also be performed by any doctor, using a unique breath collection system designed by Dr. Martin Lee of the

Great Smokies Diagnostic Laboratory (GSDL), Asheville, North Carolina. For information on breath testing for bacterial overgrowth, call GSDL at (800) 522-4762.

Treatment of gut fermentation requires alteration of dietary sugar and starch and the use of oral antimicrobials. Information on self-treatment can be obtained from two books:

The Yeast Connection Handbook by William Crook, M.D. (Professional Books, 1996), describes a treatment approach for intestinal yeast overgrowth.

Breaking the Vicious Cycle by Elaine Gottschall (Kirkton Press) describes a dietary treatment for problems associated with various types of bacterial overgrowth.

APPENDIX D

ALTERNATIVE PAIN MANAGEMENT

GENERAL INFORMATION ON CHRONIC PAIN

Periodicals

D. Kroll, Alternative therapies for pain management, *Alternative & Complementary Therapies* (Jan.–Feb. 1996), pp. 5–8.

K. White, Manual therapies. Advances in osteopathy, chiropractic, massage and other techniques. *Alternative & Complementary Therapies* (Jan.–Feb. 1996), pp. 9–15.

Reprints of these two articles are available from the publisher. Write or call Karen Ballen at Mary Ann Liebert, Inc., 2 Madison Avenue, Larchmont, NY 10538. (914) 834-3100.

Books

The Natural Way of Healing Chronic Pain, by the Natural Medicine Collective with Theresa Digerinimo, M.Ed. New York: Dell Publishing, 1995.

Healing Back Pain: The Mind-Body Connection, by John Sarno. New York: Warner Books, 1991.

Controlled studies have found that vitamins or minerals may be useful for chronic pain management, and the herb feverfew can help to prevent migraine headaches:

G. Schweiger, H. Karl, and E. Schohaber, Relapse prevention of painful vertebral syndromes in follow-up treatment with a combination of vitamins B_1, B_6, B_{12}, *Annals of the New York Academy of Science*, Vol. 585 (1990), pp. 540–42. Vitamin B_1 (thiamine 100 mg), vitamin B_6 (pyridoxine 200 mg), and vitamin B_{12} (cyanocobalamin 0.2 mg) given three times a day for six months improved mood, mobility, and pain when compared with placebo.

I. Machtey and L. Oaknine, Tocopherol in osteoarthritis: A controlled pilot study, *Journal of the American Geriatric Society*, Vol. 26 (1978), pp. 328–30. Vitamin E, 600 mg/day, produced significant pain relief when compared with placebo.

M. A. Moss, Effects of molybdenum on pain and general health: A pilot study, *Journal of Nutritional Medicine*, Vol. 5 (1995), pp. 55–61. Chronic aches and pains improved with 500 mcg per day over 28 days, when compared with placebo.

E. S. Johnson, N. P. Kadam, D. M. Hylands, and P. J. Hylands, Efficacy of feverfew as prophylactic treatment of migraine, *British Medical Journal*, Vol. 291 (1985), pp. 569–73. Feverfew (formerly *Chrysanthemum parthenium*, now classified as *Tanacetum parthenium*), 25 mg twice a day, produced migraine relief without side effects. The mechanism of action differed from that of NSAIDs. The study was done at the London Migraine Clinic.

NATURAL PRODUCTS FOR ACUTE PAIN

1. Bromelain, a mixture of enzymes from pineapple stem.

G. Tassman, J. Zafran, and G. Zayon, Evaluation of a plant proteolytic enzyme for the control of inflammation and pain, *Journal of Dental Medicine*, Vol. 19 (1964), pp. 73–77.

G. Tassman, J. Zafran, and G. Zayon, A double-blind cross-over study of a plant proteolytic enzyme in oral surgery, *Journal of Dental Medicine*, Vol. 20 (1965), pp. 51–54.

R. Howat and G. Lewis, The effect of bromelain therapy on episiotomy wounds—A double blind controlled clinical trial, *Journal of Obstetrics and Gynecology of the British Commonwealth*, Vol. 79 (1972), pp. 951–53.

G. Zatuchni and D. Colombi, Bromelain therapy for the prevention of episiotomy pain, *Obstetrics and Gynecology*, Vol. 29 (1967), pp. 275–78.

2. Curcumin, a component of curry, which has anti-inflammatory potency
equal to the stronger NSAIDs. One needs pure curcumin in capsules,
400 to 600 mg three times a day. Or turmeric, the spice from which it is
derived, 8 to 60 grams per day   .
Curcumin: A potent anti-inflammatory agent, *American Journal of Natural Medicine*, Vol. 1 (1994), pp. 10–14.

NOTES

In Restauro

1. Quoted in Ken Shulman, *Anatomy of a Restoration, the Brancacci Chapel* (New York: Walker and Company, 1991), p. 86.

2. The disparity between patients' complaints and organ pathology has been the subject of several reviews. See I. K. Zola, Culture and symptoms: an analysis of patients' presenting complaints, *American Sociology Review*, Vol. 31 (1966), pp. 615–30; H. K. Beecher, Relationship of the significance of wound to the pain experienced, *Journal of the American Medical Association*, Vol. 161 (1956), pp. 1609–13; J. Stoeckle, I. K. Zola, and G. Davidson, The quantity and significance of psychological distress in medical patients, *Journal of Chronic Diseases*, Vol. 17 (1964), pp. 959–70.

3. Some of the most stimulating published commentary on the problems inherent in the theory of diseases can be found in G. L. Engel, The need for a new medical model: a challenge for biomedicine, *Science*, Vol. 196 (1977), pp. 129–36; A. Kleinman, and L. Eisenberg, Culture, illness, and care: clinical lessons learned from anthropology and cross cultural research, *Annals of Internal Medicine*, Vol. 88 (1978), pp. 251–56; J. W. Fessel, The nature of illness and diagnosis, *American Journal of Medicine*, Vol. 75 (1983), pp. 555–60; J. Ahlqvist, Multifactorial pathogenesis: ought we to classify disease or treat the individual's causes of disease? *Medical Hypotheses*, Vol. 16 (1985), pp. 289–302; A. R. Feinstein, The intellectual crisis in clinical science: medaled models and muddled mettle, *Perspectives in Biology and Medicine*, Vol. 30 (1987), pp. 215–30; C. G. Helman, Limits of biomedical explanation, *Lancet*, Vol. 337 (1991), 1080–83.

Chapter 1: Eclipse of the Patient

1. Insightful publications concerning tribal healing practices include A. M. Kleinman, The cognitive structure of traditional medical systems, *Ethnomedicine*, Vol. 3 (1974), pp. 27–49; R. Horton, African traditional thought and Western science, *Africa*, Vol. 37 (1967), pp. 50–60; M. Martin, Native American medicine: thoughts for posttraditional healers, *Journal of the American Medical Association*, Vol. 245 (1981), pp. 141–43. Dr. Martin says: "What is the underlying reason for a ceremony? It is the belief that disease and illness are the result of a lack of harmony, balance, or equilibrium between the sick person and his surroundings. This is a modern psychosocial approach and includes attention to the patient's family support system." This process is not always benign. Tribal healers may exploit suffering to produce conformity of deviants to the group. See J. E. Cawte, Australian Aboriginal medicine before European contact, *Annals of Internal Medicine*, Vol. 82 (1975), pp. 422–23.

2. Lois M. Magner, A *History of Medicine* (New York: Marcel Dekker Inc., 1992), p. 143.

3. Giovanni Boccaccio, *Decameron*, trans. G. H. McWilliam (London: Penguin, 1972), p. 58.

4. "Epidemics, Book I," in *Hippocratic Writings*, trans. J. Chadwick and W. N. Mann, ed. G. E. R. Lloyd (London: Penguin, 1983), pp. 89–90.

5. When the microorganism of syphilis, a spiral-shaped bacterium (spirochete) called *Treponema pallidum*, was discovered a hundred years ago, it seemed reasonable to accept Fracastoro's theory that syphilis was imported into Europe from the New World by Spanish sailors. The first problem with this theory is that syphilis devastated Caribbean islanders with the same ferocity that it visited upon its victims in the Old World, an unlikely occurrence were the microbe already present in the Americas before the Spanish exploration. The second problem is that a microorganism virtually identical to *T. pallidum* causes an ancient skin disease called yaws, which had been present in the Old World since antiquity. This spirochete, called *Treponema pallidum, ssp pertenue*, is practically indistinguishable from the spirochete of syphilis. When *Treponema pertenue* enters the body through a cut or scratch on the skin, it produces a localized sore that eventually heals, leaving the recipient relatively immune to developing syphilis. Occurrence of yaws is favored by rural life. Children experience frequent cuts and scrapes on bare legs and arms, and pass the infection from one to another when sleeping together in huts and hovels or at play. Urban living limits the spread of yaws in childhood. As cities grew during the late Middle Ages, the opportunity increased for multiple sexual contacts among people who had never been exposed to yaws in childhood. In the aftermath of the Black Death, a breakdown of the social fabric increased sexual promiscuity, allowing *Treponema pallidum* to emerge as a pathogen spread by sexual contact. Entering the body through the genitals, the spirochete readily spread to the internal organs, producing a pattern of disease that had not been previously recognized. A critical mass of promiscuous individuals readily spreading the spirochete encouraged the emergence of fast-growing, more virulent strains and an epidemic disease never described before.

See Laurie Garrett's review of these developments in *The Coming Plague* (New York: Farrar, Straus and Giroux, 1994), pp. 245–47.

6. Thomas Sydenham, Medical observations concerning the history and the cure of acute diseases, in *The Works of Thomas Sydenham*, trans. R. G. Latham (Birmingham, Ala.: Classics of Medicine Library, 1979), Section 12, p. 15.

7. Philippe Pinel, *La Médecine Clinique*, 2nd ed. (Paris: J. A. Brosson, 1804), Introduction, p. xxvii.

8. Jean N. Corvisart, *An Essay on the Organic Diseases and Lesions of the Heart and Blood Vessels* (1806), trans. J. Gates (New York: Hafner, 1962), p. 25.

9. The change in medical vision engendered by the autopsy is itself dissected in detail, with some degree of obscurity, by Michel Foucault in *The Birth of the Clinic: An Archaeology of Medical Perception*, trans. A. M. Sheridan Smith (New York: Pantheon, 1973).

10. See Guenter B. Risse, A shift in medical epistemology: clinical diagnosis, 1770–1828, in *History of Diagnostics* (Proceedings of the 9th International Symposium on the Comparative History of Medicine—East and West), ed. Yosio Kawakita (Osaka, Japan: The Tanaguchi Foundation, 1987), pp. 115–48.

11. The first part of this statement is quoted in R. K. Taylor, *The Concepts of Illness, Disease and Morbus* (New York: Cambridge University Press, 1979), p. 11. The second part appeared in a manifesto written by Virchow in 1854, entitled *Specifiker und Specifisches*.

12. Epidemics, III, xii, 13, in *Hippocratic Writings*, pp. 125–26.

13. Ehrlich shared the Nobel Prize for Medicine with Élie Metchnikoff in 1908. Ironically, the two men were philosophical rivals. Ehrlich viewed immunity as the result of protective antibodies and Metchnikoff viewed immunity as resulting from the ability of white blood cells to consume and destroy bacteria. Ehrlich and Metchnikoff never agreed that their discoveries might represent complementary parts of a new integrated theory of immunity to infection.

14. People whose immune systems have successfully imprisoned the tubercle bacillus when they first encountered it are resistant to developing active disease, even when exposed anew to large quantities of living microbes from another person. See W. W. Stead, Management of health care workers after inadvertent exposure to tuberculosis: a guide for the use of preventive therapy, *Annals of Internal Medicine*, Vol. 122 (1995), pp. 906–12; G. L. Templeton, et al., The risk for transmission of *Mycobacterium tuberculosis* at the bedside and during autopsy, *Annals of Internal Medicine*, Vol. 121 (1995), pp. 922–25.

The rate at which quiescent infection is activated is only about thirty cases per hundred thousand person-years. What this means is: if two thousand people carrying TB bacteria were observed for a period of fifty years, only thirty of them would ever develop active TB. From J. A. Sbarbaro, Tuberculosis: the new challenge for the practicing physician, *Chest*, Vol. 68, Supp. 3 (1975), pp. 436–43.

When people with impaired immunity are exposed to tubercle bacilli for the first time, the rate at which they become sick is very high. Elderly residents of a nursing home, for example, who tend to have subtle deficits in immune function, develop active TB at the rate of 19 percent within a year, almost seven hundred times the rate of healthy people who are TB carriers. See J. A. Sbarbaro, Tuberculosis: yesterday, today, and tomorrow, *Annals of Internal Medicine*, Vol. 122 (1995), pp. 955–56.

15. A recent study confirms the importance of Pasteur's observation for human health. People undergoing major surgery routinely experience a lowering of body

temperature. They are also subject to infection of the surgical wound. Actively warming patients in surgery can reduce the frequency of wound infection by two thirds. See A. Kurz, D. I. Sessler, and R. Lenhardt, Perioperative normothermia to reduce the incidence of surgical-wound infection and shorten hospitalization, *New England Journal of Medicine*, Vol. 334 (1996), pp. 1209–15.

16. Quoted in W. A. Silverman, "Doing More Good Than Harm," in *Doing More Good Than Harm: The Evaluation of Health Care Interventions: Annals of the New York Academy of Medicine*, Vol. 703 (1993), p. 5.

17. S. E. Chaille, The practice of medicine as a money making occupation, *New Orleans Medical and Surgical Journal*, Vol. 49 (1897), p. 608.

18. F. Billings, Medical education, *Science*, Vol. 17 (1903), p. 763.

19. A critical discussion of the Flexner Report and its impact can be found in Paul Starr's *The Social Transformation of American Medicine: The Rise of a Sovereign Profession and the Making of a Vast Industry* (New York: Basic Books, 1984).

20. Lewis Thomas, "1937 Internship," in *The Youngest Science: Notes of a Medicine-Watcher* (New York: Viking Press, 1983).

21. T. R. Harrison, The value and limitation of laboratory tests in clinical medicine, *Journal of the Medical Association of Alabama*, Vol. 13 (1944), pp. 381–84.

22. T. M. McGill and A. R. Feinstein, A critical appraisal of the quality of quality-of-life measurements, *Journal of the American Medical Association*, Vol. 272 (1994), pp. 619–26. The patient's perspective on quality of life was invited only in 17 percent of studies that pretended to look at quality of life.

Chapter 2: Medical Odyssey

1. R. J. Goldberg et al., Cardiogenic shock after myocardial infarction: incidence and mortality from a community-wide perspective, 1975 to 1988, *New England Journal of Medicine*, Vol. 325 (1991), pp. 1117–22.

2. Farber was quoted in a *New York* magazine article, "The Best Hospitals in New York," Nov. 18, 1991, p. 44.

3. Videotapes of doctor-patient consultations reveal that the presence of an existing medical record induces doctors to look at the chart, not the patient, thereby missing important cues and opportunities to discover the patient's real concerns. See I. Njolstad, I. M. Aaraas, and S. Lundevall, Look at the patient, not the notes, *Lancet*, Vol. 340 (1992), pp. 413–14.

4. K. Adatto et al., Behavioral factors and urinary infection, *Journal of the American Medical Association*, Vol. 241 (1979), pp. 2525–26.

5. Leo Galland, Easing stress: How to help patients learn to relax, *Patient Care*, Vol. 14 (1980), pp. 138–72.

6. Leo Galland, Psychological preparation for elective surgery, *Connecticut Medicine*, Vol. 48 (1984), pp. 355–56.

7. C. Patel and W. R. North, Randomized controlled trial of yoga and biofeedback in management of hypertension, *Lancet*, Vol. ii (1975), pp. 93–95; C. Patel, 12-month follow-up of yoga and bio-feedback in the management of hypertension, *Lancet*, Vol. i (1975), pp. 62–64.

8. P. C. Weber and A. Sellmayer, Modification of the eicosanoid system and cell signalling by precursor fatty acids, *Advances in Prostaglandin Thromboxane and Leukotriene Research*, Vol. 21 (1990), pp. 217–24.

9. See B. H. Lerner, The perils of "X-ray vision": how radiographic images have historically influenced perception, *Perspectives in Biology and Medicine*, Vol. 35 (1992), pp. 382–97.

10. A doctor's decision about whether a given diagnostic test result is normal or abnormal will fluctuate with her concept of what is best for the patient and how much ambiguity he is willing to tolerate. E. D. Pellegrino, "Value Desiderata in the Logical Structuring of Computer Diagnosis," in *The Ethics of Diagnosis*, ed. J. L. Peset and D. Garcia (Dordrecht, Netherlands: Kluwer Academic Publishers, 1992), pp. 173–95.

11. Ibid.

Chapter 3: Patient–Centered Diagnosis

1. K. Kroenke, M. E. Arrington, and D. Mangelsdorff, Common symptoms in ambulatory care: incidence, evaluation, therapy and outcome, *American Journal of Medicine*, Vol. 86 (1989), pp. 262–66.

2. N. M. Hadler, Knee pain is the malady—not osteoarthritis, *Annals of Internal Medicine*, Vol. 116 (1992), pp. 598–99; N. M. Hadler, Osteoarthritis as a public health problem, *Clinics in the Rheum Diseases*, Vol. 11 (1985), pp. 175–85; F. Salaffi et al., Analysis of disability in knee osteoarthritis: relationship with age and psychological variables but not with radiographic score, *Journal of Rheumatology*, Vol. 18 (1991), pp. 1581–86; J. Dekker et al., Pain and disability in osteoarthritis: a review of biobehavioral mechanisms, *Journal of Behavioral Medicine*, Vol. 15 (1992), pp. 189–214. P. A. Kovar et al., Supervised fitness walking in patients with osteoarthritis of the knee: a randomized, controlled trial, *Annals of Internal Medicine*, Vol. 116 (1992), pp. 529–34.

3. M. Levin et al., Steroid-responsive nephrotic syndrome: a generalized disorder of membrane negative charge, *Lancet*, Vol. ii (1985), pp. 239–42.

4. Eric Cassell, *The Nature of Suffering and the Goals of Medicine* (New York: Oxford University Press, 1991).

5. A. Kleinman, L. Eisenberg, and B. Good, Culture, illness and care: clinical lessons from anthropologic and cross-cultural research, *Annals of Internal Medicine*, Vol. 88 (1978), pp. 251–58.

6. A. O'Leary, Self-efficacy and health, *Behavioral Research and Therapy*, Vol. 23 (1985), pp. 437–51; G. Holden, The relationship of self-efficacy appraisals to subsequent health related outcomes: a meta-analysis, *Social Work and Health Care*, Vol. 16 (1991), pp. 53–93.

7. D. P. Phillips, T. E. Ruth, and L. M. Wagner, Psychology and survival, *Lancet*, Vol. 342 (1993), pp. 1142–45.

8. D. P. Phillips and D. G. Smith, Postponement of death until symbolically meaningful occasions, *Journal of the American Medical Association*, Vol. 263 (1990), pp. 1947–51.

9. O'Leary, op. cit.; Holden, op. cit.; K. M. Schiaffino, T. A. Revenson, and A. Gibofsky, Assessing the impact of self-efficacy beliefs on adaptation to rheumatoid arthritis, *Arthritis Care and Research*, Vol. 4 (1991), pp. 150–57.

10. S. R. Wilson et al., A controlled trial of two forms of self-management education for adults with asthma, *American Journal of Medicine*, Vol. 94 (1993), pp. 564–76.

11. P. D. Mullen et al., Efficacy of psychoeducational interventions on pain, depression, and disability in people with arthritis: a meta-analysis, *Journal of Rheumatology*, Vol. 14, Supp. 15 (1987), pp. 33–39; K. R. Lorig, P. D. Mazonson, and H. R. Holman, Evidence suggesting that health education for self-management in patients with chronic arthritis has sustained health benefits while reducing health care costs, *Arthritis and Rheumatism*, Vol. 36 (1993), 439–46.

12. D. K. Litzelman et al., Reduction of lower extremity clinical abnormalities in patients with non–insulin dependent diabetes mellitus: a randomized, control trial, *Annals of Internal Medicine*, Vol. 119 (1993), pp. 36–41.

13. C. A. Dinarello et al., eds., *The Physiological and Pathological Effects of Cytokines* (New York: Wiley-Liss, 1990); H. Besedovsky and A. del Rey, Neuroendocrine and metabolic responses induced by interleukin-1, *Journal of Neuroscience Research*, Vol. 18 (1987), pp. 172–78; C. Dinarello and S. M. Wolff, The role of interleukin-1 in disease, *New England Journal of Medicine*, Vol. 328 (1993), pp. 106–13.

14. The white blood cells of allergic individuals actually secrete less than normal amounts of PGE when stimulated. See discussion in R. E. Rocklin et al., Altered arachidonic acid content in polymorphonuclear and mononuclear cells from patients with allergic rhinitis and/or asthma, *Lipids*, Vol. 21 (1986), pp. 17–20.

15. M. B. Sporn and A. B. Roberts, Autocrine secretion — 10 years later, *Annals of Internal Medicine*, Vol. 117 (1992), pp. 408–14.

16. B. S. McEwen and E. Stellar, Stress and the individual: mechanisms leading to disease, *Archives of Internal Medicine*, Vol. 153 (1993), pp. 2093–2101.

17. P. Chrousos, The hypothalamic-pituitary-adrenal axis and immune-mediated inflammation, *New England Journal of Medicine*, Vol. 332 (1995), pp. 1351–62.

18. E. Anggard, Nitric oxide: mediator, murderer, and medicine, *Lancet*, Vol. 343 (1994), pp. 1199–1206.

19. J. M. Hrushesky, Timing is everything, *The Sciences* (July–Aug. 1994), pp. 32–37; J. E. Muller et al., Circadian variation in the frequency of sudden cardiac death, *Circulation*, Vol. 75 (1987), pp. 131–38.

20. G. H. Tofler et al., Concurrent morning increase in platelet aggregability and the risk of myocardial infarction and sudden cardiac death, *New England Journal of Medicine*, Vol. 316 (1987), pp. 1514–18.

21. J. H. Markovitz and K. A. Matthews, Platelets and coronary heart disease: potential psychophysiologic mechanisms, *Psychosomatic Medicine*, Vol. 53 (1991), pp. 643–68.

22. S. W. Rabkin, F. A. L. Mathewson, and R. B. Tate, Chronobiology of cardiac sudden death in men, *Journal of the American Medical Association*, Vol. 244 (1980), pp. 1357–58.

23. W. Ruberman et al., Psychosocial influences on mortality after myocardial infarction, *New England Journal of Medicine*, Vol. 311 (1984), pp. 554–59; L. F. Berkman, L. Leo-Summers, and R. I. Horwitz, Emotional support and survival after myocardial infarction. *Annals of Internal Medicine*, Vol. 117 (1992), pp. 1003–9; R. B. Case et al., Living alone after myocardial infarction: impact on prognosis, *Journal of the American Medical Association*, Vol. 267 (1992), pp. 515–19.

24. R. B. Williams et al., Prognostic importance of social and economic resources among medically treated patients with angiographically documented

coronary artery disease, *Journal of the American Medical Association*, Vol. 267 (1992), pp. 520–24; R. M. Carney et al., Major depressive disorder predicts cardiac events in patients with coronary artery disease, *Psychosomatic Medicine*, Vol. 50 (1988), pp. 627–33; N. Frasure-Smith, F. Lesperance, and M. Talajic, Depression following myocardial infarction: impact on 6-month survival, *Journal of the American Medical Association*, Vol. 270 (1993), pp. 1819–25; A. P. Haines, J. D. Imeson, and T. W. Meade, Phobic anxiety and ischemic heart disease, *British Medical Journal*, Vol. 295 (1987), pp. 297–99; I. Kawachi et al., Symptoms of anxiety and risk of coronary heart disease: the Normative Aging Study, *Circulation*, Vol. 90 (1994), pp. 2225–29.

25. J. L. Levenson et al., Denial and medical outcome in unstable angina, *Psychosomatic Medicine*, Vol. 51 (1989), pp. 27–35; Markovitz and Matthews, op. cit.

26. D. Ornish et al., Can lifestyle changes reverse coronary heart disease? *Lancet*, Vol. 336 (1990), pp. 129–33.

27. R. J. Baron, Finding new models for medicine (editorial), *Journal of the American Medical Association*, Vol. 255 (1986), pp. 3404–5; D. S. Brody, Physician recognition of behavioral, psychological, and social aspects of medical care, *Archives of Internal Medicine*, Vol. 140 (1980), pp. 1286–89; D. R. Calkins et al., Failure of physicians to recognize functional disability, *Annals of Internal Medicine*, Vol. 114 (1991), pp. 451–54; B. S. Levine et al., A national survey of attitudes and practices of primary-care physicians relating to nutrition: strategies for enhancing the use of clinical nutrition in medical practice, *American Journal of Clinical Nutrition*, Vol. 57 (1993), pp. 115–19.

28. J. Schwartz et al., Particulate air pollution and hospital emergency room visits for asthma in Seattle, *American Review of Respiratory Disease*, Vol. 147 (1993), pp. 826–31; B. A. Chilmonczyk et al., Association between exposure to environmental tobacco smoke and exacerbations of asthma in children, *New England Journal of Medicine*, Vol. 328 (1993), pp. 1665–69; O. V. J. Rossi et al., Association of severe asthma attacks with weather, pollen and air pollutants, *Thorax*, Vol. 48 (1993), pp. 244–48; R. Bellomo et al., Two consecutive thunderstorm associated epidemics of asthma in the city of Melbourne, *Medical Journal of Australia*, Vol. 156 (1992), pp. 834–57; G. E. Packe and J. G. Ayres, Asthma outbreak during a thunderstorm, *Lancet*, Vol. ii (1985), pp. 199–204; P. M. O'Byrne, J. Dolovich, and F. E. Hargreave, Late asthmatic responses, *American Review of Respiratory Disease*, Vol. 136 (1987), pp. 740–51; L. E. Gelber et al., Sensitization and exposure to indoor allergens as risk factors for asthma among patients presenting to hospital, *American Review of Respiratory Disease*, Vol. 147 (1993), pp. 573–78; R. F. Lemanske, Jr., et al., Rhinovirus upper respiratory infection increases airway hyperactivity and late asthmatic reactions, *Journal of Clinical Investigation*, Vol. 83 (1989), pp. 1–10; M. J. Rumbak et al., Perception of anxiety as a contributing factor of asthma: indigent versus nonindigent, *Journal of Asthma*, Vol. 30 (1993), pp. 165–69; W. L. Eschenbacher et al., Pulmonary responses of asthmatic and normal subjects to different temperatures and humidity conditions in an environmental chamber, *Lung*, Vol. 170 (1992), pp. 51–62; D. A. Mahler, Exercise-induced asthma, *Medical Science in Sports and Exercise*, Vol. 25 (1993), pp. 554–61.

29. J. Avorn, D. E. Everitt, and M. W. Baker, The neglected medical history and therapeutic choices for abdominal pain: a nationwide study of 799 physicians and nurses, *Archives of Internal Medicine*, Vol. 151 (1991), pp. 694–98.

30. H. Offenbacher et al., Assessment of MRI criteria for a diagnosis of MS, *Neurology*, Vol. 43 (1993), pp. 905–9. The accuracy of MRI varied depending upon the criteria used and the patient's age. Positive predictive value ranged from 23 percent to 64 percent.

31. J. O. Brabander and F. Blank, Intestinal moniliasis in adults, *Canadian Medical Association Journal*, Vol. 77 (1957), pp. 478–83; J. G. Alexander, Thrush bowel infection: existence, incidence, prevention and treatment, particularly by a Lactobacillus acidophilus preparation, *Current Medicine and Drugs*, Vol. 8 (1967), pp. 3–11; J. G. Kane, J. H. Chretien, and V. F. Garagusi, Diarrhoea caused by Candida, *Lancet*, Vol. i (1976), pp. 335–36; A. Lorenz et al., Fungal infection of the small bowel mucosa, *Mykosen*, Vol. 27 (1984), pp. 506–10; M. Caselli et al., Dead fecal yeasts and chronic diarrhea, *Digestion*, Vol. 41 (1988), pp. 142–48; P. L. Danna et al., Role of Candida in pathogenesis of antibiotic-induced diarrhoea in elderly inpatients, *Lancet*, Vol. 337 (1991), pp. 511–14.

32. Leo Galland, "The Effect of Intestinal Microbes on Systemic Immunity," in R. Jenkins and P. Mowbray, *Post-Viral Fatigue Syndrome* (London: John Wiley and Sons, 1991), pp. 405–30.

33. B. Hagglof et al., The Swedish Childhood Diabetes Study: indication of severe psychological stress as a risk factor for type 1 (insulin-dependent) diabetes mellitus in childhood, *Diabetologia*, Vol. 34 (1991), pp. 579–83; B. Winsa et al., Stressful life events and Graves' disease, *Lancet*, Vol. 338 (1991), pp. 1475–79; F. Creed, Life events and appendectomy, *Lancet*, Vol. i (1981), pp. 1381–88; G. De benedittis, A. Lorenzetti, and A. Pieri, The role of stressful life events in the onset of chronic primary headache, *Pain*, Vol. 40 (1990), pp. 65–75.

34. R. W. Bartrop et al., "Depressed Lymphocyte Function After Bereavement," in *Foundations of Psychoneuroimmunology*, ed. S. Locke et al. (New York: Aldine Publishing Company, 1985), pp. 337–40; J. K. Kiecolt-Glaser and R. Glaser, Psychosocial moderators of immune function, *Annals of Behavioral Medicine*, Vol. 9 (1987), pp. 16–20.

35. Jeffrey W. Fessel, The nature of illness and diagnosis, *American Journal of Medicine*, Vol. 75 (1983), pp. 555–60.

36. T. Ronne, Measles virus infection without rash in childhood is related to disease in adult life, *Lancet*, Vol. 325 (1985), pp. 1–4.

37. J. Leor, W. K. Poole, and R. A. Kloner, Sudden cardiac death triggered by an earthquake, *New England Journal of Medicine*, Vol. 334 (1996), pp. 413–19.

38. A. Johsson and L. Hansson, Prolonged exposure to a stressful stimulus (noise) as a cause of raised blood pressure in man, *Lancet*, Vol. i (1977), pp. 86–87.

39. D. W. Phillips, Twin studies in medical research (letter), *Lancet*, Vol. 342 (1993), p. 52.

40. D. J. P. Barker et al., Weight in infancy and death from ischaemic heart disease, *Lancet*, Vol. ii (1989), pp. 577–80; D. J. P. Barker et al., Fetal and placental size and risk of hypertension in adult life, *British Medical Journal*, Vol. 301 (1990), pp. 259–62; D. J. P. Barker, *Fetal and Infants' Origins of Adult Disease* (London: British Medical Journal, 1992); G. R. Goldberg and A. Prentice, Maternal and fetal determinants of adult diseases, *Nutrition Reviews*, Vol. 52 (1994), pp. 191–200.

41. D. L. Paulhus and C. L. Martin, Predicting adult temperament from minor physical anomalies, *Journal of Personality and Social Psychology*, Vol. 50 (1986), pp. 1235–39.

42. See M. H. Swartz, M. V. Herman, and L. Teicholz, Dermatoglyphic patterns in patients with mitral valve prolapse: a clue to pathogenesis, *American Journal of Cardiology*, Vol. 38 (1976), pp. 588–93.

Chapter 4: The Four Pillars of Healing

1. C. B. Thomas, Stamina: the thread of life, *Journal of Chronic Diseases*, Vol. 34 (1981), pp. 41–44.

2. R. Dubos, Biological and social aspects of tuberculosis, *Bulletin of the New York Academy of Medicine*, Vol. 27 (1951), p. 351.

3. A. S. Kraus and A. M. Lilienfeld, Some epidemiological aspects of the high mortality rate in the young widowed group, *Journal of Chronic Diseases*, Vol. 10 (1959), pp. 207–17.

4. M. Young, B. Bernard, and G. Wallis, The mortality of widowers, *Lancet* Vol. ii, (1963), pp. 454–56.

5. J. H. Medalie and U. Goldbourt, Angina pectoris among 10,000 men II: psychosocial and other risk factors as evidenced by a multivariate analysis of five-year incidence study, *American Journal of Medicine*, Vol. 60 (1976), pp. 910–21.

6. L. F. Berkman and S. L. Syme, Social networks, host resistance, and mortality: a nine year follow-up of Alameda County residents, *American Journal of Epidemiology*, Vol. 109 (1979), pp. 186–204.

7. R. B. Williams et al., Prognostic importance of social and economic resources among medically treated patients with angiographically documented coronary artery disease, *Journal of the American Medical Association*, Vol. 267 (1992), pp. 520–24; R. B. Case et al., Living alone after myocardial infarction: impact on prognosis, *Journal of the American Medical Association*, Vol. 267 (1992), pp. 515–19; L. F. Berkman, L. Leo-Summers, and I. Horwitz, Emotional support and survival after myocardial infarction, *Annals of Internal Medicine*, Vol. 117 (1992), pp. 1003–9.

8. K. Ell et al., Social relations, social support and survival among patients with cancer, *Journal of Psychosomatic Research*, Vol. 36 (1992), pp. 1–11.

9. L. Eisenberg, What makes persons "patients" and patients "well," *American Journal of Medicine*, Vol. 69 (1980), pp. 277–86.

10. D. Spiegel et al., Effect of psychosocial treatment on survival of patients with metastatic breast cancer, *Lancet*, Vol. ii (1989), pp. 888–91.

11. F. I. Fawzy et al., Malignant melanoma: effects of an early structured psychiatric intervention, coping, and effective state on recurrence and survival 6 years later, *Archives of General Psychiatry*, Vol. 50 (1993), pp. 681–89.

12. F. I. Fawzy et al., A structured psychiatric intervention for cancer patients; II. Changes over time in immunological measures, *Archives of General Psychiatry*, Vol. 47 (1990), pp. 729–35.

13. H. C. Bucher, Social support and prognosis following first myocardial infarction, *Journal of General Internal Medicine*, Vol. 9 (1994), pp. 409–17.

14. S. Cobb, Social support as a moderator of life stress, *Psychosomatic Medicine*, Vol. 38 (1976), pp. 300–314. "Social support is defined as information leading the subject to believe that he is cared for and loved, esteemed, and a member of a network of mutual obligations. . . . Social support can protect people in crisis from

a wide range of pathological states: low birth weight, death, arthritis, tuberculosis, depression, alcoholism . . ."

15. K. B. Thomas, The placebo in general practice, *Lancet*, Vol. 344 (1994), pp. 1066–67. The author states, in conclusion: "The placebo effect in general practice is the power of the doctor alone to make the patient feel better, irrespective of medication. It is one of the most important factors in the consultation, yet generally it is neglected." See also H. Waitzkin, Doctor-patient communication: clinical implications of social scientific research, *Journal of the American Medical Association*, Vol. 252 (1984), pp. 2441–46. Patients want more information than doctors think they do. The discrepancy between physician expectations and patients' desires is especially strong for the economically disadvantaged.

16. S. H. Kaplan, S. Greenfield, and J. E. Ware, Jr., Assessing the effects of physician-patient interactions on the outcomes of chronic disease, *Medical Care*, Vol. 27, Supp. 3 (1989), pp. S110–S127. Patients coaxed by assistants to ask more questions and participate in decisions about their care fared better in the outcome of chronic conditions like high blood pressure, diabetes, and ulcers.

17. Tanya Wenman Steel, "A Nation Addicted to Junk (Shhhh!)," *New York Times*, June 7, 1995, pp. C1, C6.

18. A. K. Kant and A. Schatzkin, Consumption of energy-dense, nutrient-poor foods by the US population: effect on nutrient profiles, *Journal of the American College of Nutrition*, Vol. 13 (1994), pp. 285–91.

19. R. J. Kuczmarski et al., Increasing prevalence of overweight among U.S. adults: the national health and nutrition examination surveys, 1960 to 1991, *Journal of the American Medical Association*, Vol. 272 (1994), pp. 205–11.

20. R. M. Dougherty, A. K. H. Fong, and J. M. Iacono, Nutrient content of the diet when the fat is reduced, *American Journal of Clinical Nutrition*, Vol. 48 (1988), pp. 970–79; P. M. Emmett and K. W. Heaton, Is extrinsic sugar a vehicle for dietary fat? *Lancet*, Vol. 345 (1995), pp. 1537–40.

21. S. M. Krebs-Smith et al., Fruit and vegetable intakes of children and adolescents in the United States, *Archives of Pediatrics and Adolescent Medicine*, Vol. 150 (1996), pp. 81–86.

22. J. Hallfrisch and D. C. Muller, Does diet provide adequate amounts of calcium, iron, magnesium and zinc in a well-educated adult population? *Experimental Gerontology*, Vol. 28 (1993), pp. 473–83.

23. G. S. El-Assal, Ancient Egyptian medicine, *Lancet*, Vol. ii (1972), pp. 272–74.

24. R. Dubos, *Mirage of Health: Utopias, Progress, and Biological Change* (New York: Harper & Brothers, 1959, rpt. New Brunswick, N.J.: Rutgers University Press, 1987).

25. W. P. D. Logan, Mortality in the London fog incident, *Lancet*, Vol. 264 (1953), pp. 336–38.

26. E. T. Wilkins, Air pollution aspects of the London fog of December 1952, *Quarterly Journal Reports of the Meteorologic Society*, Vol. 80 (1952), pp. 267–71.

27. J. Schwartz and D. W. Dockery, Particulate air pollution and daily mortality in Steubenville, Ohio, *American Journal of Epidemiology*, Vol. 135 (1992), pp. 12–19; J. Schwartz and D. W. Dockery, Increased mortality in Philadelphia associated with daily air pollution concentrations, *American Review of Respiratory Dis-*

ease, Vol. 145 (1992), pp. 600–604; D. W. Dockery, J. Schwartz, and J. D. Spenger, Air pollution and daily mortality: association with particulates and acid aerosols, *Environmental Research*, Vol. 59 (1992), pp. 362–73; D. W. Dockery et al., An association between air pollution and mortality in six U.S. cities, *New England Journal of Medicine*, Vol. 329 (1993), pp. 1753–59.

28. B. D. Ostro and S. Rothschild, Air pollution and acute respiratory morbidity: an observational study of multiple pollutants, *Environmental Research*, Vol. 50 (1989), pp. 238–47; J. Schwartz et al., Particulate air pollution and hospital emergency room visits for asthma in Seattle, *American Review of Respiratory Disease*, Vol. 147 (1993), pp. 826–31.

29. New study links airborne dust to higher cancer rate for women, *Environmental Health Letter*, Vol. 30 (1991), p. 231.

30. A. Fackelmann, Air pollution boosts cancer spread, *Science News*, April 7, 1990, p. 221.

31. M. Strahilevitz, A. Strahilevitz, and J. E. Miller, Air pollutants and the admission rate of psychiatric patients, *American Journal of Psychiatry*, Vol. 136 (1979), pp. 205–7.

32. A. A. LaVerne, Nonspecific Air Pollution Syndrome (NAPS), *Behavioral Psychology*, Vol. 2 (1970), pp. 19–21.

33. Boston, Houghton Mifflin, 1962.

34. El-Assal, op. cit.

35. Élie Metchnikoff, *Prolongation of Life* (New York: G. P. Putnam's Sons, 1908). Metchnikoff, incidentally, was the younger brother of Ivan Ilyich, whose tragic story was recounted by Leo Tolstoy in *The Death of Ivan Ilyich*.

36. H. Avakian et al., Ankylosing spondylitis, HLA-B27 and Klebsiella; II. Cross-reactivity studies with human tissue typing sera, *British Journal of Experimental Pathology*, Vol. 61 (1980), pp. 92–96; R. Ebringer et al., Ankylosing spondylitis: klebsiella and HLA-B27, *Rheumatology and Rehabilitation*, Vol. 16 (1977), pp. 190–96; A. Ebringer and M. Ghuloom, Ankylosing spondylitis, HLA-B27, and klebsiella: cross reactivity and antibody studies (letter), *Annals of the Rheumatic Diseases*, Vol. 45 (1986), pp. 703–4; A. Ebringer, The relationship between Klebsiella infection and ankylosing spondylitis, *Baillieres Clinical Rheumatology*, Vol. 3 (1989), pp. 321–38; A. F. Geczy et al., Cross-reactivity of anti-Klebsiella K43 BTS 1 serum and lymphocytes of patients with ankylosing spondylitis: antipodean curiosity? (letter), *Lancet*, Vol. i (1985), p. 1169; A. F. Geczy et al., HLA-B27, molecular mimicry, and ankylosing spondylitis: popular misconceptions, *Annals of the Rheumatic Diseases*, Vol. 46 (1987), pp. 171–72; G. Husby et al., Cross-reactive epitope with Klebsiella pneumoniae nitrogenase in articular tissue of HLA-B27+ patients with ankylosing spondylitis, *Arthritis and Rheumatism*, Vol. 32 (1989), pp. 437–45; S. Khalafpour et al., Antibodies to Klebsiella and Proteus microorganisms in ankylosing spondylitis and rheumatoid arthritis patients measured by ELISA, *British Journal of Rheumatology*, Vol. 2 (1988), pp. 86–89; J. S. Sullivan et al., Cross-reacting bacterial determinants in ankylosing spondylitis, *American Journal of Medicine*, Vol. 85 (1988), pp. 54–55; A. K. Trull et al., IgA antibodies to Klebsiella pneumoniae in ankylosing spondylitis, *Scandinavian Journal of Rheumatology*, Vol. 12 (1983), pp. 249–53; J. Welsh et al., Ankylosing spondylitis, HLA-B27 and Klebsiella; I. Cross-reactivity studies with rabbit

antisera, *British Journal of Experimental Pathology*, Vol. 61 (1980), pp. 85–91; D. T. Yu, S. Y. Choo, and T. Schaack, Molecular mimicry in HLA-B27-related arthritis (see comments), *Annals of Internal Medicine*, Vol. 111 (1989), pp. 581–91.

37. R. Hallgren, S. Feltelius, and U. Lindhi, Redistribution of minerals and trace elements in chronic inflammation—a study on isolated blood cells from patients with ankylosing spondylitis, *Journal of Rheumatology*, Vol. 14 (1987), pp. 548–53; K. Svenson et al., Abnormal calcium, magnesium and zinc stores in peripheral blood cells from patients with inflammatory connective tissue disorders, *Acta Pharmacologica et Toxicologia*, Vol. 59, Supp. (1986), pp. 386–91.

Chapter 5: The First Pillar: Relationship

1. Marion H. Carter, "One Man and His Town," *McClure's Magazine*, Vol. 30 (1908), pp. 275–86.

2. R. Oppedisano, "Roseto Revisited," *The National Magazine for Italian Americans*, Feb. 1970, p. 38.

3. Stewart Wolf and John G. Bruhn, *The Power of Clan: The Influence of Human Relationships on Heart Disease* (New Brunswick, N.J.: Transaction Publishers, 1993), pp. 10–11.

4. B. Egolf et al., The Roseto effect: a 50-year comparison of mortality rates, *American Journal of Public Health*, Vol. 82 (1992), pp. 1089–92.

5. Quoted in H. M. Spiro, To hope helps, *Alternative & Complementary Therapies*, Sept.–Oct. 1995, p. 301.

6. E. V. Hersch et al., Narcotic receptor blockade and its effect on the analgesic response to placebo and ibuprofen after oral surgery, *Oral Surgery, Oral Medicine and Oral Pathology*, Vol. 75 (1993), pp. 539–46.

7. Data on the cholesterol-lowering effect of placebo can be gleaned from the Coronary Drug Project Research Group, Influence of adherence to treatment and response of cholesterol on mortality in the coronary drug project, *New England Journal of Medicine*, Vol. 303 (1980), pp. 1038–41.

8. The recent demonstration that most peptic ulcer disease is triggered by a chronic bacterial infection of the stomach makes the high rate of placebo responsiveness especially intriguing.

9. D. E. Moerman, General medical effectiveness and human biology: placebo effects in the treatment of ulcer disease, *Medical Anthropology Quarterly*, Vol. 14 (1983), pp. 13–16.

10. Variability of placebo response is reviewed in A. H. Roberts et al., The power of nonspecific effects in healing: implications for psychosocial and biological treatments, *Clinical Psychology Review*, Vol. 13 (1993), pp. 375–91.

11. H. Benson and D. P. McCalle, Angina pectoris and the placebo effect, *New England Journal of Medicine*, Vol. 300 (1979), pp. 1424–29. "Data from enthusiast's studies reveal subjective improvement in 82.4%."

12. F. J. Evans, The power of a sugar pill, *Psychology Today*, Apr. 1974. A review of the author's research.

13. J. Kleinen et al., Placebo effect in double-blind clinical trials: a review of interactions with medications, *Lancet*, Vol. 344 (1994), pp. 1347–49. For those clinical trials in which informed consent was required of the experimental subjects, there was a decreased placebo response and also a decreased difference between

active drug and placebo. The placebo/drug relationship varies from clinic to clinic. This variation may have to do with the quality of the interaction between health care providers and patients.

H. Brody, The lie that heals: the ethics of giving placebos, *Annals of Internal Medicine*, Vol. 97 (1992), pp. 112–18. The character of the doctor affects drug responses. Active drug works better when given by a caring physician. Distinction between active drug and placebo is wiped out and both are less effective when prescribed by a noncaring physician.

14. Doctors and nurses give placebos to demanding, anxious patients. They are the least likely to respond. J. S. Goodwin, J. M. Goodwin, and A. V. Vogel, Knowledge and use of placebos by house officers and nurses, *Annals of Internal Medicine*, Vol. 91 (1979), pp. 106–10.

15. L. Park and L. Covi, Nonblind placebo trial: an exploration of neurotic patients' responses to placebo when its first inert content is disclosed, *Archives of General Psychiatry*, Vol. 12 (1965), pp. 336–45.

16. L. D. Egbert et al., Reduction of postoperative pain by encouragement and instruction of patients: a study of doctor-patient rapport, *New England Journal of Medicine*, Vol. 270 (1964), pp. 825–27.

17. The Headache Study group of the University of Western Ontario. Predictors of outcome in headache patients presenting to family physicians—a one year prospective study, *Headache*, Vol. 26 (1986), pp. 285–94.

18. K. B. Thomas, The placebo in general practice, *Lancet*, Vol. 344 (1994), pp. 1066–67.

19. G. L. Engel, Psychologic stress, vasodepressor (vasovagal) syncope, and sudden death, *Annals of Internal Medicine*, Vol. 89 (1978), pp. 403–12.

20. Anatole Broyard, *Intoxicated by My Illness: And Other Writings on Life and Death* (New York: Clarkson Potter, 1992).

21. Eric Cassell, *The Nature of Suffering and the Goals of Medicine* (New York: Oxford University Press, 1991), p. 126.

22. C. Sanchez-Menegay and H. Stalder, Do physicians take into account patients' expectations? *Journal of General Internal Medicine*, Vol. 9 (1994), pp. 404–6.

23. D. M. Eisenberg et al., Unconventional medicine in the United States: prevalence, costs, and patterns of use, *New England Journal of Medicine*, Vol. 328 (1993), pp. 246–52. Twenty-two million Americans annually see an unconventional provider for a medical condition.

24. A. Ekbom et al., Ulcerative colitis and colorectal cancer: a population-based study, *New England Journal of Medicine*, Vol. 323 (1990), pp. 1228–33.

25. R. Wright and S. C. Truelove, Auto-immune reactions in ulcerative colitis, *Gut*, Vol. 7 (1966), pp. 32–40; R. Lagercrantz et al., Immunological studies in ulcerative colitis; III. Incidence of antibodies to colon-antigen in ulcerative colitis and other gastro-intestinal diseases, *Clinical and Experimental Immunology*, Vol. 1 (1966), pp. 263–76; T. Hibi et al., In vitro anticolon antibody production by mucosal or peripheral blood lymphocytes from patients with ulcerative colitis, *Gut*, Vol. 31 (1990), pp. 1371–76; E. Salem et al., Autoantibodies in amebic colitis, *Journal of the Egyptian Medical Association*, Vol. 56 (1973), pp. 113–18; J. D. Bennet, Ulcerative colitis: the result of an altered bacterial metabolism of bile acids or cholesterol, *Medical Hypotheses*, Vol. 20 (1986), pp. 125–32; J. E. Chodos, Campylobacter infection mimicking ulcerative colitis, *New York State Journal of*

Medicine (Jan. 1986), pp. 22–24; R. P. Bolton, *Clostridium difficile* and its association with inflammatory bowel disease, *IM* (Oct. 1980), pp. 19–23; R. J. A. Diepersloot et al., Acute ulcerative proctocolitis associated with primary cytomegalovirus infection, *Archives of Internal Medicine*, Vol. 150 (1990), pp. 1749–51; D. A. Burke and A. T. R. Axon, Hydrophobic adhesion of *E. coli* in ulcerative colitis, *Gut*, Vol. 29 (1988), pp. 41–43; D. A. Burke and A. T. R. Axon, Ulcerative colitis and *Escherichia coli* with adhesive properties, *Journal of Clinical Pathology*, Vol. 40 (1987), pp. 782–86; M. L. McCann et al., Clinical recovery in inflammatory bowel disease (IBD) following bowel flora replacement with *E. coli* (abstract), presentation to Society of Clinical Immunology, Chicago, Nov. 10, 1990; M. McCann, Reflorastation therapy in inflammatory bowel disease, *Interdisziplinares Symposium, Darmflora in Sybiose und Pathogenitat; Der Internist Beilage*, Vol. 33 (1992), p. 10; M. L. McCann, R. S. Abrams, and R. P. Nelson, "Treatment of Inflammatory Bowel Disease," in *Microbial Pathogenesis and Immune Response*, ed. E. W. Ades, R. F. Rest, and S. A. Morse, *Proceedings of the New York Academy of Sciences* (1994), pp. 243–45.

26. A. G. Schwartz et al., Sulfasalazine-induced exacerbation of ulcerative colitis, *New England Journal of Medicine*, Vol. 306 (1982), pp. 409–12.

27. R. Wright and S. C. Truelove, A controlled trial of various diets in ulcerative colitis, *British Medical Journal*, Vol. 2 (1965), pp. 138–41.

28. M. J. Hill et al., Faecal bile acids, dysplasia, and carcinoma in ulcerative colitis, *Lancet*, Vol. ii (1987), pp. 185–86.

29. B. M. Peskar et al., Enhanced formation of sulfitopeptide-leukotrienes in ulcerative colitis and Crohn's disease: inhibition by sulfasalzine and 5-aminosalicylic acid, *Agents and Actions*, Vol. 18 (1986), pp. 381–83.

30. H. Jick and A. M. Walker, Cigarette smoking and ulcerative colitis, *New England Journal of Medicine*, Vol. 308 (1983), pp. 1477–78.

31. Produced by Metagenics, Inc., San Clemente, California 92673.

32. S. J. Reiser, The era of the patient: using the experience of illness in shaping the missions of health care, *Journal of the American Medical Association*, Vol. 269 (1993), pp. 1012–17; H. B. Beckman and R. M. Frankel, The effect of physician behavior on the collection of data, *Annals of Internal Medicine*, Vol. 101 (1984), pp. 692–96; R. Frankel, "Talking in Interviews: A Dispreference for Patient-Initiated Questions in Physician-Patient Encounters," in *Studies in Ethnomethodology and Conversation Analysis*, No. 1, ed. G. Psathas (Washington, D.C.: The International Institute for Ethnomethodology and Conversation Analysis and University Press of America, 1990), pp. 231–62; E. E. Bartlett et al., The effects of physician communications skills on patient satisfaction; recall and adherence, *Journal of Chronic Disease*, Vol. 37 (1984), pp. 755–64; R. C. Smith and R. B. Hoppe, The patient's story: integrating the patient- and physician-centered approaches to interviewing, *Annals of Internal Medicine*, Vol. 115 (1991), pp. 470–77.

33. An excellent resource on the science and practice of caring is *The Medical Interview: Clinical Care, Education and Research*, ed. Mack Lipkin, Jr., Samuel M. Putnam, and Aaron Lazare (New York: Springer-Verlag, 1995). My analysis draws upon data presented in Chapter 3, "Therapeutic Aspects of the Clinical Encounter," by Dennis Novack, pp. 32–49, and Chapter 47, "The Patient-Centered Interview: Research Support," by Samuel M. Putnam and Mack Lipkin, Jr., pp. 530–37.

34. Beckman and Frankel, op. cit.; H. B. Beckman and R. M. Frankel, Soliciting the patient's complete agenda: a relationship to the distribution of concerns, *Clinical Research*, Vol. 33 (1985), p. 714A.

35. D. L. Roter and J. A. Hall, Physician interviewing styles and medical information obtained from patients, *Journal of General Internal Medicine*, Vol. 2 (1987), pp. 325–29.

36. R. B. Fredidin, L. Goldin, and R. R. Cecil, Patient-physician concordance in problem identification in the primary care setting, *Annals of Internal Medicine*, Vol. 93 (1980), pp. 490–93.

37. D. Tuckett et al., *Meetings Between Experts: An Approach to Sharing Ideas in Medical Consultations* (London and New York: Tavistock Publications, 1985).

38. C. Sanchez-Menegay and M. Stalder, Do physicians take into account patients' perspectives? *Journal of General Internal Medicine*, Vol. 9 (1994), pp. 404–6. No, at least in Switzerland.

39. B. M. Korsch, E. K. Gozzi, and V. Francis, Gaps in doctor-patient communication; I: Doctor-patient interaction and patient satisfaction, *Pediatrics*, Vol. 42 (1968), pp. 855–71.

40. G. H. Williams and P. H. N. Wood, Common-sense beliefs about illness: a mediating role for the doctor, *Lancet*, Vol. 328 (1986), 1435–37.

41. J. A. Hall, D. L. Roter, and N. R. Katz, Meta-analysis of correlates of provider behavior in medical encounters, *Medical Care*, Vol. 28 (1990), pp. 657–75.

42. The impact of physicians' advice on patients' self-care practices is studied in P. A. Ades et al., Predictors of cardiac rehabilitation participation in older coronary patients, *Archives of Internal Medicine*, Vol. 152 (1992), pp. 1033–35.

Physicians frequently fail to address psychosocial or behavioral problems among their patients. See D. S. Brody, Physician recognition of behavioral, psychological, and social aspects of medical care, *Archives of Internal Medicine*, Vol. 140 (1980), pp. 1286–89.

Some studies concerning the effect of patient education on medical outcomes: P. D. Mullen et al., Efficacy of psychoeducational interventions on pain, depression, and disability in people with arthritis: a meta-analysis, *Journal of Rheumatology*, Vol. 14, Supp. 15 (1987), pp. 33–39; S. R. Wilson et al., A controlled trial of two forms of self-management education for adults with asthma, *American Journal of Medicine*, Vol. 94 (1993), pp. 564–76; K. R. Lorig, P. D. Mazonson, and H. R. Holman, Evidence suggesting that health education for self-management in patients with chronic arthritis has sustained health benefits while reducing health care costs, *Arthritis and Rheumatism*, Vol. 36 (1993), pp. 439–46; D. K. Litzelman et al., Reduction of lower extremity clinical abnormalities in patients with non–insulin dependent diabetes mellitus: a randomized, control trial, *Annals of Internal Medicine*, Vol. 119 (1993), pp. 36–41.

43. H. Waitzkin, Doctor-patient communication: clinical implications of social scientific research, *Journal of the American Medical Association*, Vol. 252 (1984), pp. 2441–46.

44. Anatole Broyard, "Doctor, Talk to Me," *New York Times Magazine*, Aug. 26, 1990, p. 33.

45. V. K. Fine and M. E. Therrien, Empathy in the doctor-patient relationship: skill training for medical students, *Journal of Medical Education*, Vol. 52 (1977), pp.

752–57; A. L. Suchman and D. A. Matthews, What makes the patient-doctor relationship therapeutic? Exploring the connexional dimension of medical care, *Annals of Internal Medicine*, Vol. 108 (1988), pp. 125–30; H. Spiro, What is empathy and can it be taught? *Annals of Internal Medicine*, Vol. 116 (1992), pp. 843–46; D. Gianokos, Empathy revisited, *Archives of Internal Medicine*, Vol. 156 (1996), pp. 135–36.

46. Engel, op. cit.; "Taking hopelessness to heart," *Science News*, July 31, 1993, p. 79 (report on paper by Robert Anda in *Epidemiology*, July 1993).

47. Elisabeth Kübler-Ross, *On Death and Dying* (New York: Macmillan, 1969).

48. D. R. Calkins et al., Failure of physicians to recognize functional disability, *Annals of Internal Medicine*, Vol. 114 (1991), pp. 451–54.

49. D. S. Brody et al., The relationship between patients' satisfaction with their physicians and perceptions about interventions they desired and received, *Medical Care*, Vol. 27 (1989), pp. 1027–35.

50. S. Molde and D. Baker, Explaining primary care visits, *Image*, Vol. 17 (1985), pp. 72–76.

51. J. White, W. Levinson, and D. Roter, "Oh, by the way . . .": The closing moments of the medical visit, *Journal of General Internal Medicine*, Vol. 9 (1994), pp. 24–28.

52. S. Greenfield, S. Kaplan, and J. E. Ware, Expanding patient involvement in care: effects on patient outcomes, *Annals of Internal Medicine*, Vol. 102 (1985), pp. 520–28; S. H. Kaplan, S. Greenfield, and J. E. Ware, Assessing the effects of physician-patient interactions on the outcomes of chronic disease, *Medical Care*, Vol. 27 (1989), pp. S110–S127.

53. Bartlett et al., op. cit.

54. The Coronary Drug Project Research Group, op. cit.

55. E. J. Gallagher, C. M. Viscoli, and R. I. Horwitz, The relationship of treatment adherence to the risk of death after myocardial infarction in women, *Journal of the American Medical Association*, Vol. 270 (1993), pp. 742–44; R. I. Horwitz et al., Treatment adherence and risk of death after a myocardial infarction, *Lancet*, Vol. ii (1990), pp. 542–45; R. I. Horwitz and S. M. Horwitz, Adherence to treatment and health outcomes, *Archives of Internal Medicine*, Vol. 153 (1993), pp. 1863–68.

56. A. O'Leary, Self-efficacy and health, *Behavioral Research and Therapy*, Vol. 23 (1985), pp. 437–51; G. Holden, The relationship of self-efficacy appraisals to subsequent health related outcomes: a meta-analysis, *Social Work and Health Care*, Vol. 16 (1991), pp. 53–93.

57. Information about the effects of instruction, encouragement, and advice on perceived self-efficacy, self-care behaviors, and medical outcomes can be found in the sources listed in Note 42, this chapter.

Chapter 6: The Second Pillar: *Díaita*

1. D. W. Black and R. Fisher, Mortality in DSM-III-R schizophrenia, *Schizophrenia Research*, Vol. 7 (1986), pp. 109–16.

2. Where next with psychiatric illness? *Nature*, Vol. 336 (1988), pp. 95–96.

3. L. L. Bachrach, What we know about homelessness among mentally ill persons: an analytical review and commentary. In H. R. Lamb, L. L. Bachrach, and

F. I. Kass, eds., *Treating the Homeless Mentally Ill* (Washington, D.C.: American Psychiatric Press, 1992), pp. 13–40.

4. Research into the origins of schizophrenia has stumbled across a number of paradoxes and inconsistencies. On the one hand, the clinical manifestations of schizophrenia are fairly easy to discern. A recent review in the British journal *Lancet* assures readers that "patients with this illness look essentially the same throughout the world, and a skilled clinician can usually recognize the classic forms of the illness even when unable to speak the patient's language and conduct a full interview." [N. C. Andreasen, Symptoms, signs, and diagnosis of schizophrenia, *Lancet*, Vol. 346 (1995), pp. 466–81.] On the other hand, schizophrenia is clearly not a single disease entity.

There is no doubt that schizophrenic behavior tends to run in families. The child of a schizophrenic parent has a risk of developing schizophrenia that is fifteen times greater than the risk of schizophrenia in the population as a whole. The more relatives with schizophrenia one has and the more closely related they are, the greater one's likelihood of becoming schizophrenic. Adoption studies indicate that familial predisposition to schizophrenia is to a large extent genetic. Children who are adopted become schizophrenic at a rate that matches their biological family's rather than their adoptive family's. "Normal" children adopted by schizophrenic parents do not have increased rates of schizophrenia. [T. C. Manschreck, Schizophrenic disorders, *New England Journal of Medicine*, Vol. 305 (1981), pp. 1628–32.] On the other hand, the majority of schizophrenics have no relatives with schizophrenia. If one of two identical twins is schizophrenic, the likelihood that the other twin will be schizophrenic is a bit less than 50 percent. [P. McGuffin, M. J. Owen, and A. E. Farmer, Genetic basis of schizophrenia, *Lancet*, Vol. 346 (1995), pp. 678–82.] Since identical twins have the same genes, then the genes themselves must contribute less than half the burden of risk. Some scientists attempted to explain this discrepancy by dividing the disease into two general types: inherited and acquired. However, if a pair of identical twins is discordant for schizophrenia (i.e., one has it, the other doesn't), the likelihood that either twin will have a child with schizophrenia is 10 percent, which is far greater than the rate for parents who are not schizophrenic, indicating that something familial is passed on, even for those twin pairs in whom schizophrenia is not determined by the genes themselves.

Evidence from epidemiology supports a role for nongenetic prenatal influences on the development of schizophrenia. Maternal malnutrition during the first three months of pregnancy or influenza during the sixth or seventh month of pregnancy increases the chance that the offspring of the pregnancy will be schizophrenic. [E. S. Susser and S. P. Lin, Schizophrenia after exposure to the Dutch Hunger Winter of 1944–1945, *Archives of General Psychiatry*, Vol. 49 (1992), pp. 983–88; S. A. Mednick et al., Adult schizophrenia following prenatal exposure to an influenza epidemic, *Archives of General Psychiatry*, Vol. 45 (1988), pp. 189–92; C. E. Barr, S. A. Mednick, and P. Munk-Jorgensen, Exposure to influenza epidemics during gestation and adult schizophrenia: a 40-year study, *Archives of General Psychiatry*, Vol. 47 (1990), pp. 189–92; P. C. Sham et al., Schizophrenia following pre-natal exposure to influenza epidemics between 1939 and 1960, *British Journal of Psychiatry*, Vol. 160 (1992), pp. 461–66.] The presumed mechanism is a disturbance in the development of the brain produced by nutritional deficiency or viral infection. Schizophrenia is also more common among people born and raised in cities, the risk increasing with the size of the city. [G. Lewis et al., Schizophrenia and city life, *Lancet*, Vol. 340 (1992), pp. 137–40.] An urban upbringing increases exposure to infectious disease, drugs, childhood head trauma, and stressful life events, each of which is associated with the appearance of schizophrenia. [E. F. Torrey, Stalking the schizovirus, *Schizophrenia Bulletin*, Vol. 14 (1988), pp. 229–34; J. A. Wilcox and H. A. Nasrallah, Childhood head trauma and psychosis, *Psychiatric Research*, Vol. 21 (1987), pp. 303–7; J. H. Field, *Epidemiology of Head Injuries in England and Wales* (London: Her Majesty's Stationery Office, 1976); G. W. Brown and R. Prudo, Psychiatric disorder in a rural and an urban population, *Psychological Medicine*, Vol. 11 (1981), pp. 581–99.]

Frustrated by the failure to identify a distinct set of biochemical or pathological disturbances in the brains of schizophrenics, molecular geneticists have argued that the "fast track" to finding the cause of schizophrenia is to find the gene that creates the liability, because the gene must control the biochemical function that has gone astray. [M. Gill and C. Walsh, Molecular genetics and the major psychoses. In *Neurobiology and Psychiatry*, Vol. 2, ed. Robert Kerwin (London: Cambridge Medical Reviews, 1993), pp. 1–18.] As the twentieth century draws to a close, molecular genetics has replaced the autopsy as the biological foundation for the theory of diseases. The existence of a gene that causes a disease can be used to demonstrate that clinical diseases are indeed distinct entities that can be meaningfully described without regard to the context in which they appear or the individuals who are afflicted. Ironically, research into the molecular genetics of schizophrenia indicates that the genes associated with schizophrenia are different for different families, even though these families appear to have a strongly heritable form of the same disease. When a pair of research teams studied the DNA patterns in two families with high rates of schizophrenia among their members, they found that the genetic patterns associated with the disorder in each family group were clearly different. [R. Sherrington et al., Localization of a susceptibility locus for schizophrenia on chromosome 5, *Nature*, Vol. 10 (1988), pp. 164–67; J. L. Kennedy et al., Evidence against linkage of schizophrenia to markers on chromosome 5 in a northern Swedish pedigree, *Nature*, Vol. 10 (1988), pp. 167–70.]

5. Studies that examine the role of social stress in the aggravation of schizophrenic symptoms: I. R. H. Falloon et al., Family management in prevention of exacerbations of schizophrenia: a controlled study, *New England Journal of Medicine*, Vol. 306 (1982), pp. 1437–40; J. M. Kane and T. H. McGlashan, Treatment of schizophrenia, *Lancet*, Vol. 346 (1995), pp. 820–25.

6. W. K. Yamanka, G. W. Clemans, and M. L. Hutchinson, Essential fatty acid deficiency in humans, *Progress in Lipid Research*, Vol. 19 (1981), pp. 187–215.

7. K. K. Carroll and M. B. Davidson, The role of lipids in tumorigenesis, in *Molecular Interrelations of Nutrition and Cancer* (New York: Raven Press, 1982), pp. 237–45.

8. A. P. Simopoulos, Executive summary, *Dietary n3 and n6 Fatty Acids: Biological Effects and Nutritional Essentiality*, ed. C. Galli and A. P. Simopoulos (New York: Plenum Press, 1989); A. P. Simopoulos, n-3 fatty acids in growth and development and in health and disease; Part II. The role of n-3 fatty acids in health and disease: dietary implications, *Nutrition Today* (Mar.–Apr. 1988), pp. 10–18.

9. F. O. Obi and A. C. Nwanze, Fatty acid profiles in mental disease; Part 1. Linolenate variations in schizophrenia, *Journal of the Neurological Sciences*, Vol. 43 (1979), pp. 447–54.

10. D. O. Rudin, The major psychoses and neuroses as omega-3 essential fatty acid deficiency syndrome, *Biological Psychiatry*, Vol. 16 (1981), pp. 837–50.

11. R. M. McClain and J. M. Rohrs, Potentiation of the teratogenic effects and altered disposition of diphenylhydantoin by diet, *Toxicology and Applied Pharmacology*, Vol. 77 (1985), pp. 86–93; R. A. Karmali, Dietary n-3 and n-6 fatty acids in cancer, in *Dietary n3 and n6 Fatty Acids*, ed. Galli and Simopoulos, pp. 351–59.

12. J. J. F. Belch et al., Effects of altering dietary essential fatty acids on requirements for non-steroidal anti-inflammatory drugs in patients with rheumatoid arthritis: a double blind placebo controlled study, *Annals of the Rheumatic Diseases*, Vol. 47 (1988), pp. 96–104; P. C. Weber and A. Sellmayer, Modification of the eicosanoid system and cell signalling by precursor fatty acids, *Advances in Prostaglandin, Thromboxane and Leukotriene Research*, Vol. 21 (1990), pp. 217–24; W. F. Stenson et al., Dietary supplements with fish oil in ulcerative colitis, *Annals of Internal Medicine*, Vol. 116 (1992), pp. 609–14; J. P. Gapinski et al., Preventing restenosis with fish oils following coronary angioplasty, *Archives of Internal Medicine*, Vol. 153 (1993), pp. 1595–1601; J. J. Homan et al., Effect of dietary fish oil on renal function and rejection in cyclosporine-treated recipients of renal transplants, *New England Journal of Medicine*, Vol. 329 (1993), pp. 769–73; L. J. Appel et al., Does supplementation with "fish oil" reduce blood pressure? A meta-analysis of controlled clinical trials, *Archives of Internal Medicine*, Vol. 153 (1993), pp. 1429–38; R. Lawrence and T. Sorrell, Eicosapaentanoic acid in cystic fibrosis: evidence of a pathogenetic role for leukotriene B4, *Lancet*, Vol. 342 (1993), pp. 465–69; M. Anti et al., Effect of omega-3 fatty acids on rectal mucosal proliferation in subjects at risk for colon cancer, *Gastroenterology*, Vol. 103 (1992), pp. 883–91; T. McCaren et al., Amelioration of severe migraine by fish oil (n-3) fatty acids, *American Journal of Clinical Nutrition*, Vol. 41 (1985), p. 874.

13. D. F. Horrobin, *Prostaglandins: Physiology, Pharmacology & Clinical Significance* (Montreal: Eden Press, 1977); H. Rasmussen, *Calcium and cAMP as Synarchic Messengers* (New York: John Wiley & Sons, 1981).

14. An intriguing monograph on this subject was written by Julian Lieb, M.D., *A Medical Solution to the Health Care Crisis* (St. Louis: Warren H. Green, Inc., 1993).

15. Leo Galland, Increased requirement for essential fatty acids in atopic individuals, *Journal of the American College of Nutrition*, Vol. 5 (1986), pp. 213–28.

16. M. R. Griffin, W. A. Ray, and W. Schaffner, Nonsteroidal anti-inflammatory drug use and death from peptic ulcer in elderly persons, *Annals of Internal Medicine*, Vol. 109 (1988), pp. 359–63; I. Bjarnasson et al., NSAID induced intestinal inflammation in humans, *Gastroenterology*, Vol. 93 (1987), pp. 480–89; S. W. Shankel et al., Acute renal failure and glomerulopathy caused by nonsteroidal anti-inflammatory drugs, *Archives of Internal Medicine*, Vol. 152 (1992), pp. 986–90; J. E. Pope, J. J. Anderson, and D. T. Felson, A meta-analysis of the effects of non-steroidal anti-inflammatory drugs on blood pressure, *Archives of Internal Medicine*, Vol. 153 (1993), pp. 477–84; D. P. Meeker and H. P. Wiedemann, Drug-induced bronchospasm, *Clinical Chest Medicine*, Vol. 11 (1990), pp.

163–75; H. Katayama and A. Kawada, Exacerbation of psoriasis induced by indomethacin, *Journal of Dermatology*, Vol. 8 (1981), pp. 323–37; H. J. Kaufmann and H. L. Taubin, Nonsteroidal anti-inflammatory drugs activate quiescent inflammatory bowel disease, *Annals of Internal Medicine*, Vol. 107 (1987), pp. 513–16.

17. I. Nyman et al., Prevention of serious cardiac events by low-dose aspirin in patients with silent myocardial ischemia, *Lancet*, Vol. 340 (1992), pp. 497–501; M. J. Thun, M. M. Namboodiri, and C. W. Heath, Aspirin use and reduced risk of fatal colon cancer, *New England Journal of Medicine*, Vol. 325 (1991), pp. 1593–96; E. Schiff et al., The use of aspirin to prevent pregnancy-induced hypertension and lower the ratio of thromboxane A2 to prostacyclin in relatively high risk pregnancies, *New England Journal of Medicine*, Vol. 321 (1989), pp. 351–56; S. Uzan et al., Prevention of fetal growth retardation with low-dose aspirin: findings of the EPREDA trial, *Lancet*, Vol. 337 (1991), pp. 1427–31; J. E. Buring, R. Peto, and C. H. Hennekins, Low-dose aspirin for migraine prophylaxis, *Journal of the American Medical Association*, Vol. 264 (1990), pp. 1711–13; J. P. Kelly et al., Risk of aspirin-associated major upper-gastrointestinal bleeding with enteric-coated or buffered product, *Lancet*, Vol. 348 (1996), pp. 1413–16.

18. Recent research has found that D-cycloserine, an analogue of the amino acid serine, decreased negative symptoms in schizophrenics by an average of 21 percent. The researchers speculated that cycloserine may mimic its natural relative in restoring lines of communication between nerve cells. D. C. Goff et al., Dose-finding trial of D-cycloserine added to neuroleptics for negative symptoms in schizophrenia, *American Journal of Psychiatry*, Vol. 152 (1995), pp. 1213–15.

19. Robert Crayhon, *Robert Crayhon's Nutrition Made Simple* (New York: M. Evans and Company, 1994), p. 266.

20. A. J. Wittwer et al., Nutrient density—evaluation of nutritional attributes of foods, *Journal of Nutritional Education*, Vol. 9 (1977), pp. 26–30.

21. *Environmental Nutrition*, Vol. 18, no. 6 (June 1995), p. 5.

22. *Environmental Health Letter*, Oct. 16, 1992, p. 203.

23. Reported in *New York Times*, November 22, 1995, "Do I Dare to Eat a Strawberry?" p. C5.

24. D. S. Siscovik et al., Dietary intake and cell membrane levels of long-chain n-3 polyunsaturated fatty acids and the risk of primary cardiac arrest, *Journal of the American Medical Association*, Vol. 274 (1995), pp. 1363–67; D. Kromhout, Epidemiologic aspects of fish in the diet, *Proceedings of the Nutrition Society*, Vol. 52 (1993), pp. 437–39; D. Kromhout, E. B. Bosscheter, and C. de Lezenne Coulander, The inverse relation between fish consumption and 20-year mortality from coronary heart disease, *New England Journal of Medicine*, Vol. 312 (1985), pp. 1205–9; R. B. Shelelle et al., Fish consumption and mortality from coronary heart disease, *New England Journal of Medicine*, Vol. 313 (1985), p. 820; S. D. Kristensen et al., Fish oil and ischaemic heart disease, *British Heart Journal*, Vol. 70 (1993), pp. 212–15; J. E. Kinsella, B. Lokesh, and R. A. Stone, Dietary n-3 polyunsaturated fatty acids and amelioration of cardiovascular disease: possible mechanisms, *American Journal of Clinical Nutrition*, Vol. 52 (1990), pp. 1–28; S. O. Keli, E. J. M. Feskens, and D. Kromhout, Fish consumption and risk of stroke: the Zutphen Study, *Stroke*, Vol. 25 (1994), pp. 328–32; R. F. Gillum, M. E. Mussolino, and J. H. Madans, The relationship between fish consumption and stroke incidence: The

NHANES I Epidemiologic Follow-up Study, *Archives of Internal Medicine*, Vol. 156 (1996), pp. 537–42.

25. *Nutrition Action Healthletter*, Oct. 1988, pp. 5–7.

26. Leon Jaroff, "Is Your Fish Really Foul?" *Time*, June 29, 1992, pp. 70–71.

27. N. E. Skakkebaek and N. Keiding, Changes in semen and the testis, *British Medical Journal*, Vol. 309 (1994), pp. 1316–17; D. Forman and H. Moller, Testicular cancer, *Cancer Surveys*, Vols. 19–20 (1994), pp. 323–41; S. E. Rier et al., Endometriosis in Rhesus monkeys (*Macaca mullatta*) following chronic exposure to 2,3,7,8-tetrachlorodibenzo-p-dioxin, *Fundamental and Applied Toxicology*, Vol. 21 (1993), pp. 433–41.

28. B. Carlsen et al., Evidence for decreasing quality of semen during the past 50 years, *British Medical Journal*, Vol. 305 (1992), pp. 609–13; J. Auger et al., Decline in semen quality among fertile men in Paris during the past 20 years, *New England Journal of Medicine*, Vol. 332 (1995), pp. 281–85; D. S. Irvine, Falling sperm quality, *British Medical Journal*, Vol. 309 (1994), p. 476; Male reproductive health and environmental oestrogens (editorial), *Lancet*, Vol. 345 (1995), pp. 933–35.

29. G. R. N. Jones, Polychlorinated biphenyls: where do we stand now? *Lancet*, Vol. ii (1989), pp. 791–94; Janet Raloff, Dioxin: is everyone contaminated? *Science News*, Vol. 128 (July 13, 1985), pp. 26–29; Janet Raloff, Beyond estrogens: why unmasking hormone-mimicking pollutants proves so challenging, *Science News*, Vol. 148 (July 15, 1995), pp. 44–46; Cynthia Washam, Is the breast still best? E. *The Environmental Magazine*, Vol. 6 (Dec. 1995), pp. 46–47. Also see: *Intolerable Risk: Pesticides in Our Children's Food* (New York: Natural Resources Defense Council, 1989).

30. T. Inasmasu et al., Mercury concentration change in human hair after the ingestion of canned tuna fish, *Bulletin of Environmental Contamination and Toxicology*, Vol. 37 (1986), pp. 475–81.

31. Quoted in Janet Raloff, Mercurial risks from acid's reign: tainted fish may pose a serious human health hazard, *Science News*, Vol. 139 (1991), pp. 152–56.

32. "Is Our Fish Fit to Eat?" *Consumer Reports*, Feb. 1992, pp. 103–14. This report contains excellent tips on buying fresh fish and storing it safely.

33. I. Bou-Holaighi et al., The relationship between neurally mediated hypotension and the chronic fatigue syndrome, *Journal of the American Medical Association*, Vol. 274 (1995), pp. 961–67.

34. M. B. Katan, Exit *trans* fatty acids, *Lancet*, Vol. 346 (1995), pp. 1245–46. An editorial summary of recent evidence, occasioned by new regulations in Holland that will effectively limit the exposure of the population to partially hydrogenated vegetable oils.

35. Quoted by Marian Burros in *New York Times*, Nov. 15, 1995, in an article entitled "Additives in Advice on Food," p. C4, discussing the contributions made by the food industry to the American Dietetics Association.

36. H. S. Garewal and A. T. Diplock, How "safe" are antioxidant vitamins? *Drug Safety*, Vol. 13 (1995), pp. 8–14. High safety profile of vitamins A, C, E. Only problem is possible increase in efficacy of anticoagulant drugs with vitamin E, necessitating more careful monitoring in patients taking anticoagulants.

37. J. Booyens et al., Some effects of the essential fatty acids linoleic acid and alpha-linolenic acid and of their metabolites gamma-linolenic acid, arachidonic

acid, eicosapentaenoic acid, docosahexaenoic acid, and of prostaglandins A1 and E1 on the proliferation of human osteogenic sarcoma cells in culture, *Prostaglandins and Leukotrienes in Medicine*, Vol. 15 (1984), pp. 15–33; M. E. Begin et al., Differential killing of human carcinoma cells supplemented with n-3 and n-6 polyunsaturated fatty acids, *Journal of the National Cancer Institute*, Vol. 77 (1986), pp. 1053–62; N. Dippenaar et al., The reversibility of cancer: evidence that malignancy in melanoma cells is gamma-linolenic acid deficiency-dependent, *South African Medical Journal*, Vol. 62 (1982), pp. 505–9.

38. D. F. Horrobin, Gamma linolenic acid: an intermediate in essential fatty acid metabolism with potential as an ethical pharmaceutical and as a food, *Reviews in Contemporary Pharmacotherapy*, Vol. 1 (1990), pp. 1–45; L. Leventhal, E. G. Boyce, and R. B. Zurier, Treatment of rheumatoid arthritis with gammalinolenic acid, *Annals of Internal Medicine*, Vol. 119 (1993), pp. 867–73; J. Puolakka et al., Biochemical and clinical effects of treating the premenstrual syndrome with prostaglandin synthesis precursors, *Journal of Reproductive Medicine*, Vol. 30 (1985), pp. 149–53.

39. R. L. Swank and B. L. Dugan, Effect of low saturated fat diet in early and late cases of multiple sclerosis, *Lancet*, Vol. 336 (1990), pp. 37–39. Other researchers have shown favorable effects of EFA-rich oils on the course of MS: R. H. Dworkin et al., Linoleic acid and multiple sclerosis: a re-analysis of three double-blind trials, *Neurology*, Vol. 34 (1984), pp. 1441–45; D. Bates et al., A double-blind controlled trial of n-3 polyunsaturated fatty acids in the treatment of multiple sclerosis, *Journal of Neurology, Neurosurgery and Psychiatry*, Vol. 52 (1989), pp. 18–22.

40. W. A. Sibley et al., *Therapeutic Claims in Multiple Sclerosis*, Third Edition (New York: Demos Publications, 1992).

41. Patients with MS often have low levels of vitamin B_{12} in blood, which may aggravate their neurological symptoms. E. H. Reynolds et al., Vitamin B_{12} metabolism in multiple sclerosis, *Archives of Neurology*, Vol. 49 (1992), pp. 649–52.

42. M. Schechter, E. Kaplinsky, and B. Rabinowitz, The rationale for magnesium supplementation in acute myocardial infarction, *Archives of Internal Medicine*, Vol. 152 (1992), pp. 2189–96; B. M. Altura, Calcium antagonist properties of magnesium: implications for antimigraine actions, *Magnesium and Trace Elements*, Vol. 4 (1985), pp. 169–75.

43. L. Cohen and R. Kitzes, Characterization of the magnesium status of elderly people with congestive heart failure, hypertension and diabetes mellitus by the magnesium-load test, *Magnesium-Bulletin*, Vol. 15 (1993), pp. 105–9; H. F. Schimatschek and H. G. Classen, Epidemiologic studies on the frequency of hypomagnesemia and hypocalcemia in children with functional disorders and neurasthenia, *Magnesium-Bulletin*, Vol. 15 (1993), pp. 85–104; T. J. Romano and J. W. Stiller, Magnesium deficiency in fibromyalgia syndrome, *Journal of Nutritional Medicine*, Vol. 4 (1994), pp. 165–67; V. Gallai et al., Magnesium content of mononuclear blood cells in migraine patients, *Headache*, Vol. 34 (1994), pp. 160–65; J. Britton et al., Dietary magnesium, lung function, wheezing, and airway hyperresponsiveness in a random adult population sample, *Lancet*, Vol. 344 (1994), pp. 357–62; J. C. M. Witteman et al., Reduction of blood pressure with oral magnesium supplementation in women with mild to moderate hypertension, *American Journal of Clinical Nutrition*, Vol. 60 (1994), pp. 129–35; V. Holm, Further studies of the concentration of magnesium ion (Mg++) in blood from pa-

tients with autoimmune diseases, *Danish Medical Bulletin*, Vol. 30 (1983), pp. 180–84; P. McNair et al., Hypomagnesemia, a risk factor in diabetic retinopathy, *Diabetes*, Vol. 27 (1978), pp. 1075–77; R. B. Singh et al., Effect of dietary minerals on incidence of sudden cardiac death, *Trace Elements in Medicine*, Vol. 7 (1990), pp. 19–24; G. E. Burch and T. D. Giles, The importance of magnesium in cardiovascular disease, *American Heart Journal*, Vol. 94 (1977), pp. 649–57; L. M. Resniock et al., Divalent cations in essential hypertension: relations between serum ionized calcium, magnesium and plasma renin activity, *New England Journal of Medicine*, Vol. 309 (1983), pp. 888–91; K. Koto et al., Magnesium deficiency detected by intravenous loading test in variant angine pectoris, *American Journal of Cardiology*, Vol. 65 (1990), pp. 709–12; K. S. Kubena, The role of magnesium in immunity, *Journal of Nutritional Immunology*, Vol. 2 (1993), pp. 107–26.

44. K. J. Morgan et al., Magnesium and calcium dietary intakes of the U.S. population, *Journal of the American College of Nutrition*, Vol. 4 (1985), pp. 195–206; I. J. Lichton, Dietary intake levels and requirements for Mg and Ca for different segments of the U.S. population, *Magnesium and Trace Minerals*, Vol. 8 (1989), pp. 117–23.

45. K. L. Woods et al., Intravenous magnesium sulphate in suspected acute myocardial infarction: results of the second Leicester Intravenous Magnesium Intervention Trial (LIMIT-2), *Lancet*, Vol. 339 (1992), pp. 1553–58; E. M. Skobeloff et al., Intravenous magnesium sulfate for the treatment of acute asthma in the emergency department, *Journal of the American Medical Association*, Vol. 262 (1989), pp. 1210–13; H. Okayama et al., Treatment of status asthmaticus with intravenous magnesium sulphate, *Journal of Asthma*, Vol. 28 (1991), pp. 11–17.

46. Leo Galland, Magnesium, stress and neuropsychiatric disorders, *Magnesium and Trace Elements*, Vol. 10 (1991), pp. 287–301.

47. A. Gaby and J. Wright, Nutrients and osteoporosis, *Journal of Nutritional Medicine*, Vol. 1 (1990), pp. 63–72.

48. J. F. Fries et al., Running and the development of disability with age, *Annals of Internal Medicine*, Vol. 121 (1994), pp. 502–9 (mortality much lower in runners); J. K. McNeil, E. M. LeBlanc, and M. Joyner, The effect of exercise on depressive symptoms in the moderately depressed elderly, *Psychology and Aging*, Vol. 6 (1991), pp. 487–88; D.-M. C. Lockett and J. F. Campbell, The effects of aerobic exercise on migraine, *Headache*, Vol. 32 (1992), pp. 152–56; L. Nelson et al., Effect of changing levels of physical activity on blood-pressure and haemodynamics in essential hypertension, *Lancet*, Vol. ii (1986), pp. 473–76; I.-M. Lee, C. Hsieh, and R. S. Paffenbarger, Exercise intensity and longevity in men: the Harvard alumni health study, *Journal of the American Medical Association*, Vol. 273 (1995), pp. 1179–84 (vigorous activity increases longevity); M. Pahor et al., Physical activity and risk of severe gastrointestinal hemorrhage in older persons, *Journal of the American Medical Association*, Vol. 272 (1994), pp. 595–99 (less risk of hemorrhage in those with regular physical activity).

49. L. Sandvik et al., Physical fitness as a predictor of mortality among healthy, middle-aged Norwegian men, *New England Journal of Medicine*, Vol. 328 (1993), pp. 533–37.

50. R. R. Pate et al., Physical activity and public health, *Journal of the American Medical Association*, Vol. 273 (1995), pp. 402–6.

51. R. S. Paffenberger et al., The association of changes in physical-activity level and other lifestyle characteristics with mortality among men, *New England Journal of Medicine*, Vol. 328 (1993), pp. 538–45.

52. J. A. McCubbin et al., Aerobic fitness and opioidergic inhibition of cardio-vascular stress reactivity, *Psychophysiology*, Vol. 29 (1992), pp. 687–97.

53. R. N. Lemaitre et al., Leisure-time physical activity and the risk of non-fatal myocardial infarction in post-menopausal women, *Archives of Internal Medicine*, Vol. 155 (1995), pp. 2302–8.

54. Y. Schoenfeld et al., Walking: a method for rapid improvement of physical fitness, *Journal of the American Medical Association*, Vol. 243 (1980) pp. 2062–63.

55. J. M. Krueger et al., Sleep, microbes and cytokines, *Neuroimmunomodula-tion*, Vol. 1 (1994), pp. 100–109.

56. "Fail to snooze, immune cells lose." Reported in *Science News*, Jan. 7, 1995, p. 11.

57. R. Hyman et al., The effects of relaxation training on clinical symptoms: a meta-analysis, *Nursing Research*, Vol. 38 (1989), pp. 216–20.

58. G. S. Everly and H. Benson, Disorders of arousal and the relaxation response: speculations on the nature and treatment of stress-related disorders, *International Journal of Psychosomatics*, Vol. 36 (1989), pp. 15–21.

59. J. W. Hoffman et al., Reduced sympathetic nervous system responsivity associated with the relaxation response, *Science*, Vol. 215 (1982), pp. 190–92.

60. M. R. Ford et al., Quieting response training: long-term evaluation of a clinical biofeedback practice, *Biofeedback and Self-Regulation*, Vol. 8 (1983), pp. 265–78.

Chapter 7: The Third Pillar: Your Environment

1. This case was published in the *Journal of the American Medical Association*, Vol. 235 (1976), pp. 398–401, by R. D. Stewart and C. L. Hake from the department of environmental medicine at the Medical College of Wisconsin, under the title "Paint-remover hazard."

2. M. A. Carome and J. Moore, Nephrotic syndrome in adults: a diagnostic and management challenge, *Postgraduate Medicine*, Vol. 92 (1992), pp. 209–20.

3. This issue has been most explored by investigations of the incongruities between the degree of distress or symptom severity reported by patients and the ability of physicians to find "objective" corollaries. A. Kleinman and L. Eisenberg, Culture, illness, and care: clinical lessons learned from anthropology and cross cultural research, *Annals of Internal Medicine*, Vol. 88 (1978), pp. 251–57; I. K. Zola, Culture and symptoms: an analysis of patients' presenting complaints, *American Sociological Review*, Vol. 31 (1966), pp. 615–30; H. K. Beecher, Relationship of the significance of wound to the pain experienced, *Journal of the American Medical Association*, Vol. 161 (1956), pp. 1609–13; J. Stoeckle, I. K. Zola, and G. Davidson, The quantity and significance of psychological distress in medical patients, *Journal of Chronic Diseases*, Vol. 17 (1964), pp. 959–70.

4. M. Chan-Yeung, Occupational asthma, *Chest*, Vol. 88 (1990), pp. 148S–161S.

5. After identifying a high frequency of kidney diseases among dry cleaners, a European team concluded, ". . . solvent-exposed subjects . . . need to be monitored

for the possible development of chronic renal [kidney] diseases." A. Mutti et al., Nephropathies and exposure to perchloroethylene in dry-cleaners, *Lancet*, Vol. 340 (1992), pp. 189–93. Exposure to formaldehyde, a component of many adhesives, can cause kidney damage and nephrotic syndrome. P. Breysse et al., Membranous nephropathy and formaldehyde exposure, *Annals of Internal Medicine*, Vol. 120 (1994), pp. 396–97. Also see J. G. Abuolo, Renal failure caused by chemicals, foods, plants, animal venoms and misuse of drugs, *Archives of Internal Medicine*, Vol. 150 (1990), pp. 505–9.

6. D. H. Sandberg et al., Severe steroid-responsive nephrosis associated with hypersensitivity, *Lancet*, Vol. 309 (1977), pp. 388–91; H. Howanietz and G. Lubec, Idiopathic nephrotic syndrome, treated with steroids for five years, found to be allergic reaction to pork, *Lancet*, Vol. 326 (1985), p. 450; R. Genova et al., Food allergy in steroid-resistant nephrotic syndrome, *Lancet*, Vol. 330 (1987), pp. 1315–16.

Also see: G. Lagrue and J. Laurent, Is lipod nephrosis an "allergic" disease? *Transplantation Proceedings*, Vol. 14 (1982), pp. 485–88; G. Lagrue et al., Basophile sensitization for food allergens in idiopathic nephrotic syndrome, *Nephron*, Vol. 42 (1986), pp. 123–27; J. Laurent et al., Is adult idiopathic nephrotic syndrome food allergy? Value of oligoantigenic diets, *Nephron*, Vol. 47 (1987), pp. 7–11.

7. This is a hypoallergenic food, produced from nutritionally supplemented white rice powder, designed by Jeffrey Bland, Ph.D., of HealthComm, Inc., Gig Harbor, Washington, distributed by Metagenics, Inc., San Clemente, California.

8. D. A. Schwartz et al., The occupational history in the primary care setting, *American Journal of Medicine*, Vol. 90 (1991), pp. 315–27.

9. P. J. Landrigan, Commentary: Environmental disease—a preventable epidemic, *American Journal of Public Health*, Vol. 82 (1992), pp. 941–43.

10. *Indoor Air Pollutants: Exposure and Health Effects* (Copenhagen: World Health Organization, 1983).

11. W. M. Alberts, Building-related illness: what it is, what you can do, *Journal of Respiratory Diseases*, Vol. 15 (1994), pp. 899–912.

12. E. F. Banaszak, W. H. Thiede, and J. N. Fink, Hypersensitivity pneumonitis due to contamination of an air conditioner, *New England Journal of Medicine*, Vol. 283 (1970), pp. 271–76; J. M. Samet, M. C. Marbury, and J. D. Spengler, Health effects and sources of indoor air pollution, *American Review of Respiratory Diseases*, Vol. 137 (1988), pp. 221–42.

13. S. Burge et al., Sick building syndrome: a study of 4373 office workers, *Annals of Occupational Hygiene*, Vol. 31 (1987), pp. 493–504; P. Skov, O. Valbjorn, and Danish Indoor Climate Study Group, The "sick" building syndrome in the office environment: the Danish Town Hall study, *Environment International*, Vol. 13 (1987), pp. 339–49; D. Norback, I. Michel, and J. Widstrom, Indoor air quality and personal factors related to sick building syndrome, *Scandinavian Journal of Work and Environmental Health*, Vol. 16 (1990), pp. 121–28; J. E. Woods, Cost avoidance and productivity in owning and operating buildings, *Occupational Medicine*, Vol. 4 (1989), pp. 753–70; H. I. Hall et al., Influence of building-related symptoms on self-reported productivity, in *Healthy Buildings* (Atlanta: American Society of Heating, Refrigeration, and Air-Conditioning Engineers, 1991), pp. 33–35; L. Preller et al., Sick leave due to work-related health complaints among office workers in the Netherlands, in D. J. Walkinshaw, ed., *Proceedings of the Fifth In-*

ternational Conference on Air Quality and Climate, Vol. 1 (Toronto: Canadian Mortgage and Housing, July 29–Aug. 1, 1990), pp. 227–30.

14. R. Menzies et al., The effect of varying levels of outdoor-air supply on the symptoms of sick building syndrome, *New England Journal of Medicine*, Vol. 328 (1993), pp. 821–27.

15. M. J. Hodgson, Buildings & health, *Health & Environment Digest*, Vol. 7 (1993), pp. 1–3; D. Norback, M. Torgen, and C. Edling, Volatile organic compounds, respiratory dust and personal factors related to the prevalence and incidence of SBS in primary schools, *British Journal of Industrial Medicine*, Vol. 47 (1990), pp. 733–41; M. J. Hodgson et al., Symptoms and microenvironmental measures in non-problem buildings, *Journal of Occupational Medicine*, Vol. 35 (1991), pp. 527–33; M. Hodgson, Field studies on the sick building syndrome, in *Sources of Indoor Air Contaminants: Characterizing Emissions and Health Impacts*, W. G. Tucker et al., eds., *Annals of the New York Academy of Sciences*, Vol. 641 (1992), pp. 21–36.

16. M. J. Mendell and A. H. Smith, Consistent pattern of elevated symptoms in air-conditioned office buildings: a reanalysis of epidemiologic studies, *American Journal of Public Health*, Vol. 80 (1990), pp. 1193–99.

17. *Occupational Health and Safety*, Jan. 1996, pp. 13–14. Reported in *ACTS Facts*, the monthly newsletter of Arts, Crafts and Theater Safety, 181 Thompson Street, New York, NY 10012-2586, March 1996.

18. R. C. Anderson, Toxic emissions from carpets, *Journal of Nutritional & Environmental Medicine*, Vol. 5 (1995), pp. 375–86.

19. K. R. Smith, Total exposure assessment: Part 1. Implications for the United States, *Environment*, Vol. 30 (1988), pp. 10–15, 33–38; K. R. Smith, Looking for pollution where the people are, *Asia Pacific Issues*, East-West Center, Honolulu, Jan. 10, 1994, pp. 1–8.

20. S. D. Platt et al., Damp housing, mould growth and symptomatic health state, *British Medical Journal*, Vol. 198 (1989), pp. 1673–78.

21. T. A. E. Platts-Mills et al., Reduction of bronchial hyperreactivity during prolonged allergen avoidance, *Lancet*, Vol. 320 (1982), pp. 675–78; R. Sporik et al., Exposure to house-dust mite allergen (*Der p* I) and the development of asthma in childhood: a prospective study, *New England Journal of Medicine*, Vol. 323 (1990), pp. 502–7.

22. A. P. Verhoeff et al., Damp housing and childhood respiratory symptoms: the role of sensitization to dust mites and molds, *American Journal of Epidemiology*, Vol. 141 (1995), pp. 103–10.

23. W. A. Croft, B. B. Jarvis, and C. S. Yatawara, Airborne outbreak of trichothecene toxicosis, *Atmosphere and Environment*, Vol. 20 (1986), pp. 549–52.

24. B. B. Wray and K. G. O'Steen, Mycotoxin-producing fungi from house associated with leukemia, *Archives of Environmental Health*, Vol. 30 (1975), pp. 571–73; J. Aleksandrowicz and B. Smyk, The association of neoplastic diseases and mycotoxins in the environment, *Texas Reports of Biological Medicine*, Vol. 31 (1973), pp. 715–26.

25. "Molds: The Fungus Among Us," *Nutrition Action Healthletter*, Center for Science in the Public Interest, Washington, DC, Nov. 1991, pp. 5–7.

26. C. G. Rousseaux, The hazards of fungi to man, *Clinical Ecology*, Vol. 6 (1990), pp. 11–15; J. L. Richard, Experimental evidence for mycotoxin-induced immunomodulation, *Environmental Medicine*, Vol. 9 (1986), pp. 94–112.

27. R. K. Ross et al., Urinary aflatoxin biomarkers and risk of hepatocellular carcinoma, *Lancet,* Vol. 339 (1992), pp. 943–46.

28. *Nutrition Action Healthletter,* Center for Science in the Public Interest, Nov. 1991, pp. 5–7.

29. W. O. Caster et al., Dietary aflatoxins, intelligence and school performance in Southern Georgia, *International Journal of Vitamin and Nutrition Research,* Vol. 56 (1986), pp. 291–95; B. Jarvis, The occurrence of mycotoxins in UK foods, *Food Technology in Australia,* Vol. 34 (1982), pp. 508–14.

30. M. Lappé, *Breakout: The Evolving Threat of Drug-Resistant Disease* (San Francisco: Sierra Club Books, 1995), chapter 11, "Evolution and Asthma," pp. 193–208.

31. M. L. Burr, ed., *Epidemiology of Clinical Allergy,* (Basel: Karger, 1993).

32. M. Profet, The function of allergy: immunological defense against toxins, *Quarterly Review of Biology,* Vol. 66 (1991), pp. 23–51.

33. H. S. Kaufman and J. R. Hobbs, Immunologic deficiencies in an atopic population, *Lancet,* Vol. ii (1970), pp. 1061–63; C. R. Stokes, B. Taylor, and M. W. Turner, Association of house-dust and grass-pollen allergies with specific IgA antibody deficiency, *Lancet,* Vol. ii (1974), pp. 485–88; A. G. Siccardi et al., Defective bactericidal reaction by the alternative pathway of complement in atopic patients, *Infection and Immunity,* Vol. 33 (1981), pp. 710–13; O. Strannegard and I.-L. Strannegard, T lymphocyte abnormalities in atopic disease, *Immunology and Allergy Practice,* Vol. 5 (1983), pp. 382–88.

34. Leo Galland, Increased requirements for essential fatty acids in atopic individuals, *Journal of the American College of Nutrition,* Vol. 5 (1986), pp. 213–28; R. E. Rocklin et al., Altered arachidonic acid content in polymorphonuclear and mononuclear cells from patients with allergic rhinitis and/or asthma, *Lipids,* Vol. 21 (1986), pp. 17–20; I.-L. Strannegard and O. Strannegard, Stimulatory and inhibitory effects of cyclic AMP on lymphocytes from atopic children, *International Archives of Allergy and Applied Immunology,* Vol. 58 (1979), pp. 167–74.

35. K. A. Fackelman, Do antihistamines spur cancer growth? *Science News,* Vol. 25 (May 21, 1994), p. 145.

36. For a long time, asthma was divided into two different diseases: "extrinsic" asthma, which was caused by environmental allergy, and "intrinsic" asthma, which was not. Over the past several years it has become clear that most asthma in adults as well as children has an allergic basis, and that the distinction between "intrinsic" and "extrinsic" varieties is spurious. B. Burrows et al., Association of asthma with serum IgE levels and skin-test reactivity to allergens, *New England Journal of Medicine,* Vol. 329 (1989), pp. 271–77; J. N. Kalliel et al., High frequency of atopic asthma in a pulmonary clinic population, *Chest,* Vol. 96 (1989), pp. 1336–40.

37. J. W. Yuninger et al., A community-based study of the epidemiology of asthma: incidence rates, 1964–1983, *American Review of Respiratory Diseases,* Vol. 146 (1992), pp. 888–94; R. Evans et al., National trends in the morbidity and mortality of asthma in the US: prevalence, hospitalization and death from asthma over two decades: 1965–1984, *Chest,* Vol. 91 (1987), pp. 65S–74S; K. B. Weiss and D. K. Wagener, Changing patterns of asthma mortality: identifying target populations at high risk, *Journal of the American Medical Association,* Vol. 264 (1990), pp. 1683–92.

38. E. R. McFadden and I. A. Gilbert, Asthma, *New England Journal of Medicine*, Vol. 327 (1992), pp. 1928–37.

39. G. J. Blauw and R. G. J. Westendorp, Asthma deaths in New Zealand: whodunnit? *Lancet*, Vol. 345 (1995), pp. 2–3.

40. E. A. Mitchell, Is current treatment increasing asthma morbidity and mortality? *Thorax*, Vol. 44 (1989), pp. 81–84; M. R. Sears et al., Regular inhaled beta-agonist treatment in bronchial asthma, *Lancet*, Vol. 336 (1990), pp. 1391–96; C. P. Van Schayck et al., Bronchodilator treatment in moderate asthma or chronic bronchitis: continuous or on demand? *British Medical Journal*, Vol. 303 (1991), pp. 1426–31; E. Dompeling et al., Slowing the deterioration of asthma and chronic obstructive pulmonary disease observed during bronchodilator therapy by adding inhaled cortico-steroids: a 4-year prospective study, *Annals of Internal Medicine*, Vol. 118 (1993), pp. 770–78.

41. W. O. Spitzer et al., The use of B-agonists and the risk of death and near death from asthma, *New England Journal of Medicine*, Vol. 326 (1992), pp. 501–6; E. D. Robin, Death from bronchial asthma, *Chest*, Vol. 93 (1988), pp. 614–18.

42. D. G. Kern and H. Frumkin, Asthma in respiratory therapists, *Annals of Internal Medicine*, Vol. 110 (1989), pp. 767–73.

43. Inhaled cortisone preparations, which are the present fad in asthma therapy, are absorbed into the body and, with long-term use, may produce the same undesirable side effects as oral cortisone, especially in children. I. J. M. Doull, N. J. Freezer, and S. T. Holgate, Growth of asthmatic children on inhaled corticosteroids, *American Review of Respiratory Disease*, Vol. 147 (1993), p. A265; O. D. Wolthers and S. Pedersen, Growth of asthmatic children during treatment with budesonide: a double blind trial, *British Medical Journal*, Vol. 303 (1991), pp. 163–65; M. Ip et al., Decreased bone mineral density in premenopausal asthma patients receiving long-term inhaled steroids, *Chest*, Vol. 105 (1994), pp. 1722–27; W. H. Nicolaizik et al., Endocrine and lung function in asthmatic children on inhaled corticosteroids, *American Journal of Respiratory and Critical Care Medicine*, Vol. 150 (1994), pp. 624–28; S. Capwell et al., Purpura and dermal thinning associated with high dose inhaled corticosteroids, *British Medical Journal*, Vol. 300 (1990), pp. 1548–51.

44. L. Nilsson and B. Bjorksten, Factors which promote or prevent allergy, *Monographs in Allergy*, Vol. 31 (1993), pp. 190–210.

45. N. A. Molfino et al., Effect of low concentrations of ozone on inhaled allergen responses in asthmatic subjects, *Lancet*, Vol. 338 (1991), pp. 199–203; J. L. Devalia et al., Effect of nitrogen dioxide and sulphur dioxide on airway response of mild asthmatic patients to allergen inhalation, *Lancet*, Vol. 344 (1994), pp. 1668–71; B. D. Ostro et al., Indoor air pollution and asthma: results from a panel study, *American Journal of Respiratory and Critical Care Medicine*, Vol. 149 (1994), pp. 1400–1406; A. Newman-Taylor, Environmental determinants of asthma, *Lancet*, Vol. 345 (1995), pp. 296–99; J. M. Samet, The impact of indoor air pollution on allergic and respiratory diseases, *Masters in Allergy*, Vol. 2 (1991), pp. 17–21.

46. C. A. Herbert et al., Effect of mite antigen on permeability of bronchial mucosa, *Lancet*, Vol. ii (1990), p. 1132.

47. L. S. Greene, Asthma and oxidant stress: nutritional, environmental and genetic risk factors, *Journal of the American College of Nutrition*, Vol. 14 (1995), pp. 317–24.

48. P. Burney, A diet rich in sodium may potentiate asthma, *Chest*, Vol. 91 (1987), pp. 143S–147S.

49. J. Schwartz and S. Weiss, Dietary factors and their relationship to respiratory symptoms: the Second National Health and Nutrition Examination Survey, *American Journal of Epidemiology*, Vol. 132 (1990), pp. 67–76.

50. J. Stone et al., Reduced selenium status of patients with asthma, *Clinical Science*, Vol. 77 (1989), pp. 495–500; D. Pearson et al., Selenium status in relation to reduced glutathione peroxidase activity in aspirin-sensitive asthma, *Clinical and Experimental Allergy*, Vol. 21 (1991), pp. 203–8; A. Flatt et al., Reduced selenium in asthmatic subjects in New Zealand, *Thorax*, Vol. 45 (1990), pp. 95–99; L. Hasselmark et al., Lowered platelet glutathione peroxidase activity in patients with intrinsic asthma, *Allergy*, Vol. 45 (1990), pp. 523–27.

51. L. Hasselmark et al., Selenium supplementation in intrinsic asthma, *Allergy*, Vol. 48 (1993), pp. 30–36.

52. D. T. Janerich et al., Lung cancer and exposure to tobacco smoke in the household, *New England Journal of Medicine*, Vol. 323 (1990), pp. 632–36. Seventeen percent of lung cancers were attributed to secondhand smoke.

53. Home carpets: shoeing in toxic pollution, *Science News*, Vol. 138 (1990), p. 86; J. W. Roberts and D. E. Camann, Pilot study of a cotton glove press test for assessing exposure to pesticides in house dust, *Bulletin of Environmental Contamination and Toxicology*, Vol. 43 (1989), pp. 717–24.

54. H. A. Burge et al., Prevalence of microorganisms in domestic humidifiers, *Applied Environmental Microbiology*, Vol. 39 (1980), pp. 840–44.

55. T. Godish, *Indoor Air Pollution Control* (Chelsea, Mich.: Lewis Publishers, 1989), pp. 41–42; T. L. Vaughan et al., Formaldehyde and cancers of the pharynx, sinus and nasal cavity: residential exposure, *International Journal of Cancer*, Vol. 38 (1986), pp. 685–88.

56. Godish, op. cit., pp. 123–27.

57. C. J. Wechsler, Indoor-outdoor relationships for non-polar organic constituents of aerosol particles, *Environmental Science and Technology*, Vol. 18 (1984), pp. 648–52.

58. R. D. Morris et al., Chlorination, chlorination by-products, and cancer: a meta-analysis, *American Journal of Public Health*, Vol. 82 (1992), pp. 955–63; K. P. Cantor et al., Bladder cancer, drinking water source, and tap-water consumption: a case-controlled study, *Journal of the National Cancer Institute*, Vol. 79 (1987), pp. 1269–79; J. E. Vena et al., Drinking water, fluid intake, and bladder cancer in western New York, *Archives of Environmental Health*, Vol. 48 (1993), pp. 191–98. Experimental data on THMs as carcinogens: J. K. Dunnick and R. L. Melnick, Assessment of the carcinogenic potential of chlorinated water: experimental studies of chlorine, chloramine, and trihalomethanes, *Journal of the National Cancer Institute*, Vol. 85 (1993), pp. 817–22.

59. J. B. Andelman, Human exposures to volatile halogenated organic chemicals in indoor and outdoor air, *Environmental Health Perspectives*, Vol. 62 (1985), pp. 313–18.

60. K. Tennakone and S. Wickramanayake, Aluminum leaching from cooking utensils, *Nature*, Vol. 325 (1987), pp. 270–72.

61. J. M. H. Howard, Clinical import of small increases in serum aluminum, *Clinical Chemistry*, Vol. 30 (1984), pp. 1722–23.

62. C. N. Martyn et al., Geographical relationship between Alzheimer's disease and aluminum in drinking water, *Lancet*, Vol. i (1989), pp. 59–62.

63. American Academy of Pediatrics, "Lead Poisoning: Next Focus of Environmental Action," statement issued Jan. 1991.

64. S. Davies, Lead and disease, *Nutrition and Health*, Vol. 2 (1983), pp. 135–45 (a comprehensive review); H. L. Needleman et al., The long-term effects of exposure to low doses of lead in childhood: an 11-year follow-up report, *New England Journal of Medicine*, Vol. 322 (1990), pp. 83–88; H. Hu et al., The relationship between bone lead and hemoglobin, *Journal of the American Medical Association*, Vol. 272 (1994), pp. 1512–17; J. A. Staeessen et al., Impairment of renal function with increasing blood lead concentrations in the general population, *New England Journal of Medicine*, Vol. 327 (1992), pp. 151–56; H. G. Preuss, A review of persistent, low-grade lead challenge: neurological and cardiovascular consequences, *Journal of the American College of Nutrition*, Vol. 12 (1993), pp. 246–54.

65. E. Charney et al., Childhood lead poisoning: a controlled trial of the effect of dust-control measures on blood lead levels, *New England Journal of Medicine*, Vol. 309 (1983), pp. 1089–93.

66. Lead-contaminated drinking water in bulk-storage water tanks—Arizona and California, 1993, *Morbidity and Mortality Weekly Reports*, Vol. 43 (Oct. 24, 1994), pp. 751, 757–58.

67. M. N. Meah et al., Lead and tin in canned food: results of the UK Survey 1983–1987, *Food Additives & Contaminants*, Vol. 8 (1991), pp. 485–96; D. S. Forsyth, R. W. Dabeka, and C. Cleroux, Organic and total lead in selected fresh and canned seafood products, *Food Additives & Contaminants*, Vol. 8 (1991), pp. 477–84.

Chapter 8: The Fourth Pillar: Detoxification

1. L. Galland and S. Barrie, Intestinal dysbiosis and the causes of disease, *Journal of Advancement in Medicine*, Vol. 6 (1993), pp. 67–82.

2. U. Pirzer et al., Reactivity of infiltrating T lymphocytes with microbial antigens in Crohn's disease, *Lancet*, Vol. 338 (1991), pp. 1238–40.

3. A. Fox, Role of bacterial debris in inflammatory diseases of the joint and eye, *APMIS*, Vol. 98 (1990), pp. 957–68; J. A. Mills, Do bacteria cause chronic arthritis? *New England Journal of Medicine*, Vol. 320 (1989), pp. 245–46.

4. J. O. W. Brabinder and F. Blank, Intestinal moniliasis in adults, *Canadian Medical Association Journal*, Vol. 77 (1957), pp. 478–83; J. G. Kane, J. H. Chretien, and V. F. Garagusi, Diarrhoea caused by Candida, *Lancet*, Vol. i (1976), pp. 335–36; S. A. Alam, M. Tahir, and M. N. De, Candida as a cause of diarrhea in children, *Bangladesh Medical Research Council Bulletin*, Vol. 3 (1977), pp. 32–36; P. L. Danna et al., Role of candida in pathogenesis of antibiotic-associated diarrhoea in elderly inpatients, *Lancet*, Vol. 337 (1991), pp. 511–14.

5. I reviewed and analyzed the world literature on *Candida* allergy in "The Effects of Intestinal Microbes on Systemic Immunity," in *Post-Viral Fatigue Syndrome*, ed. R. Jenkins and P. Mowbray (Chichester: John Wiley & Sons, 1991), pp. 405–30.

6. P. G. Miotti et al., Age-related rate of seropositivity of antibody to *Giardia lamblia* in four diverse populations, *Journal of Clinical Microbiology*, Vol. 24 (1986), pp. 972–75.

7. C. L. Chappell and C. C. Matson, *Giardia* antigen detection in patients with chronic gastrointestinal disturbances, *Journal of Family Practice*, Vol. 35 (1992), pp. 49–53.

8. P. H. Levine et al., Clinical, epidemiologic, and virologic studies in four clusters of the chronic fatigue syndrome, *Archives of Internal Medicine*, Vol. 152 (1992), pp. 1611–16.

9. Leo Galland et al., Giardia lamblia infection as a cause of chronic fatigue, *Journal of Nutritional Medicine*, Vol. 1 (1990), pp. 27–32.

10. P. S. Millard et al., An outbreak of cryptosporidiosis from fresh-pressed apple cider, *Journal of the American Medical Association*, Vol. 272 (1994), pp. 1592–96; J. M. McAnulty, D. W. Fleming, and A. H. Gonzalez, A community-wide outbreak of cryptosporidiosis associated with swimming at a wave pool, *Journal of the American Medical Association*, Vol. 272 (1994), pp. 1597–1600.

11. *In the Drink* (Washington, D.C.: Environmental Working Group, 1995). This report may be ordered from Environmental Working Group (a nonprofit research organization), 1718 Connecticut Avenue N.W., Suite 600, Washington, DC 20009, (202) 667-6982.

12. A. Schepers, Study warns: don't take safe water for granted, *Environmental Nutrition*, Vol. 16 (1993), p. 2. Contact the National Resources Defense Council, 40 West 20th Street, New York, NY 10011, for a full copy of their report, *Think Before You Drink* (cost: $8.95).

13. S. T. Goldstein et al., Cryptosporidiosis: an outbreak associated with drinking water despite state-of-the-art water treatment, *Annals of Internal Medicine*, Vol. 124 (1996), pp. 459–68.

14. E. A. Deitch, The role of intestinal barrier failure and bacterial translocation in the development of systemic infection and multiple organ failure, *Archives of Surgery*, Vol. 125 (1990), pp. 403–4; M. P. Hazenberg et al., Are intestinal bacteria involved in the etiology of rheumatoid arthritis? Review article, *APMIS*, Vol. 100 (1992), pp. 1–9; T. J. Peters and I. Bjarnason, Uses and abuses of intestinal permeability measurements, *Canadian Journal of Gastroenterology*, Vol. 2 (1988), pp. 127–32; P. J. Rooney, R. T. Jenkins, and W. W. Buchanan, A short review of the relationship between intestinal permeability and inflammatory joint disease, *Clinical and Experimental Rheumatology*, Vol. 8 (1990), pp. 75–83; W. A. Walker, Antigen absorption from the small intestine and gastrointestinal disease, *Pediatric Clinics of North America*, Vol. 22 (1975), pp. 731–46; P. Bloembergen et al., Endotoxin-induced auto-immunity in mice; I. Time and dose dependence of production and serum levels of antibodies against bromelain-treated mouse erythrocytes and circulating immune complexes, *International Archives of Allergy and Applied Immunology*, Vol. 84 (1987), pp. 291–97; P. Bloembergen et al., Endotoxin-induced auto-immunity in mice; II. Reactivity of LPS-hyporesponsive and C5-deficient animals, *International Archives of Allergy and Applied Immunology*, Vol. 86 (1988), pp. 370–74; P. Bloembergen et al., Endotoxin-induced auto-immunity in mice; III. Comparison of different endotoxin preparations, *International Archives of Allergy and Applied Immunology*, Vol. 92 (1990), pp. 124–30.

15. D. C. Whitcomb and G. D. Block, Association of acetaminophen hepato-toxicity with fasting and ethanol use, *Journal of the American Medical Association*, Vol. 272 (1994), pp. 1845–50. Describes the depletion of antioxidants that accompanies increased detoxification activity and its harmful effects on the liver.

16. K. E. Anderson, Dietary regulation of cytochrome P450, *Annual Review of Nutrition*, Vol. 11 (1991), pp. 141–67; A. J. Paine, Excited states of oxygen in biology: their possible involvement in cytochrome P450 linked oxidations as well as in the induction of the P450 system by many diverse compounds, *Biochemical Pharmacology*, Vol. 27 (1978), pp. 1805–13.

17. J. M. Braganza et al., Lipid-peroxidation (free-radical-oxidation) products in bile from patients with pancreatic disease, *Lancet*, Vol. ii (1983), pp. 375–78; J. M. Braganza, Pancreatic disease: a casualty of hepatic "detoxification"? *Lancet*, Vol. ii (1983), pp. 1000–1002.

18. K. D. Katz et al., Intestinal permeability in patients with Crohn's disease and their healthy relatives, *Gastroenterology*, Vol. 97 (1989), pp. 927–31; A. D. Pearson et al., Intestinal permeability in children with Crohn's disease and coeliac disease, *British Medical Journal*, Vol. 285 (1982), pp. 20–21; L. Pironi et al., Relationship between intestinal permeability to [51Cr]EDTA and inflammatory activity in asymptomatic patients with Crohn's disease, *Digestive Diseases and Sciences*, Vol. 35 (1990), pp. 582–88; P. Munkholm et al., Intestinal permeability in patients with Crohn's disease and ulcerative colitis and their first degree relatives, *Gut*, Vol. 35 (1994), pp. 68–72; D. Hollander et al., Increased intestinal permeability in patients with Crohn's disease and their relatives: a possible etiologic factor, *Annals of Internal Medicine*, Vol. 105 (1986), pp. 883–85; K. Teahon et al., Intestinal permeability in patients with Crohn's disease and their first degree relatives, *Gut*, Vol. 33 (1992), pp. 320–23; E. Barau and C. Dupont, Modifications of intestinal permeability during food provocation procedures in pediatric irritable bowel syndrome, *Journal of Pediatric Gastroenterology and Nutrition*, Vol. 11 (1990), pp. 72–77; R. Paganelli et al., Intestinal permeability in irritable bowel syndrome: effect of diet and sodium cromoglycate administration, *Annals of Allergy*, Vol. 64 (1990), pp. 377–80.

19. Rooney, Jenkins, and Buchanan, op. cit.; R. T. Jenkins et al., Increased intestinal permeability in patients with rheumatoid arthritis: a side-effect of oral non-steroidal anti-inflammatory drug therapy? *British Journal of Rheumatology*, Vol. 26 (1987), pp. 103–7; H. Mielants, Reflections on the link between intestinal permeability and inflammatory joint disease (letter; comment), *Clinical and Experimental Rheumatolology*, Vol. 8 (1990), pp. 523–24; A. J. Morris et al., Increased intestinal permeability in ankylosing spondylitis—primary lesion or drug effect? (see comments), *Gut*, Vol. 32 (1991), pp. 1470–72; M. D. Smith, R. A. Gibson, and P. M. Brooks, Abnormal bowel permeability in ankylosing spondylitis and rheumatoid arthritis, *Journal of Rheumatology*, Vol. 12 (1985), pp. 299–305; L. Skoldstam and K. E. Magnusson, Fasting, intestinal permeability, and rheumatoid arthritis, *Rheumatic Disease Clinics of North America*, Vol. 17 (1991), pp. 363–71.

20. L. Juhlin and C. Vahlquist, The influence of treatment on fibrin microclot generation in psoriasis, *British Journal of Dermatology*, Vol. 108 (1983), pp. 33–37; L. Juhlin and G. Michaelsson, Fibrin microclot formation in patients with acne, *Acta Dermatologica Venereologica*, Vol. 63 (1983), pp. 538–40; I. Hamilton et al., Small intestinal permeability in dermatological disease, *Quarterly Journal of Med-*

icine, Vol. 56 (1985), pp. 559–67; P. W. Belew et al., Endotoxemia in psoriasis (letter), *Archives of Dermatology*, Vol. 118 (1982), pp. 142–43; P. Jacobson, R. Baker, and M. Lessof, Intestinal permeability in patients with eczema and food allergy, *Lancet*, Vol. i (1981), pp. 1285–86; K. Falth-Magnusson et al., Gastrointestinal permeability in children with cow's milk allergy: effect of milk challenge and sodium cromoglycate as assessed with polyethyleneglycols (PEG 400 and PEG 1000), *Clinics in Allergy*, Vol. 16 (1986), pp. 543–51; K. Falth-Magnusson et al., Gastrointestinal permeability in atopic and non-atopic mothers, assessed with different-sized polyethyleneglycols (PEG 400 and PEG 1000), *Clinics in Allergy*, Vol. 15 (1985), pp. 565–70; K. Falth-Magnusson et al., Intestinal permeability in healthy and allergic children before and after sodium-cromoglycate treatment assessed with different-sized polyethyleneglycols (PEG 400 and PEG 1000), *Clinics in Allergy*, Vol. 14 (1984), pp. 277–86.

21. D. R. Mack et al., Correlation of intestinal lactulose permeability with exocrine pancreatic dysfunction, *Journal of Pediatrics*, Vol. 120 (1992), pp. 696–701.

22. S. Batash et al., Intestinal permeability in HIV infection: proper controls are necessary (letter), *American Journal of Gastroenterology*, Vol. 87 (1992), p. 680; S. G. Lim et al., Intestinal permeability and function in patients infected with human immunodeficiency virus: a comparison with coeliac disease, *Scandinavian Journal of Gastroenterology*, Vol. 28 (1993), pp. 573–80; R. E. Tepper et al., Intestinal permeability in patients infected with human immunodeficiency virus, *American Journal of Gastroenterology*, Vol. 89 (1994), pp. 878–82.

23. R. Lahesmaa-Rantala et al., Intestinal permeability in patients with yersinia triggered reactive arthritis, *Annals of the Rheumatic Diseases*, Vol. 50 (1991), pp. 91–94; R. Serrander, K. E. Magnusson, and T. Sundqvist, Acute infections with Giardia lamblia and rotavirus decrease intestinal permeability to low–molecular weight polyethylene glycols (PEG 400), *Scandinavian Journal of Infectious Disease*, Vol. 16 (1984), pp. 339–44; R. Serrander et al., Acute yersinia infections in man increase intestinal permeability for low–molecular weight polyethylene glycols (PEG 400), *Scandinavian Journal of Infectious Disease*, Vol. 18 (1986), pp. 409–13; Lim et al., op. cit.; I. Bjarnason, R. Wise, and T. Peters, The leaky gut of alcoholism: possible route of entry for toxic compounds, *Lancet*, Vol. i (1984), pp. 79–82; B. S. Worthington, L. Meserole, and J. A. Syrotuck, Effect of daily ethanol ingestion on intestinal permeability to macromolecules, *American Journal of Digestive Diseases*, Vol. 23 (1978), pp. 23–32; I. Bjarnason et al., Effect of non-steroidal anti-inflammatory drugs on the human small intestine, *Drugs*, Vol. 1 (1986), pp. 35–41; Jenkins et al., op. cit.

24. C. Andre, Food allergy: objective diagnosis and test of therapeutic efficacy by measuring intestinal permeability, *Presse Medicale*, Vol. 15 (1986), pp. 105–8; C. Andre, F. Andre, and L. Colin, Effect of allergen ingestion challenge with and without cromoglycate cover on intestinal permeability in atopic dermatitis, urticaria and other symptoms of food allergy, *Allergy*, Vol. 9 (1989), pp. 47–51; C. Andre et al., Measurement of intestinal permeability to mannitol and lactulose as a means of diagnosing food allergy and evaluating therapeutic effectiveness of disodium cromoglycate, *Annals of Allergy*, Vol. 59 (1987), pp. 127–30; E. Barau and C. Dupont, Allergy to cow's milk proteins in mother's milk or in hydrolyzed cow's milk infant formulas as assessed by intestinal permeability measurements, *Allergy*, Vol. 49 (1994), pp. 295–98.

25. The name given this condition is *reactive arthritis*. The name presupposes that the arthritis is a reaction to an infection that has occurred somewhere in the body, usually in the intestine. A condition very much like reactive arthritis also occurs in patients with chronic bowel inflammation of unknown cause, such as Crohn's disease. K. Granfors et al., Salmonella lipopolysaccharide in synovial cells from patients with reactive arthritis, *Lancet*, Vol. 335 (1990), pp. 685–88; O. Maki-Ikola and K. Granfors, Salmonella-triggered reactive arthritis, *Lancet*, Vol. 339 (1992), pp. 1096–98; K. Granfors et al., Yersinia antigens in synovial fluid cells from patients with reactive arthritis, *New England Journal of Medicine*, Vol. 320 (1989), pp. 216–21; A. Fox, op. cit.; P. E. Philips, The role of infectious agents in the spondylo-arthropathies, *Scandinavian Journal of Rheumatology*, Vol. 17 (1988), pp. 435–43.

26. The name given this condition is *ankylosing spondylitis*. Ankylosing spondylitis is defined by its clinical characteristics. It is very strongly associated with a particular gene that regulates part of the immune response pattern of the individual.

27. K. D. Katz and D. Hollander, Intestinal mucosal permeability and rheumatological diseases, *Bailliere's Clinical Rheumatology*, Vol. 3 (1989), pp. 271–84; G. R. Davies, M. E. Wilkie, and D. S. Rampton, Effects of metronidazole and misoprostol on indomethacin-induced changes in intestinal permeability, *Digestive Diseases and Sciences*, Vol. 38 (1993), pp. 417–25; I. Bjarnason et al., Effect of prostaglandin on indomethacin-induced increased intestinal permeability in man, *Scandinavian Journal of Gastroenterology*, Supplement, Vol. 164 (1989), pp. 97–102; I. Bjarnason et al., Misoprostol reduces indomethacin-induced changes in human small intestinal permeability, *Digestive Diseases and Sciences*, Vol. 34 (1989), pp. 407–11; I. Bjarnason et al., Metronidazole reduces intestinal inflammation and blood loss in non-steroidal anti-inflammatory drug induced enteropathy, *Gut*, Vol. 33 (1992), pp. 1204–8.

28. R. Balfour Sartor, Importance of intestinal mucosal immunity and luminal bacterial cell wall polymers in the aetiology of inflammatory joint diseases, *Balliere's Clinical Rheumatology*, Vol. 3 (1989), pp. 223–45; Rooney, Jenkins, and Buchanan, op. cit.

29. M. Dearlove et al., The effect of non-steroidal anti-inflammatory drugs on faecal flora and bacterial antibody levels in rheumatoid arthritis, *British Journal of Rheumatology*, Vol. 31 (1992), pp. 443–47; A. Ebringer et al., Antibodies to Proteus in rheumatoid arthritis, *Lancet*, Vol. ii (1985), pp. 305–7.

30. M. P. Hazenberg et al., Are intestinal bacteria involved in the etiology of rheumatoid arthritis? *APMIS*, Vol. 100 (1992), pp. 1–9.

31. Bjarnason et al., "Metronidazole."

32. These publications indicate that patients with a diagnosis of chronic rheumatoid arthritis may improve with the use of a variety of different antibiotics. The authors' explanations for why the antibiotics are beneficial differ from one another's and from mine: G. S. Alarcon and I. S. Mikhail, Antimicrobials in the treatment of rheumatoid arthritis and other arthritides: a clinical perspective, *American Journal of the Medical Sciences*, Vol. 309 (1994), pp. 201–9; T. M. Brown, The puzzling problem of the rheumatic diseases, *Maryland State Medical Journal* Vol. 2 (1956), pp. 88–109; E. M. Caperton et al., Ceftriaxone therapy of chronic inflammatory arthritis: a double-blind placebo controlled trial, *Archives of Internal Med-*

icine, Vol. 150 (1990), pp. 1677–82; T. M. Brown et al., Antimycoplasma approach to the mechanism and the control of rheumatoid disease, in *Inflammatory Diseases and Copper*, ed. J. R. J. Sorenson (Clifton, N.J.: Humana Press, 1982); D. Porter et al., Prospective trial comparing the use of sulphasalazine and auranofin as second line drugs in patients with rheumatoid arthritis, *Annals of the Rheumatic Diseases*, Vol. 51 (1992), pp. 461–64; D. R. Porter and H. A. Capell, The use of sulphasalazine as a disease modifying antirheumatic drug, *Bailliere's Clinical Rheumatology*, Vol. 4 (1990), pp. 535–51; P. K. Pybus, Metronidazole in rheumatoid arthritis, *South African Medical Journal*, (Feb. 20, 1982), pp. 261–62; B. C. Tilley et al., Minocycline in rheumatoid arthritis: a 48-week, double-blind, placebo-controlled trial, *Annals of Internal Medicine*, Vol. 122 (1995), pp. 81–89; J. A. Wojtulewski, P. J. Gow, and J. Waller, Clotrimazole in rheumatoid arthritis, *Annals of the Rheumatic Diseases*, Vol. 39 (1980), pp. 469–72; M. Kloppenburg et al., Antibiotics as disease modifiers in arthritis, *Clinics in Experimental Rheumatology*, Vol. 11, Supp. 8 (1993), pp. S113–S115.

33. J. Kjeldsen-Kragh et al., Controlled trial of fasting and one-year vegetarian diet in rheumatoid arthritis, *Lancet*, Vol. 338 (1991), pp. 899–902.

34. T. Sundqvist et al., Influence of fasting on intestinal permeability and disease activity in patients with rheumatoid arthritis, *Scandinavian Journal of Rheumatology*, Vol. 11 (1982), p. 33; L. Skoldstam and K.-E. Magnusson, Fasting, intestinal permeability and rheumatoid arthritis, *Rheumatic Disease Clinics of North America*, Vol. 17 (1991), pp. 363–71.

35. R. Peltonen et al., Changes of faecal flora in rheumatoid arthritis during fasting and one-year vegetarian diet, *British Journal of Rheumatology*, Vol. 33 (1994), pp. 638–43.

36. U. Fagiolo et al., Intestinal permeability and antigen absorption in rheumatoid arthritis, *International Archives of Allergy and Applied Immunology*, Vol. 89 (1989), pp. 98–102.

37. C. O'Farrelly, D. Melcher, and R. Price, *Lancet*, Vol. ii (1988), pp. 819–22; C. O'Farrelly et al., IgA rheumatoid factor and IgG dietary protein antibodies are associated in rheumatoid arthritis, *Immunological Investigations*, Vol. 18 (1989), pp. 753–64.

38. L. G. Darlington and N. W. Ramsey, Review of dietary therapy for rheumatoid arthritis, *British Journal of Rheumatology*, Vol. 32, Supp. 6 (1993), pp. 507–14; M. A. van de Laar and J. K. van der Korst, Food intolerance in rheumatoid arthritis, I. A double blind controlled trial of the clinical effects of elimination of milk allergens and azo dyes, *Annals of the Rheumatic Diseases*, Vol. 51 (1992), pp. 298–302; M. A. van de Laar et al., Food intolerance in rheumatoid arthritis; II. Clinical and histological aspects, *Annals of the Rheumatic Diseases*, Vol. 51 (1992), pp. 303–6; C. H. Little, A. G. Stewart, and M. R. Fennessy, Platelet serotonin release in rheumatoid arthritis: a study in food-intolerant patients, *Lancet*, Vol. ii (1983), pp. 297–99; L. G. Darlington, N. W. Ramsey, and J. R. Mansfield, Placebo-controlled, blind study of dietary manipulation therapy in rheumatoid arthritis, *Lancet*, Vol. i (1986), pp. 236–38; D. Beri et al., Effects of dietary restrictions on disease activity in rheumatoid arthritis, *Annals of the Rheumatic Diseases*, Vol. 47 (1988), pp. 69–72; A. I. Parkes and G. R. V. Hughes, Rheumatoid arthritis and food: a case study, *British Medical Journal*, Vol. 282 (1981), pp. 2027–29; R. M. Stroud, The effect of fasting followed by specific food challenges in rheumatoid arthritis,

in *Current Topics in Rheumatology,* ed. B. H. Hahn, F. C. Arnett, and T. M. Zizic (Kalamazoo, Mich.: Upjohn, 1983), pp. 145–57; R. Williams, Rheumatoid arthritis and food: a case study, *British Medical Journal,* Vol. 283 (1981), p. 563; R. S. Panush, Delayed reactions to foods: food allergy and rheumatic disease, *Annals of Allergy,* Vol. 56 (1986), pp. 500–503.

39. D. L. Scott et al., Long-term outcome of treating rheumatoid arthritis: results after 20 years, *Lancet,* Vol. i (1987), 1108–11; S. Gabriel and H. S. Luthra, Rheumatoid arthritis: can the long-term outcome be altered? *Mayo Clinic Proceedings,* Vol. 63 (1988), pp. 58–68.

40. A. L. Parke, Gastrointestinal disorders in rheumatic diseases, *Current Opinion in Rheumatology,* Vol. 4 (1992), pp. 68–75.

41. A. C. Jordan, *Chronic Intestinal Stasis: A Radiologic Study* (London: Oxford Medical Publishers, 1923). Quoted in J. L. Smith and Sir Arbuthnot Lane, Chronic intestinal stasis, and autointoxication, *Annals of Internal Medicine,* Vol. 86 (1982), pp. 365–69.

42. R. J. Playford et al., Effect of luminal growth factor preservation on intestinal growth, *Lancet,* Vol. 341 (1993), pp. 843–48.

43. J. A. Vanderhoof et al., Effect of dietary menhaden oil on normal growth and development and on ameliorating mucosal injury in rats, *American Journal of Clinical Nutrition,* Vol. 54 (1991), pp. 346–50.

44. J. M. Braganza et al., Lipid-peroxidation (free-radical-oxidation) products in bile from patients with pancreatic disease, *Lancet,* Vol. ii (1983), pp. 375–78; J. M. Braganza, Pancreatic disease: a casualty of hepatic "detoxification"? *Lancet,* Vol. ii (1983), pp. 1000–1002 (Braganza's research indicates that high intake of polyunsaturated fatty acids increases the free radical content of bile); J. M. Stark and S. K. Jackson, Sensitivity to endotoxin is induced by increased membrane fatty-acid unsaturation and oxidant stress, *Journal of Medical Microbiology,* Vol. 32 (1990), pp. 217–21 (tissue damage produced by the endotoxin released from normal intestinal bacteria is increased in an environment where free radical activity is high).

45. G. Spaeth et al., Food without fiber promotes bacterial translocation from the gut, *Surgery,* Vol. 108 (1990), pp. 240–46.

46. E. Lanza et al., Dietary fiber intake in the US population, *American Journal of Clinical Nutrition,* Vol. 46 (1987), pp. 790–97.

47. I. H. Ullrich, Evaluation of a high-fiber diet in hyperlipidemia: a review, *Journal of the American College of Nutrition,* Vol. 6 (1987), pp. 19–25; J. W. Anderson et al., Hypocholesterolemic effect of different bulk-forming hydrophilic fibers as adjuncts to dietary therapy in mild to moderate hypercholesterolemia, *Archives of Internal Medicine,* Vol. 151 (1991), pp. 1597–1602.

48. M. H. Davidson et al., The hypocholesterolemic effects of B-glucan in oatmeal and oat bran: a dose controlled study, *Journal of the American Medical Association,* Vol. 265 (1991), pp. 1833–39; J. W. Anderson et al., Oat bran cereal lowers serum total and LDL cholesterol in hypercholesterolemic men, *American Journal of Clinical Nutrition,* Vol. 52 (1990), pp. 495–99; L. Van Horn et al., Effects on serum lipids of adding instant oats to usual American diets, *American Journal of Public Health,* Vol. 81 (1991), pp. 183–88; C. M. Ripsin et al., Oat products and lipid lowering: a meta-analysis, *Journal of the American Medical Association,* Vol. 267 (1992), pp. 3317–26.

49. D. Royall, T. M. S. Wolever, and K. N. Jeejeebhoy, Clinical significance of colonic fermentation, *American Journal of Gastroenterology*, Vol. 85 (1990), pp. 1307–12; D. J. A. Jenkins, The link between colon fermentation and systemic disease, *American Journal of Gastroenterology*, Vol. 84 (1989), pp. 1362–64.

50. Fermentable fibers and vitamin B_{12} dependency, *Nutrition Reviews*, Vol. 49 (1991), pp. 119–20; I. R. Rowland and A. K. Mallett, Dietary fibre and the gut microflora — their effects on toxicity, in *New Concepts and Developments in Toxicology*, ed. P. L. Chambers, P. Gehring, and F. Sakai (New York: Elsevier Science Publishers [Biomedical Division], 1986), pp. 125–38; R. W. Chadwick et al., Role of the gastrointestinal mucosa and microflora in the bioactivation of dietary and environmental mutagens and carcinogens, *Drug Metabolism Reviews*, Vol. 24 (1992), pp. 425–92.

51. B. Eisenhans and W. F. Caspary, Differential changes in the urinary excretion of two orally administered polyethylene glycol markers (PEG 900 and PEG 4000) in rats after feeding various carbohydrate gelling agents, *Journal of Nutrition*, Vol. 119 (1989), pp. 380–87; C. P. Gyory and G. W. Chang, Effects of bran, lignin and deoxycholic acid on the permeability of the rat cecum and colon, *Journal of Nutrition*, Vol. 113 (1983), pp. 2300–2307; S. Y. Shiau and G. W. Chang, Effects of certain dietary fibers on apparent permeability of the rat intestine, *Journal of Nutrition*, Vol. 116 (1986), pp. 223–32.

52. J. R. Lupton and L. R. Jacobs, Fiber supplementation results in expanded proliferative zones in rat gastric mucosa, *American Journal of Clinical Nutrition*, Vol. 46 (1987), pp. 980–84; Rowland and Mallett, op. cit.; R. W. Chadwick et al., Role of the gastrointestinal mucosa and microflora in the bioactivation of dietary and environmental mutagens and carcinogens, *Drug Metabolism Reviews*, Vol. 24 (1992), pp. 425–92.

53. B. H. Ershoff, Antitoxic effects of plant fiber, *American Journal of Clinical Nutrition*, Vol. 27 (1974), pp. 1395–98; D. P. Rose et al., High-fiber diet reduces serum estrogen concentrations in premenopausal women, *American Journal of Clinical Nutrition*, Vol. 54 (1991), pp. 520–25.

54. W. C. Willett and B. MacMahon, Diet and cancer — an overview; I and II, *New England Journal of Medicine*, Vol. 310 (1984), pp. 633–38 and 697–703; P. Van 'T Veer et al., Dietary fiber, beta-carotene and breast cancer: results from a case-control study, *International Journal of Cancer*, Vol. 4 (1990), pp. 825–28; H. Adlercreutz et al., Excretion of the lignans enterolactone and enterodiol and of equol in omnivorous and vegetarian postmenopausal women and in women with breast cancer, *Lancet*, Vol. ii (1982), pp. 1295–98.

55. J. J. DeCosse, H. H. Miller, and M. L. Lesser, Effect of wheat fiber and vitamins C and E on rectal polyps in patients with familial adenomatous polyposis, *Journal of the National Cancer Institute*, Vol. 81 (1989), pp. 1290–97; D. W. Heitman and I. L. Cameron, Reduction of colon cancer risk by dietary cellulose, *Journal of the National Cancer Institute*, Vol. 82 (1990), pp. 1154–55.

56. D. P. Burkitt, A. R. P. Walker, and N. S. Painter, Dietary fiber and disease, *Journal of the American Medical Association*, Vol. 229 (1974), pp. 1068–74; D. Kromhout, E. B. Bosschieter, and E. de Lezenne Coulander, Dietary fibre and 10-year mortality from coronary heart disease, cancer and all causes: the Zutphen study, *Lancet*, Vol. ii (1982), pp. 518–21.

57. J. P. Guggenbichler, Adherence as major pathogenetic mechanisms of E. coli in enteric infections and modes to block adherance, *Infection*, Vol. 17 (1983), pp. 173–77; I. Ofek et al., Anti–*Escherichia coli* adhesion activity of cranberry and blueberry juices, *New England Journal of Medicine*, Vol. 324 (1991), p. 1599; D. Zopf and S. Roth, Oligosaccharide anti-infective agents, *Lancet*, Vol. 347 (1996), pp. 1017–21.

58. T. Fukushi, Studies on edible rice bran oils; Part 3: Antioxidant effects of oryzanol, *Reports of the Hokkaido Institute of Public Health*, Vol. 16 (1966), p. 111; K. Yagi and N. Ohishi, Action of ferulic acid and its derivatives as anti-oxidants, *Journal of Nutritional Science and Vitaminology*, Vol. 205 (1979), pp. 127–35.

59. K. M. Shahani and A. D. Ayebo, Role of dietary lactobacilli in gastrointestinal microecology, *American Journal of Clinical Nutrition*, Vol. 33 (1980), pp. 2448–57; B. R. Goldin and S. L. Gorbach, Alterations of the intestinal microflora by diet, oral antibiotics, and *Lactobacillus*: Decreased production of free amines from aromatic nitro compounds, azo dyes, and glucuronides, *Journal of the National Cancer Institute*, Vol. 73 (1981), pp. 689–95; S. L. Gorbach, Lactic acid bacteria and human health, *Annals of Medicine*, Vol. 22 (1990), pp. 37–41; S. E. Gilliland, Health and nutritional benefits from lactic acid bacteria, *FEMS Microbiology Reviews*, Vol. 87 (1990), pp. 175–88; T. Mitsuoka, Bifidobacteria and their role in human health, *Journal of Industrial Microbiology*, Vol. 6 (1990), pp. 263–68; N. Kulkarni and B. S. Reddy, Inhibitory effect of *Bifidobacterium longum* cultures on the azoxymethane-induced aberrant crypt foci formation and fecal bacterial B-glucuronidase, *Proceedings of the Society of Experimental Biology and Medicine*, Vol. 207 (1994), pp. 278–83; S. Siitonen et al., Effect of Lactobacillus GG yoghurt in prevention of antibiotic associated diarrhoea, *Annals of Medicine*, Vol. 22 (1990), pp. 57–59; E. Salminen et al., Preservation of intestinal integrity during radiotherapy using live Lactobacillus acidophilus cultures, *Clinical Radiology*, Vol. 39 (1988), pp. 435–37; P. J. Oksanen et al., Prevention of travellers' diarrhoea by Lactobacillus GG, *Annals of Medicine*, Vol. 22(1) (1990), pp. 53–56; S. L. Gorbach, T. W. Chang, and B. Goldin, Successful treatment of relapsing Clostridium difficile colitis with Lactobacillus GG, *Lancet*, Vol. ii (1987), p. 1519; S. Yamazaki et al., Immunologic responses to monoassociated *Bifidobacterium longum* and their relation to prevention of bacterial invasion, *Immunology*, Vol. 56 (1985), pp. 43–50; G. W. Elmer, C. M. Surawicz, and L. V. McFarland, Biotherapeutic agents: a neglected modality for the treatment and prevention of selected intestinal and vaginal infections, *Journal of the American Medical Association*, Vol. 275 (1996), pp. 870–76.

60. T. Mitsuoka, Bifidobacterium microecology, in *Les Laits Fermentes: Actualité de la Recherche* (Paris: John Libbey Eurotext Ltd., 1989), pp. 41–48.

61. G. R. Gibson and M. B. Roberfroid, Dietary modulation of the human colonic microbiota: introducing the concept of prebiotics, *Journal of Nutrition*, Vol. 125 (1995), pp. 1401–12; T. Mitsuoka, H. Hidaka, and T. Eida, Effect of fructooligosaccharides on intestinal flora, *Die Nahrung*, Vol. 31 (1987), pp. 427–36; C. H. Williams, S. A. Witherly, and R. K. Buddington, Influence of dietary neosugar on selected bacterial groups of the human faecal microflora, *Microbial Ecology in Health and Disease*, Vol. 7 (1994), pp. 91–97.

62. R. K. Buddington et al., Dietary supplement of neosugar alters the fecal flora and decreases activities of some reductive enzymes in human subjects, *American Journal of Clinical Nutrition*, Vol. 63 (1996), pp. 709–16.

63. E. Hilton et al., Ingested yogurt as prophylaxis for chronic candidal vaginitis, *Annals of Internal Medicine*, Vol. 116 (1992), pp. 353–57; D. J. Drutz, *Lactobacillus* prophylaxis for *Candida* vaginitis, *Annals of Internal Medicine*, Vol. 116 (1992), pp. 419–20.

64. A. Schauss, Lactobacillus acidophilus: method of action, clinical application, and toxicity data, *Journal of Advancement in Medicine*, Vol. 3 (1990), pp. 163–78; M. L. Johansson et al., Administration of different lactobacillus strains in fermented oatmeal soup: In vivo colonization of human intestinal mucosa and effect on the indigenous flora, *Applied & Environmental Microbiology*, Vol. 59 (1993), pp. 15–20.

65. C. M. Surawicz et al., Treatment of recurrent Clostridium difficile colitis with vancomycin and Saccharomyces boulardii, *American Journal of Gastroenterology*, Vol. 84 (1989), pp. 1285–87; C. M. Surawicz et al., Prevention of antibiotic-associated diarrhea by Saccharomyces boulardii: a prospective study, *Gastroenterology*, Vol. 96 (1989), pp. 981–88; J.-P. Buts et al., Stimulation of secretory IgA and secretory component of immunoglobulins in small intestine of rats treated with Saccharomyces boulardii, *Digestive Diseases and Sciences*, Vol. 35 (1990), pp. 251–56.

66. A complete discussion and set of references appears in *Textbook of Natural Medicine*, ed. J. E. Pizzorno and M. T. Murray (Seattle: John Bastyr College Publications, 1987), Vol. 1, section V, pp. 1–7. Also see: K. S. Farbman et al., Antibacterial activity of garlic and onions: a historical perspective, *Pediatric Infectious Disease Journal*, Vol. 12 (1993), pp. 613–14; Z. R. Lun et al., Antiparasitic effect of diallyl trisulfide (Dasuansu) on human and animal pathogenic protozoa (Trypanosoma sp., Entamoeba histolytica and Giardia lamblia) in vitro, *Annals of the Belgian Society of Tropical Medicine*, Vol. 74 (1994), pp. 51–59; P. V. Venugopal and T. V. Venugopal, Antidermatophytic activity of garlic (Allium sativum) in vitro, *International Journal of Dermatology*, Vol. 34 (1995), pp. 278–79; S. T. Pai and M. W. Platt, Antifungal effects of Allium sativum (garlic) extract against the Aspergillus species involved in otomycosis, *Letters in Applied Microbiology*, Vol. 20 (1995), pp. 14–18.

67. A. Leung, *Encyclopedia of Common Natural Ingredients Used in Foods, Drugs and Cosmetics* (New York: John Wiley & Sons, 1980), pp. 246–47; S. B. Vahora, M. Rizwan, and J. A. Khan, Medicinal uses of common Indian vegetables, *Planta Medica*, Vol. 23 (1973), pp. 381–93; E. I. Elnima et al., The antimicrobial activity of garlic and onion extracts, *Pharmazie*, Vol. 38 (1983), pp. 747–48; A. N. Zohri, K. Abdel-Gawad, and S. Saber, Antibacterial, antidermatophytic and antitoxigenic activities of onion (Allium cepa L.) oil, *Microbiology Research*, Vol. 150 (1995), pp. 167–72.

68. Leung, op. cit., pp. 313–14; V. J. Lutomski, B. Kedzia, and W. Debska, Effect of an alcohol extract and active ingredients from Curcuma longa on bacteria and fungi, *Planta Medica*, Vol. 26 (1974), pp. 17–19; F. Kiuchi et al., Nematocidal activity of turmeric: synergistic action of curcuminoids, *Chemical and Pharmacological Bulletin* (Tokyo), Vol. 41 (1993), pp. 1640–43.

69. P. Schulick, *Ginger: Common Spice & Wonder Drug* (Brattleboro, Vt.: Herbal Free Press, 1994).

70. L. B. Bullerman, Inhibition of aflatoxin production by cinnamon, *Journal of Food Science*, Vol. 39 (1974), pp. 1163–65.

71. R. C. Beier, Natural pesticides and bioactive compounds in food, *Review of Environmental Contamination and Toxicity*, Vol. 113 (1990), pp. 47–137. The purpose of this review is to emphasize the potential toxicity of plant foods and herbal preparations. Its author finds little evidence of toxicity for onion, garlic, rosemary, and sage.

72. H. C. Chen, M. D. Chang, and T. J. Chang [Antibacterial properties of some spice plants before and after heat treatment], *Chung Hua Min Kuo Wei Sheng Wu Chi Mien I Hsueh Tsa Chih*, Vol. 18 (1985), pp. 190–95.

73. Grapefruit juice interactions with drugs, *The Medical Letter on Drugs and Therapeutics*, Vol. 37 (1995), pp. 73–74.

74. L. L. von Moltke et al., Inhibition of terfenadine metabolism *in vitro* by azole antifungal agents and by selective serotonin reuptake inhibitor antidepressants: relation to pharmacokinetic interactions *in vivo*, *Journal of Clinical Psychopharmacology*, Vol. 16 (1996), pp. 104–12; S. H. Preskorn, Reducing the risk of drug-drug interactions: a goal of rational drug development, *Journal of Clinical Psychiatry*, Vol. 57, Supp. 1 (1996), pp. 3–6.

75. For those who desire it, here is a technical description of free-radical formation: All chemical compounds are composed of two or more basic elements (such as carbon and hydrogen), which are joined together by a chemical bond. Elements are able to form bonds because every atom of every element contains a portion that is electrically charged; this part of the atom is called an *electron*. Electrons are constantly moving, sometimes leaving the atoms to which they belong to pair with the electrons of other atoms. When all the electrons in an element such as copper move in one direction, we call their flow *electricity*. Stable compounds, like water, are formed when two types of atoms bond together by sharing electrons as pairs. If a single electron is lost from an electron pair, the remaining electron becomes unstable and searches its environment for another electron with which it can pair, snatching that electron away from another compound, damaging the second compound and leaving it with an unpaired, unstable electron that is now searching its environment for another electron to mate with, initiating a chain reaction. A compound or element with an unpaired electron that is searching for a mate is called a "free radical." Oxygen is an element that is always hungry for electrons and constantly snatches them away from other substances. The process of electron-snatching is called "oxidation," and it is vital for the existence of life on earth. Oxidation readily produces free radicals, and the body uses the energy inherent in free radicals to build up its own cellular energy supplies and to chemically alter toxins. Free radicals are not easily controlled, however. They pair promiscuously with any electron they can attract and are capable of damaging the body's membranes and enzymes. DNA, the substance of which genes are made, is especially vulnerable to free-radical attack. To protect against this damage, the body contains a defense system composed of antioxidants. Antioxidants are electron rich. They interrupt the free-radical chain reaction by supplying extra electrons.

76. W. M. H. Behan, I. A. R. More, and P. O. Behan, Mitochondrial abnormalities in the postviral fatigue syndrome, *Acta Neuropathologica*, Vol. 83 (1991), pp. 61–65. See also *Mitochondrial Disorders in Neurology*, ed. A. H. V. Schapira and S. DiMauro (Oxford: Butterworth Heinemann, 1994). The increasing diversity and prevalence of mitochondrial dysfunctions is described.

77. R. J. Shamberger, S. A. Tytko, and C. A. Willis, Antioxidants and cancer, *Archives of Environmental Health*, Vol. 30 (1976), pp. 231–35; J. T. Salonen et al., Risk of cancer in relation to serum concentrations of selenium and vitamins A and E, *British Medical Journal*, Vol. 290 (1985), pp. 417–20; S. Graham, Epidemiology of retinoids and cancer, *Journal of the National Cancer Institute*, Vol. 73 (1984), pp. 1423–28 (high intake of vitamin A from vegetable sources protects against cancers of the lung, larynx, mouth, cervix, and bladder, but increases risk of prostate cancer); R. A. Shakman, Nutritional influences on the toxicity of environmental pollutants, *Archives of Environmental Health*, Vol. 28 (1974), pp. 105–13; G. Block, B. Patterson, and A. Subar, Fruit, vegetables, and cancer prevention, *Nutrition & Cancer*, Vol. 18 (1992), pp. 1–29; T. Byers and G. Perry, Dietary carotenes, vitamin C, and vitamin E as protective antioxidants in human cancers, *Annual Review of Nutrition*, Vol. 12 (1992), pp. 139–59; J. H. Weisburger, Nutritional approach to cancer prevention with emphasis on vitamins, antioxidants, and carotenoids, *American Journal of Clinical Nutrition*, Vol. 53 (1991), pp. 226S–237S; W. C. Willet et al., Prediagnostic serum selenium and risk of cancer, *Lancet*, Vol. ii (1983), pp. 130–34; N. J. Temple and T. K. Basu, Does beta-carotene prevent cancer? A critical appraisal, *Nutrition Research*, Vol. 8 (1988), pp. 183–91. The anticancer activity of beta-carotene does not depend upon its conversion to vitamin A.

78. L. M. Canfield, N. I. Krinsky, and J. A. Olson, eds., *Carotenoids and Human Health, Annals of the New York Academy of Sciences*, Vol. 691 (1993), 300 pp., conference proceedings; C. Grubbs et al., Effect of canthaxanthin on chemically induced mammary carcinogenesis, *Oncology*, Vol. 48 (1991), pp. 239–45; R. Ziegler et al., Diet and the risk of vulvar cancer, *American Journal of Epidemiology*, Vol. 132 (1990), pp. 778–84. *Alpha*-carotene but not *beta*-carotene in the diet appears to protect against vulvar cancer.

79. B. Havsteen, Flavonoids, a class of natural products of high pharmacological potency, *Biochemical Pharmacology*, Vol. 32 (1983), pp. 1141–48.

Also see *Plant Flavonoids in Biology and Medicine*, ed. V. Cody, E. Middleton, Jr., and J. B. Harborne, *Progress in Clinical and Biological Research*, Vol. 213 (1986), and *Plant Flavonoids in Biology and Medicine II*, ed. V. Cody, E. Middleton, Jr., J. B. Harborne, and A. Beretz, *Progress in Clinical and Biological Research*, Vol. 280 (1988). Both volumes are published by Alan R. Liss, New York.

80. See *Preventive Medicine*, Vol. 21, Nos. 3 and 4 (May and July, 1992), for the proceedings of the International Symposium on the Physiological and Pharmacological Effects of *Camellia sinesis* (Tea): Implications for Cardiovascular Disease, Cancer, and Public Health, held in New York City, March 4–5, 1991.

Black tea is much lower in protective flavonoids than green tea. Black tea leaves are produced from green tea leaves by a process of bacterial fermentation which destroys most of the beneficial compounds.

81. T. Y. Aw and D. P. Jones, Nutrient supply and mitochondrial function, *Annual Review of Nutrition*, Vol. 9 (1989), pp. 229–51; *Biochemical and Clinical Aspects of Coenzyme O*, ed. K. Folkers and Y. Yamamura (Amsterdam: Elsevier/North Holland Biomedical Press, Vol. 1, 1977, Vol. 2, 1980, Vol. 3, 1981); K. Tadakashi et al., Effects of Coenzyme Q10 on exercise tolerance in chronic stable angina pectoris, *American Journal of Cardiology*, Vol. 56 (1985), pp. 247–51; R. Nakamura et al., Deficiency of Coenzyme Q in gingiva of patients with periodontal disease, *International Journal for Vitamin and Nutrition Research*, Vol. 43

(1973), pp. 84–92; T. Matsumura et al., Evidence for enhanced treatment of peri-odontal disease by therapy with Coenzyme Q, *International Journal for Vitamin and Nutrition Research*, Vol. 43 (1973), pp. 536–48; T. Yamagami, N. Shibata, and K. Folkers, Bioenergetics in clinical medicine: studies on Coenzyme Q10 and es-sential hypertension, *Research Communications in Chemical Pathology and Phar-macology*, Vol. 11 (1975), pp. 273–87; T. Yamagami, N. Shibata, and K. Folkers, Bioenergetics in clinical medicine VIII: administration of Coenzyme Q10 to pa-tients with essential hypertension, *Research Communications in Chemical Pathol-ogy and Pharmacology*, Vol. 14 (1976), pp. 721–27; T. Kishi et al., Bioenergetics in clinical medicine XI: studies on Coenzyme Q and diabetes mellitus, *Journal of Medicine*, Vol. 7 (1976), pp. 307–21.

82. D. H. Barch, Esophageal cancer and microelements, *Journal of the Ameri-can College of Nutrition*, Vol. 8 (1989), pp. 99–107.

83. P. S. Guzelian, Environmental toxins and the liver, *Practical Gastroen-terology*, Vol. 5, No. 4 (July–Aug. 1981), pp. 26–30; J. S. Bland and J. A. Bralley, Nu-tritional upregulation of hepatic detoxification enzymes, *Journal of Applied Nutrition*, Vol. 44 (1992), pp. 1–15; A. P. Kulkarni and E. Hodgson, The metabo-lism of insecticides: the role of monooxygenase enzymes, *Annual Review of Phar-macology and Toxicology*, Vol. 24 (1982), pp. 19–42; K. E. Anderson and A. Kappas, Dietary regulation of cytochrome P450, *Annual Review of Nutrition*, Vol. 11 (1991), pp. 141–67.

84. D. P. Jones et al., Glutathione in foods listed in the National Cancer Insti-tute's health habits and history food frequency questionnaire, *Nutrition & Cancer*, Vol. 17 (1992), pp. 57–75.

85. C. J. Johnston, C. G. Meyer, and J. C. Srilakshmi, Vitamin C elevates red blood cell glutathione in healthy adults, *American Journal of Clinical Nutrition*, Vol. 58 (1993), pp. 103–5.

86. D. C. Whitcomb and G. F. Block, Association of acetaminophen hepato-toxicity with fasting and ethanol use, *Journal of the American Medical Association*, Vol. 272 (1994), pp. 1845–50.

87. M. Ruprah, T. G. K. Mant, and R. J. Flanagan, Acute carbon tetrachloride poisoning in 19 patients: implications for diagnosis and treatment, *Lancet*, Vol. i (1985), pp. 1027–29.

88. P. F. Guengerich, Effects of nutritive factors on metabolic processes in-volving bioactivation and detoxification of chemicals, *Annual Review of Nutrition*, Vol. 4 (1984), pp. 207–31; J. L. Stoewsand, J. L. Anderson, and L. Munson, Protec-tive effects of dietary brussels sprouts against mammary carcinogenesis in Sprague-Dawley rats, *Cancer Letters*, Vol. 39 (1987), pp. 199–207; Z. Yuesheng et al., A major inducer of anticarcinogenic protective enzymes from broccoli: isolation and elucidation of structure, *Proceedings of the National Academy of Sciences*, Vol. 89 (1992), pp. 2399–2403.

89. A. W. Smith et al., Effects of flavonoids on the metabolism of xenobiotics, in *Plant Flavonoids in Biology and Medicine. Biochemical, Pharmacological, and Structure-Activity Relationships*, ed. V. Cody, E. Middleton, Jr., and J. B. Harborne (New York: Alan R. Liss, 1986), pp. 195–210.

90. H. Wagner, Antihepatotoxic flavonoids, in *Plant Flavonoids in Biology and Medicine*, op. cit., pp. 545–58.

91. R. Campos et al., *Plant Flavonoids in Biology and Medicine II. Biochemical, Cellular and Medicinal Properties* (New York: Alan R. Liss, 1988), pp. 375–78.

92. H. A. Salmi and S. Sarna, Effect of silymarin on chemical, functional, and morphological alteration of the liver. A double-blind controlled study, *Scandinavian Journal of Gastroenterology*, Vol. 17 (1982), pp. 417–21.

93. Intestinal toxins, absorbed from an overly permeable gut, burden the liver in exactly the same way that environmental pollutants burden it. The effects are additive. See J. P. Nolan, Intestinal endotoxins as mediators of hepatic injury—an idea whose time has come again, *Hepatology*, Vol. 10 (1989), pp. 887–91.

94. Bjarnason, Wise, and Peters, op.cit.; B. S. Worthington, L. Meserole, and J. A. Syrotuck, Effect of daily ethanol ingestion on intestinal permeability to macromolecules, *American Journal of Digestive Diseases*, Vol. 23 (1978), pp. 23–32.

95. R. A. Giannella, S. A. Broitman, and N. Zamcheck, Gastric acid barrier to ingested microorganisms: studies *in vivo* and *in vitro*, *Gut*, Vol. 13 (1972), pp. 251–56.

96. K. R. Neal, Omeprazole as a risk factor for Campylobacter gastroenteritis: a case-control study, *British Medical Journal*, Vol. 312 (1996), pp. 414–15.

97. O. Nyran et al., Absence of therapeutic benefit from antacids or cimetidine in non-ulcer dyspepsia, *New England Journal of Medicine*, Vol. 314 (1986), pp. 339–44.

98. Jonathan Dahl, "You Want Seconds at the Salad Bar. Better Think It Over," *The Wall Street Journal*, Apr. 16, 1986.

99. J. A. Vanderhoof et al., Effects of berberine, a plant alkaloid, on the growth of anaerobic protozoa in axenic culture, *Tokai Journal of Experimental and Clinical Medicine*, Vol. 15 (1990), pp. 417–23; S. Gupte, Use of berberine in treatment of giardiasis, *American Journal of Diseases of Childhood*, Vol. 129 (1975), p. 866; G. H. Rabbani et al., Randomized controlled trial of berberine sulfate therapy for diarrhea due to enterotoxigenic Escherichia coli and Vibrio cholerae, *Journal of Infectious Diseases*, Vol. 155 (1987), pp. 979–84; T. V. Subbaiah and A. H. Amin, Effect of berberine sulphate on Entamoeba histolytica, *Nature*, Vol. 215 (1967), pp. 527–28.

Chapter 9: Plagues Revisited

1. *Newsweek*, May 22, 1995.

2. Quoted in R. L. Berkelman and J. M. Hughes, The conquest of infectious diseases: who are we kidding? *Annals of Internal Medicine*, Vol. 119 (1993), pp. 426–27.

3. See the excellent introduction by Mary Wilson of the Harvard School of Public Health to *Disease in Evolution: Global Changes and Emergence of Infectious Diseases*, ed. M. E. Wilson, R. Levins, and A. Spielman, *Annals of the New York Academy of Sciences*, Vol. 740 (1994), pp. 1–12.

4. Research into the adaptive value of fever and the danger of suppressing fever is discussed in *Why We Get Sick: The New Science of Darwinian Medicine*, by R. M. Nesse and G. C. Williams (New York: Times Books, 1994), pp. 27–29.

5. A fine technical description of the cellular response to pneumococci can be found in E. I. Tuomanen, R. Austria, and H. R. Masure, Pathogenesis of pneu-

mococcal infection, *New England Journal of Medicine*, Vol. 332 (1995), pp. 1280–84.

6. Voltaire, *Lettres Philosophiques*, Lettre XI.

7. Varying accounts of the history of smallpox inoculation can be found in Lois M. Magner, *A History of Medicine* (New York: Marcel Dekker, Inc., 1992), pp. 240–41; James H. Cassedy, *Medicine in America: A Short History* (Baltimore: The Johns Hopkins University Press, 1991), pp. 16–17; Lucien Craps, From the origins of immunology to the first vaccines, *Immunology and Allergy Practice*, Vol. 15 (1993), pp. 16–19.

8. A fascinating, detailed discussion of the rise of polio is presented by Arno Karlen in *Man and Microbes* (New York: Jeremy P. Tarcher/Putnam, 1995), pp. 149–54.

9. Measles, cholera, typhoid, and influenza have ebbed and flowed, with little impact from medical intervention. D. Thomson, The ebb and flow of infection, *Journal of the American Medical Association*, Vol. 235 (1976), pp. 269–72.

10. Data are presented in E. H. Kass, The history of the specialty of infectious diseases in the United States, *Annals of Internal Medicine*, Vol. 106 (1987), pp. 745–56; Also see R. C. Lewontin, *Biology as Ideology* (New York: HarperPerennial, 1992).

11. G. D. Hussey et al., The effect of Edmonton-Zagreb and Schwartz measles vaccines on immune responses in infants, *Journal of Infectious Diseases*, Vol. 173 (1996), pp. 1320–26; S. E. Starr, Novel mechanism of immunosuppression after measles, *Lancet*, Vol. 348 (1996), pp. 1257–58.

12. A. Sommer, Vitamin A, infectious disease, and childhood mortality: a 2-cents solution? *Journal of Infectious Diseases*, Vol. 167 (1993), pp. 1003–7; W. W. Fawzi et al., Vitamin A supplementation and child mortality, *Journal of the American Medical Association*, Vol. 269 (1993), pp. 898–903; A. C. Arrieta et al., Vitamin A levels in children with measles in Long Beach, California, *Journal of Pediatrics*, Vol. 121 (1992), pp. 75–78; F. A. C. S. Campos, H. Flores, and B. A. Underwood, Effect of an infection on vitamin A status of children as measured by the relative dose response (RDR), *American Journal of Clinical Nutrition*, Vol. 46 (1987), pp. 91–94; A. J. G. Barclay, A. Foster, and A. Sommer, Vitamin A supplements and mortality related to measles: a randomized clinical trial, *British Medical Journal*, Vol. 294 (1987), pp. 294–96.

13. Frank Ryan, *The Forgotten Plague: How the Battle Against Tuberculosis Was Won—and Lost* (Boston: Little, Brown and Company, 1992), p. 8.

14. Data are presented in Kass, op. cit. See also *The White Plague: Tuberculosis, Man, Society*, by René Dubos and Jean Dubos (New Brunswick, N.J.: Rutgers University Press, 1987).

15. It is of interest that leprosy, which results from infection with a relative of the tubercle bacillus called *Mycobacterium leprae*, is treated as effectively by a high-protein diet enriched with the amino acid L-tryptophan as by antibiotics. J. Mauron et al., The use of an amino acid as a precursor of a bioactive metabolite in combatting an infectious disease: the efficacy of a tryptophan-enriched diet in the treatment of leprosy, *Amino Acids*, Vol. 2 (1992), pp. 255–69.

16. See "Causes and Their Effects," in Lewontin, op. cit., pp. 41–57. He describes the relationship between death rate, diet, and gender in nineteenth-century England. Also: *The Origins of Human Disease*, by Thomas McKeon (Ox-

ford: Basil Blackwell, 1988). He argues that increased protein intake due to improved methods of animal husbandry and increased consumption of meat and dairy products began to decrease mortality from infectious diseases by the late eighteenth century.

17. Ryan, op. cit., p. 3.

18. A. Rouillon, S. Perdrizet, and R. Parrot, Transmission of tubercle bacilli: the effects of chemotherapy, *Tubercle*, Vol. 57 (1976), pp. 275–99; S. Grzybowski, Ontario studies of tuberculin sensitivity, *Canadian Journal of Public Health*, Vol. 56 (1965), pp. 181–92.

19. A. Kocki, The global tuberculosis situation and the new control strategy of the World Health Organization, *Tubercle*, Vol. 71 (1990), pp. 1–6; M. C. Raviglione, D. E. Snider, and A. Kochi, Global epidemiology of tuberculosis. Morbidity and mortality of a worldwide epidemic, *Journal of the American Medical Association*, Vol. 273 (1995), pp. 220–26.

20. *Tuberculosis in New York City: 1992: Information Summary* (New York: New York City Department of Health, 1993); P. J. Dolin, M. C. Raviglione, and A. Kochi, Global tuberculosis incidence and mortality during 1990–2000, *Bulletin of the World Health Organization*, Vol. 72 (1994), pp. 213–20.

21. G. Myers, K. MacInnes, and L. Myers, Phylogenetic moments in the AIDS epidemic, in *Emerging Viruses*, ed. S. B. Morse (New York: Oxford University Press, 1993), pp. 120–37. Discusses the presumed origin of human immunodeficiency virus in Africa.

22. Quoted by Laurie Garrett in *The Coming Plague* (New York: Farrar, Straus, Giroux, 1994), p. 333.

23. A. R. Lifson, Preventing HIV: have we lost our way? *Lancet*, Vol. 343 (1994), pp. 1306–7; A. R. Lifson, Preventing AIDS: have we lost our way? *Lancet*, Vol. 346 (1995), pp. 262–63; World Health Organization, The current global situation of the HIV/AIDS pandemic, *Weekly Epidemiology Record*, Vol. 70 (1995), pp. 5–8; Centers for Disease Control and Prevention, Acquired immunodeficiency syndrome—United States, 1994, *Morbidity and Mortality Weekly Reports*, Vol. 44 (1995), pp. 64–67.

24. World Health Organization, Acquired immune deficiency syndrome (AIDS): interim proposal for a WHO staging system for HIV infection and disease, *Weekly Epidemiology Record*, Vol. 65 (1990), pp. 221–28.

25. For a detailed discussion of the way in which disease definition shapes the way a disease is understood and studied and the lack of specificity of any of the manifestations of HIV disease, see: R. S. Root-Bernstein, *Rethinking AIDS: The Tragic Cost of Premature Consensus* (New York: The Free Press, 1993).

P. H. Duesberg, AIDS acquired by drug consumption and other noncontagious risk factors, *Pharmaceutics and Therapy*, Vol. 55 (1992), pp. 201–77. Duesberg's thesis that AIDS results from the use of immune-suppressive drugs, not HIV infection, is an intellectual tour de force but is contradicted by most research findings. In supporting his own thesis, however, Duesberg does a thorough job of discrediting Root-Bernstein's thesis, that infections other than HIV may cause AIDS.

For a refutation of Duesberg, see M. T. Shechter et al., HIV-1 and the etiology of AIDS, *Lancet*, Vol. 341 (1993), pp. 658–59; S. C. Darby et al., Mortality in the complete population of UK haemophiliacs before and after HIV infection, *Nature*, Vol. 377 (1995), pp. 79–82.

26. M. S. Cohen et al., A new deal in HIV prevention: lessons from the global approach, *Annals of Internal Medicine*, Vol. 120 (1994), pp. 340–41.

27. T. J. Coates et al., HIV prevention in developed countries, *Lancet*, Vol. 348 (1996), pp. 1143–48.

28. J. A. Levy, Surrogate markers in AIDS research. Is there truth in numbers? *Journal of the American Medical Association*, Vol. 276 (1996), pp. 161–62.

29. A. S. Fauci, AIDS in 1996. Much accomplished, much to do, *Journal of the American Medical Association*, Vol. 276 (1996), pp. 155–56.

30. D. M. Thea et al., Plasma cytokines, cytokine antagonists, and disease progression in African women infected with HIV-1, *Annals of Internal Medicine*, Vol. 124 (1996), pp. 757–62; M. M. Lederman, Host-directed and immune-based therapies for human immunodeficiency virus infection, *Annals of Internal Medicine*, Vol. 122 (1995), pp. 218–22; J. A. Levy, HIV research: a need to focus on the right target, *Lancet*, Vol. 345 (1995), pp. 1619–21; J. K. Greenson et al., AIDS enteropathy: occult enteric infections and duodenal mucosal alterations in chronic diarrhea, *Annals of Internal Medicine*, Vol. 114 (1991), pp. 366–72. Small intestinal damage occurred in patients with AIDS who did not have diarrhea or evidence of intestinal infection. Activation of the immune system — without infection — damages the small intestine, because the cytokines released by immune activation are toxic.

31. "Opportunistic infections are responsible for much of the morbidity and mortality in AIDS patients. . . ." K. A. Sepkowitz and D. Armstrong, Treatment of opportunistic infections in AIDS, *Lancet*, Vol. 346 (1995), pp. 588–89; C. Whalen et al., Accelerated course of human immunodeficiency virus infection after tuberculosis, *American Journal of Respiratory and Critical Care Medicine*, Vol. 151 (1995), pp. 129–35. Tuberculosis accelerates the progression toward AIDS.

Intestinal parasites are responsible for much of the intestinal damage and malabsorption associated with AIDS: D. P. Kotler et al., Small intestinal injury and parasitic diseases in AIDS, *Annals of Internal Medicine*, Vol. 113 (1990), pp. 444–49; D. P. Kotler et al., Effects of enteric parasitoses and HIV infection upon small intestinal structure and function in patients with AIDS, *Journal of Clinical Gastroenterology*, Vol. 16 (1993), pp. 10–15. Damage to the small intestine was associated primarily with the presence of intestinal parasites, not with the presence of HIV itself in cells of the small intestine.

In addition, Kaposi's sarcoma (KS) has been associated with one old, well-studied virus, *cytomegalovirus*, and one newly described virus, *human herpesvirus-8* (HHV-8), both of which are commonly encountered in people who do not have HIV infection: J. E. Gallant et al., Risk factors for Kaposi's sarcoma in patients with advanced Human Immunodeficiency Virus disease treated with zidovudine, *Archives of Internal Medicine*, Vol. 154 (1994), pp. 566–72; P. S. Moore and Y. Chang, Detection of herpesvirus-like DNA sequences in Kaposi's sarcoma in patients with and those without HIV infection, *New England Journal of Medicine*, Vol. 332 (1995), pp. 1181–85.

Lymphoid cancers among people with AIDS are also strongly associated with HHV-8: E. Cesarman et al., Kaposi's sarcoma-associated herpesvirus-like DNA sequences in AIDS-related body-cavity-based lymphomas, *New England Journal of Medicine*, Vol. 332 (1995), pp. 1186–91; D. S. Karcher and S. Alkan, Herpes-like DNA sequences, AIDS-related tumors, and Castleman's disease, *New England Journal of Medicine*, Vol. 333 (1995), pp. 797–98.

32. H. Grosshurth et al., Impact of improved treatment of sexually transmitted diseases on HIV infection in rural Tanzania: randomized controlled trial, *Lancet*, Vol. 346 (1995), pp. 530–36.

33. R. D. Semba et al., Maternal vitamin A deficiency and mother-to-child transmission of HIV-1, *Lancet*, Vol. 343 (1994), pp. 1593–97. Also of note: administration of vitamin A to babies born to women with HIV improves the health of those babies during the first year of life, even if the women were not vitamin A deficient. A. Coutsoudis, R. Bobat, and H. Coovadia, The effects of vitamin-A supplementation on the morbidity of children born to HIV-infected women, *American Journal of Public Health*, Vol. 85 (1995), pp. 1076–81.

34. D. L. Archer and W. H. Glinsmann, Enteric infections and other cofactors in AIDS, *Immunology Today*, Vol. 6 (1985), pp. 292–95; Z. C. Chen et al., Mitogenic factor for T inducer/helper cells in *Entamoeba histolytica* extracts, *Acta Academiae Medicinae Wuhan*, Vol. 5 (1985), pp. 213–16; S. Croxson et al., *Entamoeba histolytica* antigen-specific induction of Human Immunodeficiency Virus replication, *Journal of Clinical Microbiology*, Vol. 26 (1988), pp. 292–94.

35. H. W. Murray et al., T4+ cell production of interferon gamma and the clinical spectrum of patients at risk for and with acquired immunodeficiency, *Archives of Internal Medicine*, Vol. 148 (1988), pp. 1613–16. Gamma-interferon is a chemical produced by white blood cells, a *cytokine* that is a critical component in the defense against viral infection. Asymptomatic, HIV-negative homosexual men made only half the level of gamma-interferon produced by healthy heterosexual men.

Also: D. P. Kotler, J. V. Scholes, and A. R. Tierney, Intestinal plasma cell alterations in acquired immunodeficiency syndrome, *Digestive Diseases and Sciences*, Vol. 32 (1987), pp. 129–38. Intestinal biopsies of asymptomatic homosexual men without HIV show an increase in the density of IgM-plasma cells but not of IgA-plasma cells when compared to a heterosexual control group. This suggests ongoing immune stimulation in the gastrointestinal tract of the homosexual group.

36. The role of blood transfusion and hemophilia as independent promoters of immune dysfunction is thoroughly reviewed by Duesberg and by Root-Bernstein in their cited works. One does not have to accept their thesis that HIV infection is the result of AIDS, not its cause, to appreciate the validity of their data. In addition, see: J. R. Cerhan et al., Transfusion history and cancer risk in older women, *Annals of Internal Medicine*, Vol. 119 (1993), pp. 8–15. Previous blood transfusion increases the risk of cancers of the lymph system and the kidneys.

37. J. K. Kreiss et al., Nontransmission of T-cell subset abnormalities from hemophiliacs to their spouses, *Journal of the American Medical Association*, Vol. 251 (1984), pp. 1450–54.

38. D. K. Henderson et al., Risk for occupational transmission of human immunodeficiency virus type 1 (HIV-1) associated with clinical exposure: a prospective evaluation, *Annals of Internal Medicine*, Vol. 113 (1990), pp. 740–46; M. Clerici et al., HIV-specific T-Helper activity in seronegative health care workers exposed to contaminated blood, *Journal of the American Medical Association*, Vol. 271 (1994), pp. 42–46.

39. S. Rowland-Jones et al., HIV-specific cytotoxic T-cells in HIV-exposed but uninfected Gambian women, *Nature Medicine*, Vol. 1 (1995), pp. 59–64; K. R. Fowke et al., Cellular immune responses correlate with protection against HIV-1

among women resistant to infection, Proceedings of the Fifth Annual Conference on HIV/AIDS Research, Winnipeg, Manitoba, June 8–11, 1995.

40. Y. Cao et al., Virologic and immunologic characterization of long-term survivors of human immunodeficiency virus type 1 infection, *New England Journal of Medicine*, Vol. 332 (1995), pp. 201–8; G. Pantaleo et al., Studies in subjects with long-term nonprogressive human immunodeficiency virus infection, *New England Journal of Medicine*, Vol. 332 (1995), pp. 209–16.

41. B. Abrams, D. Duncan, and I. Hertz-Picciotto, A prospective study of dietary intake and acquired immune deficiency syndrome in HIV-seropositive homosexual men, *Journal of the Acquired Immune Deficiency Syndromes*, Vol. 6 (1993), pp. 949–58; R. J. Jariwalla, Micro-nutrient imbalance in HIV infection and AIDS: relevance to pathogenesis and therapy, *Journal of Nutritional & Environmental Medicine*, Vol. 5 (1995), pp. 297–306; B. Halliwell and C. Cross, Reactive oxygen species, antioxidants and acquired immunodeficiency syndrome. Sense or speculation? *Archives of Internal Medicine*, Vol. 151 (1991), pp. 29–31; H. Garewal et al., A preliminary trial of beta-carotene in subjects infected with the human immunodeficiency virus, *Journal of Nutrition*, Vol. 122 (1992), pp. 728–32. Beta-carotene at a dose of sixty milligrams per day improves the activity of antiviral lymphocytes in people with HIV infection.

S. Harakeh, R. J. Jariwalla, and L. Pauling, Suppression of Human Immunodeficiency Virus replication by ascorbate in chronically and acutely infected cells, *Proceedings of the National Academy of Science*, Vol. 87 (1990), pp. 7245–49. Levels of vitamin C that could be achieved in humans by taking supplements at doses of ten thousand milligrams or more per day inhibited HIV-replication in T-helper cells.

42. A. H. Coulter, Vitamin and antioxidant protocols in HIV Disease, *Alternative & Complementary Therapies* (June–July 1995), pp. 208–11.

43. G. Ironson et al., Distress, denial and low adherence to behavioral interventions predict faster disease progression in gay men infected with human immunodeficiency virus, *International Journal of Behavioral Medicine*, Vol. 1 (1994), pp. 90–105; B. Bower, Depression, early death noted in HIV cases, *Science News*, Vol. 142 (1992), p. 53.

44. See discussion in Marc Lappé's *Breakout*, p. 103. For a fascinating presentation on the effect of human behavior on microbial virulence, see Nesse and Williams, *Why We Get Sick*. Their discussion of AIDS appears on p. 61. A similar mechanism may have caused the appearance of and spread of syphilis during the late fifteenth century. See Note 5, Chapter One.

45. L. Garrett, Nosocomial amplifiers of microbial emergence, in Wilson, Levins, and Spielman, eds., op. cit., pp. 389–95; L. Garrett, *The Coming Plague* (New York: Farrar, Strauss, Giroux, 1994), pp. 100–106.

46. A. Fleming, On the antibacterial action of cultures of a Penicillium, with special reference to their use in the isolation of *H. influenzae*, *British Journal of Experimental Pathology*, Vol. 10 (1929), pp. 226–36.

47. H. A. Berman and L. Weinstein, Antibiotics and nutrition, *American Journal of Clinical Nutrition*, Vol. 24 (1971), pp. 260–64.

48. See S. B. Levy, G. B. FitzGerald, and A. B. Macone, Changes in intestinal flora of farm personnel after introduction of a tetracycline-supplemented feed on a farm, *New England Journal of Medicine*, Vol. 295 (1976), pp. 583–88. See also:

S. B. Levy, Environmental reservoirs of antibiotic resistance, *Health & Environment Digest*, Vol. 7, No. 7 (Nov. 1993), pp. 4–5.

49. L. Weinstein, The spontaneous occurrence of new bacterial infections during the course of treatment with streptomycin or penicillin, *American Journal of Medical Science*, Vol. 214 (1947), pp. 56–65. Possibly the first report.

50. B. N. Doebbeling et al., Comparative efficacy of alternative hand-washing agents in reducing nosocomial infections in intensive care units, *New England Journal of Medicine*, Vol. 327 (1992), pp. 88–93. In reviewing this article for *Journal Watch*, Aug. 1, 1992 (Vol. 10, No. 3, p. 24), Anthony Komaroff of Harvard Medical School states: "Although this study was designed to compare two hand-washing regimens, its main messages are that despite intensive education, health workers still don't get it, and that our patients are suffering the consequences."

51. J. G. Morris et al., Enterococci resistant to multiple antimicrobial agents, including vancomycin: establishment of endemicity in a university medical center, *Annals of Internal Medicine*, Vol. 123 (1995), pp. 250–59.

52. D. M. Berwick, The threat of antibiotic resistance grows, *Journal Watch*, Vol. 15 (1994), pp. 6–7; A. Tomasz, The pneumococcus at the gates, *New England Journal of Medicine*, Vol. 333 (1995), pp. 514–15; J. Hofmann et al., The prevalence of drug-resistant *Streptococcus pneumoniae* in Atlanta, *New England Journal of Medicine*, Vol. 333 (1995), pp. 481–86; R. F. Breitman et al., Emergence of drug-resistant pneumococcal infections in the United States, *Journal of the American Medical Association*, Vol. 271 (1994), pp. 1831–35; G. M. Caputo, P. C. Appelbaum, and H. C. Liu, Infections due to penicillin-resistant pneumococci: clinical, epidemiologic, and microbiologic features, *Archives of Internal Medicine*, Vol. 153 (1993), pp. 1301–10.

53. L. F. McCaig and J. M. Hughes, Trends in antimicrobial drug prescribing among office-based physicians in the United States, *Journal of the American Medical Association*, Vol. 273 (1995), pp. 214–19.

54. See R. Gonzales and M. Sande, What will it take to stop physicians from prescribing antibiotics in acute bronchitis? *Lancet*, Vol. 345 (1995), pp. 665–66; P. H. Orr et al., Randomized placebo-controlled trials of antibiotics for acute bronchitis: a critical review of the literature, *Journal of Family Practice*, Vol. 36 (1993), pp. 507–12.

55. J. M. Gwaltney et al., Computed tomographic study of the common cold, *New England Journal of Medicine*, Vol. 330 (1994), pp. 25–29.

56. W. Huck et al., Cefaclor vs. amoxicillin in the treatment of acute, recurrent, and chronic sinusitis, *Archives of Family Medicine*, Vol. 2 (1993), pp. 497–503.

57. A. W. Dohlman et al., Subacute sinusitis: are antimicrobials necessary? *Journal of Allergy and Clinical Immunology*, Vol. 91 (1993), pp. 1015–23.

58. R. M. Rosenfeld et al., Clinical efficacy of antimicrobial drugs for acute otitis media: metaanalysis of 5400 children from thirty-three randomized trials, *Journal of Pediatrics*, Vol. 124 (1994), pp. 355–67.

59. F. L. van Buchem, J. A. Knottnerus, and M. F. Peeters, Otitis media in children (letter), *New England Journal of Medicine*, Vol. 333 (1995), p. 1151. The Dutch policy was prompted by research reported in 1981: F. L. van Buchem, J. H. M. Dunk, and M. A. van't Hof, Therapy of acute otitis media: myringotomy, antibiotics, or neither? *Lancet*, Vol. ii (1981), pp. 883–87.

60. R. L. Williams et al., Use of antibiotics in preventing recurrent acute otitis media and in treating otitis media with effusion: a meta-analytic attempt to resolve the brouhaha, *Journal of the American Medical Association*, Vol. 270 (1993), pp. 1344–51.

61. T. M. Nsouli et al., Role of food allergy in serous otitis media, *Annals of Allergy*, Vol. 73 (1994), pp. 215–19. Although these authors described children with chronic fluid in the ear, rather than patients with established infection, others have found that almost all children with fluid in the ear harbor pathogenic bacteria in the fluid: J. C. Post et al., Molecular analysis of bacterial pathogens in otitis media with effusion, *Journal of the American Medical Association*, Vol. 273 (1995), pp. 1598–1604.

62. Reviews on the relationship between nutrition and immunity include R. K. Chandra, Immunodeficiency in undernutrition and overnutrition, *Nutrition Reviews*, Vol. 39 (1981), pp. 225–31; *Single Nutrients and Immunity*, Supplement to the *American Journal of Clinical Nutrition* (Feb. 1982), pp. 417–68; L. C. Corman, Effects of specific nutrients on the immune response: selected clinical applications, *Medical Clinics of North America*, Vol. 69 (1985), pp. 759–90.

63. A. Ryan, L. Craig, and S. Finn, Nutrient intakes and dietary patterns of older Americans: a national study, *Journal of Gerontology*, Vol. 47 (1992), pp. M145–M150. Consumption of vitamins A and E and zinc were low for 40 percent of men and women over the age of sixty-five; J. D. Bogden et al., Zinc and immunocompetence in the elderly: baseline data on zinc nutriture and immunity in unsupplemented subjects, *American Journal of Clinical Nutrition*, Vol. 46 (1987), pp. 101–9.

64. S. J. Wayne et al., Cell-mediated immunity as a predictor of morbidity and mortality in subjects over 60, *Journals of Gerontology*, Vol. 45 (1990), pp. M45–M48.

65. S. M. Meydani, Vitamin/mineral supplementation, the aging immune response, and risk of infection, *Nutrition Reviews*, Vol. 51 (1993), pp. 106–15.

66. L. C. Rall and S. M. Meydani, Vitamin B6 and immune competence, *Nutrition Reviews*, Vol. 51 (1993), pp. 217–25; R. R. Watson et al., Effect of beta-carotene on lymphocyte subpopulations in elderly humans: evidence for a dose-response relationship, *American Journal of Clinical Nutrition*, Vol. 53 (1991), pp. 90–94; A. Peretz et al., Lymphocyte response is enhanced by supplementation of elderly subjects with selenium-enriched yeast, *American Journal of Clinical Nutrition*, Vol. 53 (1991), pp. 1323–28; S. M. Meydani et al., Vitamin E supplementation enhances cell-mediated immunity in healthy elderly subjects, *American Journal of Clinical Nutrition*, Vol. 52 (1990), pp. 557–63.

67. W. J. Rea and H.-C. Liang, Effects of pesticides on the immune system, *Journal of Nutritional Medicine*, Vol. 2 (1991), pp. 399–410; A. Broughton, J. D. Thrasher, and R. Madison, Chronic health effects and immunological alterations associated with exposure to pesticides, *Comments in Toxicology*, Vol. 4 (1990), pp. 59–71; N. I. Kerkvliet, Halogenated aromatic hydrocarbons (HAH) as immunotoxicants, *Progress in Clinical and Biological Research*, Vol. 161 (1984), pp. 369–87.

68. R. Lipkin, Vegemania: scientists tout the health benefits of saponins, *Science News*, Vol. 148 (Dec. 9, 1995), pp. 392–93.

69. J. Barone, J. R. Hebert, and M. M. Reddy, Dietary fat and natural-killer-cell activity, *American Journal of Clinical Nutrition*, Vol. 50 (1989), pp. 861–67; Effects of dietary fats on virus-induced autoimmune disease, *Nutrition Reviews*, Vol. 41 (1983), pp. 128–30.

70. U. N. Das et al., Free radicals, lipid peroxidation and essential fatty acids in patients with pneumonia, septicemia and collagen vascular diseases, *Journal of Nutritional Medicine*, Vol. 3 (1992), pp. 117–27; M. Fletcher and V. Ziboh, Effects of dietary supplementation with eicosapentaenoic acid or gamma-linolenic acid on neutrophil fatty acid composition and activation responses, *Inflammation*, Vol. 14 (1990), pp. 585–97.

71. (Impact, Sandoz Nutrition, Minneapolis). Lymphocyte responsiveness was enhanced by this diet.

72. A. Venuta et al., Essential fatty acids: the effects of dietary supplementation among children with recurrent respiratory infections, *Journal of International Medical Research*, Vol 24 (1996), pp. 325–30.

73. D. S. Kelley et al., Dietary alpha-linolenic acid and immune competence in humans, *American Journal of Clinical Nutrition*, Vol. 53 (1991), pp. 40–46; Fletcher and Ziboh, op. cit.

74. T. R. Kramer et al., Increased vitamin E intake restores fish-oil-induced suppressed blastogenesis of mitogen-stimulated T lymphocytes, *American Journal of Clinical Nutrition*, Vol. 54 (1991), pp. 896–902.

75. Vitamin E (400 mg/day) may improve or inhibit PMN function, depending on the individual. Vitamin E enhances opsonization by normal PMNs but slightly reduces microbial killing.

76. A. Bendich and L. J. Machlin, Safety of oral intake of vitamin E, *American Journal of Clinical Nutrition*, Vol. 48 (1988), pp. 612–19. This review from the research department at Hoffman-LaRoche, where most of the world's vitamin E is produced, indicates that doses as high as 3,200 units per day have been shown safe in human studies.

77. A. Bendich, Vitamin E status of U.S. children, *Journal of the American College of Nutrition*, Vol. 11 (1992), pp. 441–44.

78. J. S. Vobecky et al., Nutritional influences on humoral and cell-mediated immunity in healthy infants, *Journal of the American College of Nutrition*, Vol. 3 (1984), p. 265.

79. A. Sherman, Influence of iron on immunity and disease resistance, *Annals of the New York Academy of Science*, Vol. 587 (1990), pp. 140–46; J. H. Brock, Iron and immunity, *Journal of Nutritional Immunology*, Vol. 2 (1993), pp. 47–106.

80. R. K. Chandra and A. K. Saraya, Impaired immunocompetence associated with iron deficiency, *Journal of Pediatrics*, Vol. 86 (1975), pp. 899–902; J. Fletcher et al., Mouth lesions in iron-deficient anemia. Relationship to Candida albicans in saliva and to impairment of lymphocyte transformation, *Journal of Infectious Disease*, Vol. 131 (1975), pp. 44–50; R. G. Strauss, Iron deficiency, infections, and immune function: a reassessment, *American Journal of Clinical Nutrition*, Vol. 31 (1978), pp. 660–66.

81. B. Borch-Johnson et al., Bioavailability of daily low-dose iron supplements in menstruating women with low iron stores, *European Journal of Clinical Nutrition*, Vol. 44 (1990), pp. 29–34.

82. M. C. Weijmer, H. Neering, and C. Welten, Preliminary report: furunculosis and hypoferraemia, *Lancet*, Vol. 336 (1990), pp. 464–66.

83. P. Idjradinata, W. E. Watkins, and E. Pollitt, Adverse effects of iron supplementation on weight gain of iron-replete young children, *Lancet*, Vol. 343 (1994), pp. 1252–54.

84. Nesse and Williams, *Why We Get Sick*, p. 29.

85. P. Johnson et al., Zinc bioavailability from beef served with various carbohydrates or beverages, *Nutrition Research*, Vol. 10 (1990), pp. 155–62.

86. G. C. Sturniolo et al., Inhibition of gastric acid secretion reduces zinc absorption in man, *Journal of the American College of Nutrition*, Vol. 10 (1991), pp. 372–75.

87. G. Pulverer et al., Adequate function of the immune system and physiological microflora are closely correlated, *Pneumonoligia i Alergologia Polska*, Vol. 59 (1991), pp. 65–72; C. DeSimone et al., Probiotics and stimulation of the immune response, *European Journal of Clinical Nutrition*, Vol. 45, Supp. 2 (1991), pp. 32–34.

88. O. Kandil et al., Garlic and the immune systems in humans: its effect of natural killer cells, *Federation Proceedings*, Vol. 46 (1987), p. 1222; T. H. Abdullah, D. V. Kirkpatrick, and J. Carter, Enhancement of natural killer cell activity in AIDS with garlic, *Deutsche Zeitschrift für Onkologie*, Vol. 21 (1989), pp. 52–54.

89. C. S. Johnston, J. S. Martin, and X. Cai, Antihistamine effect of supplemental ascorbic acid and neutrophil chemotaxis, *Journal of the American College of Nutrition*, Vol. 11 (1992), pp. 172–76.

90. S. Kaspar et al., Immunological correlates of seasonal fluctuations in mood and behavior and their relationship to phototherapy, *Psychiatry Research*, Vol. 36 (1991), pp. 253–64.

91. P. W. Jannace et al., Effects of oral soy phosphatidylcholine on phagocytosis, arachidonate concentrations, and killing by human polymorphonuclear leukocytes, *American Journal of Clinical Nutrition*, Vol. 56 (1992), pp. 599–603.

92. C. D. Graber et al., Immunomodulating properties of dimethylglycine in humans, *Journal of Infectious Diseases*, Vol. 143 (1981), pp. 101–5.

93. M. T. Murray, Echinacea: pharmacology and clinical applications, *American Journal of Natural Medicine*, Vol. 2 (1995), pp. 18–25; also see M. T. Murray, *Natural Alternatives to Over-the-Counter and Prescription Drugs* (New York: Morrow, 1994).

94. S. B. Mossad et al., Zinc gluconate lozenges for treating the common cold. A randomized, double-blind, placebo-controlled study, *Annals of Internal Medicine*, Vol. 125 (1996), pp. 81–88.

95. Y. Ying-zhen et al., Effect of Astragalus membranaceous on natural killer cell activity and induction of alpha- and gamma-interferon in patients with Coxsackie B viral myocarditis, *Chinese Medical Journal*, Vol. 103 (1990), pp. 304–7.

96. E. J. Lien, Fungal metabolites and Chinese herbal medicine as immune stimulants, *Progress in Drug Research*, Vol. 34 (1990), pp. 395–420.

97. J. Lapides, Pathophysiology of urinary tract infections, *University of Michigan Medical Center Journal*, Vol. 39 (1973), pp. 103–12.

98. D. Zafriri et al., Inhibitory activity of cranberry juice on adherence of type I and type P fimbriated Escherichia coli to eucaryotic cells, *Antimicrobial Agents and Chemotherapy*, Vol. 33 (1989), pp. 92–98; J. Avorn et al., Reduction of bacteri-

uria and pyuria after ingestion of cranberry juice, *Journal of the American Medical Association*, Vol. 271 (1994), pp. 751–54.

99. V. Frohne, Untersuchungen zur frage der hardesifirzierenden wirkungen von barentraubenblatt-extracten, *Planta Medica*, Vol. 18 (1970), pp. 1–25.

100. G. Reid et al., Is there a role for lactobacilli in prevention of urogenital and intestinal infections? *Clinical Microbiology Review*, Vol. 3 (1990), pp. 335–44.

101. J. A. McGroarty et al., Influence of the spermicidal compound nonoxynol-9 on the growth and adhesion of urogenital bacteria in vitro, *Current Microbiology*, Vol. 21 (1990), pp. 447–51.

102. W. E. Stamm and T. M. Hooten, Management of urinary tract infections in adults, *New England Journal of Medicine*, Vol. 329 (1985), pp. 1328–34.

103. S. Cohen, D. A. J. Tyrrell, and A. P. Smith, Psychological stress and susceptibility to the common cold, *New England Journal of Medicine*, Vol. 325 (1991), pp. 606–12; S. Cohen and G. M. Williamson, Stress and infectious disease in humans, *Psychological Bulletin*, Vol. 109 (1991), pp. 5–24; R. J. Meyer and R. J. Haggerty, Streptococcal infections in families: factors altering individual susceptibility, in *Foundations of Psychoneuroimmunology*, ed. S. Locke et al. (New York: Aldine Publishing Company, 1985), pp. 307–17.

104. D. J. Longo, G. A. Clum, and N. J. Yaeger, Psychosocial treatment for recurrent genital herpes, *Journal of Consulting and Clinical Psychology*, Vol. 56 (1988), pp. 61–66.

105. H. Hall, L. Minnes, and K. Olness, The psychophysiology of voluntary immunomodulation, *International Journal of Neuroscience*, Vol. 69 (1993), pp. 221–34.

Epilogue: Each Patient Is a Work of Art

1. Eric Cassell, *The Nature of Suffering and the Goals of Medicine* (New York: Oxford University Press, 1991), p. 138.

2. S. E. Bedell et al., Incidence and characteristics of preventable iatrogenic cardiac arrests, *Journal of the American Medical Association*, Vol. 265 (1991), pp. 2815–20.

3. L. L. Leape, Error in medicine, *Journal of the American Medical Association*, Vol. 272 (1994), pp. 1851–57.

4. D. M. Eisenberg et al., Unconventional medicine in the United States: prevalence, costs, and patterns of use, *New England Journal of Medicine*, Vol. 328 (1993), pp. 246–52. Twenty-two million Americans annually see an unconventional provider for a medical condition.

INDEX

A
Academy for Integrated Medical Studies
  (AIMS), 49
acetaminophen, 209, 211
acrylic adhesives, 161–63
adrenaline, 57, 59, 61, 151, 159
Aesculapius, 6
aflatoxins, 169
AIDS, 58, 219, 226–30, 243
alcohol consumption, 209, 211, 212
allergies, 59, 60, 64, 164
  asthma. *See* asthma
  fibromyalgia and, 184–85
  home allergens, control of, 255–57
  mold and dust mites, 168–69, 255–57
  origins and reasons for, 170–71
Alliance for the Prudent Use of Antibiotics,
  237–38
alternative medicine, 19, 111–12, 185, 265–67
aluminum, 178–79
Alzheimer's disease, 178–79
American Medical Association (AMA), 19, 20
American medicine, 19–20
  alternatives sought, 19, 111–12
  changes in (1970's), 38–39
  Flexner Report on medical education,
    20–21, 22
  health care industry, expansion of, 22–24,
    38–39
  insurance companies, effect of, 22–24, 39

life-prolonging technology, 38–39
  specialization, 39
  testing, addiction to, 22, 47–48, 53
  women physicians, 20
ammonia, 177
amoebic infection, 112–16, 184–85
angina, 60, 87
ankylosing spondylitis (AS), 96–101
Annals of Internal Medicine, 45, 200
antecedents to illness
  congenital factors, 73, 74, 76–77
  developmental factors, 74, 75, 77
  diathesis, knowledge of, 73–75
  genes and destiny, 76–77
  repeated exposures, 75
antibiotics, 213, 226
  birth and explosion of, 232–33
  cautions regarding, 237–38
  chronic illness after, 70–71
  food supply, entering, 233–34
  questioning need for, 235–38
  resistance, increase in, 234–35
antihistamines, 171, 204
antinutrients, 142–44
antioxidants, 205–8
  EFA, balance with, 144–50
  free radicals and, 204–8
antisepsis, 15–16
Archives of Pathological Anatomy (Virchow), 14
arginine, 61

About the Author

LEO GALLAND, M.D., is a pioneer and leader in the emerging field of integrated medicine, which brings alternative and conventional therapies together. He is internationally known for his work in nutrition, intestinal health, and detoxification. Graduating with Honors from Harvard University, Dr. Galland went to New York University where he received his medical doctorate and trained in internal medicine at the Bellevue Hospital-New York University Medical Center. He has held faculty positions at Rockefeller University, Albert Einstein College of Medicine, the State University of New York at Stony Brook, and at the University of Connecticut. Dr. Galland served as the director of medical research at the Gesell Institute of Human Development in New Haven. In 1989 he received the Harold W. Harper Memorial Award in Preventive Medicine from the American College of Advancement in Medicine. Dr. Galland is the author of numerous scientific articles describing the importance of magnesium, essential fatty acids, and normal intestinal ecology for health, and has devolped the concept of patient-centered diagnosis. His previous book, the highly acclaimed *Superimmunity for Kids*, was published in 1988. He is the director of the Foundation for Integrated Medicine and maintains a private consulting practice in New York City, where he lives with his wife, Christina, and their sons.

About the Type

This book was set in Electra, a typeface designed for Linotype by W. A. Dwiggins, the renowned type designer (1880-1956). Electra is a fluid typeface, avoiding the contrasts of thick and thin strokes that are prevalent in most modern typefaces.